W9-AGL-108

MILADY

SKIN CARE AND COSMETIC INGREDIENTS

DICTIONARY

FOURTH EDITION

M. VARINIA MICHALUN

AND

JOSEPH C. DINARDO

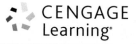

Australia • Brazil • Mexico • Singapore • United Kingdom • United States

CENGAGE
Learning·

Skin Care and Cosmetic Ingredients Dictionary, Fourth Edition

M. Varinia Michalun

Joseph C. DiNardo

Executive Director:
Sandra L. Bruce

Product Director:
Corina Santoro

Product Manager:
Philip I. Mandl

Associate Content Developer:
Sarah Prediletto

Director, Marketing & Training: Gerard McAvey

Community Manager:
Matthew McGuire

Senior Production Director:
Wendy Troeger

Production Manager:
Sherondra Thedford

Art and Cover Direction, Production Management, and Composition: PreMediaGlobal

Cover Image: ©ElenaGaak/ Shutterstock.com

© 2015, 2010, 2001, 1993 Milady, a part of Cengage Learning

ALL RIGHTS RESERVED. No part of this work covered by the copyright herein may be reproduced, transmitted, stored, or used in any form or by any means graphic, electronic, or mechanical, including but not limited to photocopying, recording, scanning, digitizing, taping, Web distribution, information networks, or information storage and retrieval systems, except as permitted under Section 107 or 108 of the 1976 United States Copyright Act, without the prior written permission of the publisher.

For product information and technology assistance, contact us at **Cengage Learning Customer & Sales Support, 1-800-354-9706.**
For permission to use material from this text or product, submit all requests online at **www.cengage.com/ permissions.** Further permissions questions can be e-mailed to **permissionrequest@cengage.com.**

Library of Congress Control Number: 2013951170

ISBN: 978-1-285-06079-8

Milady
5 Maxwell Drive
Clifton Park, NY 12065-2919
USA

Cengage Learning is a leading provider of customized learning solutions with office locations around the globe, including Singapore, the United Kingdom, Australia, Mexico, Brazil, and Japan. Locate your local office at **international.cengage.com/region.**

Cengage Learning products are represented in Canada by Nelson Education, Ltd.

For your lifelong learning solutions, visit **milady.cengage.com**

Purchase any of our products at your local college store or at our preferred online store **www.cengagebrain.com.**

Visit our corporate website at **cengage.com**

Notice to the Reader
Publisher does not warrant or guarantee any of the products described herein or perform any independent analysis in connection with any of the product information contained herein. Publisher does not assume, and expressly disclaims, any obligation to obtain and include information other than that provided to it by the manufacturer. The reader is expressly warned to consider and adopt all safety precautions that might be indicated by the activities described herein and to avoid all potential hazards. By following the instructions contained herein, the reader willingly assumes all risks in connection with such instructions. The publisher makes no representations or warranties of any kind, including but not limited to, the warranties of fitness for particular purpose or merchantability, nor are any such representations implied with respect to the material set forth herein, and the publisher takes no responsibility with respect to such material. The publisher shall not be liable for any special, consequential, or exemplary damages resulting, in whole or part, from the readers' use of, or reliance upon, this material.

Printed in the United States of America
11 12 13 14 22 21 20 19

Contents

Author Biography

M. Varinia Michalun has specialized in international cosmetics marketing and new product development and has lectured on cosmetic ingredients and product use to professionals in the United States, Europe, Australia, New Zealand, and Asia. Her experience also includes skin care salon management, and aesthetics education. She has authored articles for industry magazines, provides expertise to beauty journalist, is a contributor for *Milady Standard Esthetics: Advanced* and co-author of *Skin Care and Cosmetic Ingredients Dictionary.*

Mr. DiNardo has 37 years of experience in the skin care field. He is a highly respected product formulator, well versed in all aspects of regulatory and safety affairs, clinical research and international product registration. Chief Scientific Officer—Emeritus for Pharma Cosmetix Research and a former Vice President of Research & Development for Revlon-Almay Inc., Mr. DiNardo was the VP of R&D for Almay Hypoallergenic Cosmetics and spent many years leading research for the development of products dedicated to atopic dermatitis.

His professional affiliations include the Personal Care Products Council (formerly known as the Cosmetic, Toiletry & Fragrance Association), the Society of Toxicology, and he is a former Chairman of the Carolina Chapter of the Society of Cosmetic Chemists.

Mr. DiNardo has published several articles and abstracts in the areas of Photobiology, Reproductive Toxicology, General Toxicology, Contact Dermatitis, Regulatory Affairs, Comedogenicity, Alpha Hydroxy Acid Safety & Efficacy, and General Anti-oxidant Research.

He possesses a Master of Science degree in Toxicology from St. John's University with his undergraduate degree in Biology from Mercy College in New York.

Acknowledgments

The author and publisher would like to thank the following professionals for their assistance and expertise in the preparation of the final product.

Afsheen Ather, Parama Center for Health and Wellness, The Esthetic Institute, Director of Aesthetics

Casey Durrett, Paul Mitchell the School, Licensed Esthetician, Instructor

Amber Falls, Marinello School of Beauty, Esthetic Instructor

Patrice Ann Hredzak, Director of Esthetics

Fredrick J. Laurino, House of Heavilin of Kansas, Inc. CEO

Lynn Maestro, IBSG, LLC. Director of Marketing and Education

Fumi Ozaki, "O" de Kirei, Owner

Janet Prediletto, LPN. Janet Prediletto Professional Aesthetics, LTD, Owner, Medical Aesthetician

Jennifer Schrodt, University of Nebraska, Post-Secondary Education

Paula Di Marco Young, BS, RN. Young Medical Spa® & Dr. TattAway® Laser Tattoo and Hair Removal, Co-Owner, Registered Nurse, Certified Laser Operator/Aesthetician

Foreword

This book is now in its fourth edition, and the skin care and cosmetic industry has undergone significant changes since the first volume was published in 1993. More is known about how the skin works, how cosmetic ingredients interact with each other, and how they work with the skin's own chemical composition. This increase in understanding, however, has not been matched with greater simplicity. In fact, the cosmetic industry is more complicated and confusing than ever, and cosmetic ingredients remain a mystery to most consumers and professionals. Information tools, particularly those available on the Internet, can provide what appear to be ready answers to such questions as *What is this ingredient?; Where does it come from?; What does it do?; Who uses it in their products?* These tools, however, do not provide insight into other questions, for instance *Does this product really do what it claims?; Is it worth the price being asked?* Nor do they often clarify chemical terms, government regulations, and cosmetic-industry labeling practices. This book was originally written as a tool to help cosmetic users navigate these questions and concerns, and to develop their own well-reasoned conclusions regarding skin care ingredients and cosmetic products.

This edition remains true to the original intent. However, it is similar to and different from its predecessors. As in previous editions, it begins with a basic explanation of skin anatomy and physiology as this is critical for understanding product performance. This section is intended to provide general information on the skin and its functions, and it is written to support the spirit of the book as a dictionary and not a reference text on skin care. Like past editions it includes information on skin types, conditions and problems, as well a chapter (Chapter 4) defining common terms used in skin care formulation. Part II, the alphabetical listing of ingredients, has also been updated. The number of new ingredients available, especially botanicals, is vast, and we have incorporated those that appear to be very frequently used or for which an appropriate amount of reliable data are available.

At the same time, this edition has undergone significant revisions. For example, there are now sections on adverse reactions, product testing, and claim substantiation; and we have done our best to ensure that ingredients are listed by their International Nomenclature of Cosmetic Ingredients (INCI) name, with cross-references to other names when appropriate. It is also the first edition to be written without Natalia Michalun—without her energy and her vast knowledge and commitment to professional skin care. I am extremely grateful to Joseph C. DiNardo for joining me in this project and inspiring new directions while remaining true to its original purpose. His immense experience, patience, humor, and style have combined to make a fresh and strong volume.

Many U.S. and European sources of information were used for this edition, and we are grateful to all of them. Our reviewers have been invaluable and we wish to express our most sincere appreciation for their efforts. Finally our appreciation goes to Maria Lynch, Sarah Prediletto, and Philip Mandl of Cengage Learning for their continued support of this dictionary.

We hope that in this volume you find answers to the many skin care cosmetic ingredient questions that estheticians and cosmetic consumers share.

Dedication

*Natalia Michalun dedicated more than half of her
life to the esthetics and cosmetic industry.
With her knowledge, enthusiasm, and energy she
inspired professionals around the world to
provide the best in skincare.
We dedicate this edition to her.*

PART I

The Skin and Cosmetics

PART I

The Skin and Cosmetics

Introduction

How we treat our skin is part of living a healthy life. The skin is the body's largest organ. It has been called the body's armor because it keeps all the organs and muscles safe from the elements outside the body that can cause harm—like the sun's rays, bacteria, insects, and irritating chemicals. In addition, the skin helps in regulating a number of the body's functions, including temperature and eliminating toxic chemicals. Its most important role by far, though, is to keep the body's water from evaporating. When we are born, 90 percent of our body is made up of water; as we age it reduces to 70 percent and might even drop as low as 50 percent in our later years. Without healthy, intact skin covering our body we would die.

Given the skin's importance to our survival, it is essential that we learn how to take care of it, not only so that we look beautiful, but so we can also live long, healthy lives. From this perspective, it is important that all skincare professionals, from estheticians to physicians, have a good understanding of skin structure (anatomy) and function (physiology), skin types and conditions, as well as what happens when cosmetics or other products are applied to the skin. The same understanding is also important for cosmetic consumers, particularly given the amount of information and misinformation about cosmetics currently available. That is the purpose of this book—to better inform skincare professionals and their clients about how and why a product impacts the skin, and the purpose and function of individual ingredients in a cosmetic formulation.

Before moving into a discussion of the skin—its anatomy, physiology, typing and common problems—and its interaction with cosmetic ingredients and products, it may be helpful to concentrate a moment on the history of cosmetic ingredients and regulation. Cosmetics and the cosmetic industry are heading in directions that will be of great benefit to skin care professionals and cosmetic users, but in order to understand what these directions mean, it is important to understand the links between the past and the present.

Historically, people used common or everyday substances for beautifying, healing, soothing, or creating other effects. Cleopatra was well known for using sour milk on her skin. Today, we know that sour milk contains high levels of lactic acid, commonly referred to as an alpha hydroxy acid (AHA). In modern times, AHAs are considered to have launched the cosmeceutical revolution and represent the skincare ingredient category with the most significant impact on the cosmetic industry. In the second decade of the 2000s, sales of AHA-based products contributed well over a billion dollars a year to the anti-aging skincare market. Perhaps more importantly, however, this revolution changed how we look at skincare, and how we perceive the interaction of ingredients with the skin's anatomy and physiology—not bad for a thought that started out with sour milk!

There are other interesting stories about how and why a variety of ingredients are used in skincare formulas. Most, if not all, come from folklore, often based on observation and passed down from generation to generation for hundreds if not thousands of years: rub the juice from the aloe plant on a burn and the skin will not blister; an extract from chamomile applied to irritated skin will have a calming effect; apply tea tree oil to acne skin. Scientists have examined such stories and have explored why these effect the skin. Today, they are able to isolate and develop purified versions of a botanical's specific chemical constituents that have therapeutic value, creating versions that can be stronger and more effective for healing various skin care problems than the original treatment. This marks the beginning of the "synthetic versus natural" debate, a topic that is explored in more detail in Chapter 3.

The use of folklore as a basis for skincare and color cosmetics is also what launched government regulations in the cosmetic industry. In the 1930s (and before) there were many traveling shows that sold magical elixirs and lotions claiming to cure all varieties of aliments. Two major incidents occurred that caused the U.S. Congress to give the Food and Drug Administration (FDA) power over food, drug, and cosmetic products in 1938. The first was a magical "feel good" elixir that killed several people after they drank it. The main ingredient turned out to be anti-freeze, commonly used today in car radiators and chemically known as ethylene glycol. The second was a mascara called "Lash Lure." It promised to stain eyelashes, so that it did not have to be used frequently. It also caused a dozen women to go blind and one to die. The product contained an ingredient called paraphenylenediamine or PPD, a very common ingredient that today is used safely in hair dyes, PPD may cause an allergic reaction in some people.

These incidents were the "straw that broke the camel's back" and the FDA was charged with developing guidelines to protect consumers from food, drug, and cosmetic products that were potentially harmful. One of the first things that the FDA did was to place the responsibility of proving product safety on the manufacturer. If the manufacturer did not test the product and demonstrate that it was safe, then a warning label was placed on the product stating: "Warning: The safety of this product has not been determined."

For the first time, the FDA also defined the terms drug and cosmetic. A drug was defined as "a substance that altered the structure or function of the body." A cosmetic was defined as "any product, except soap, intended to be applied to the human body for cleansing, beautifying, promoting attractiveness, or altering appearances." These definitions were part of the 1938 Food, Drug and Cosmetic Act and are still used by the FDA to regulate the cosmetic industry. While this appears straightforward, our understanding of the skin's anatomy, physiology, chemical composition, and relationship to cosmetic ingredients has vastly improved since 1938. Thus, using a definition that is over 70 years old to govern cosmetic chemistry, a science that changes dramatically every few years, has significant consequences.

In 1938, skin was commonly considered a dead tissue, and thought to be almost completely impermeable. Keeping it clean and applying makeup to "alter the appearance" was more than an adequate way to describe what a cosmetic product should do. However, in the 1980s doctors Van Scott and Yu patented AHA technology. In their patent, they illustrated that these ingredients could thin very thick skin by exfoliation, plump up skin by increasing the water-binding materials naturally found in skin called humectants (e.g., hyaluronic acid), and help minimize lines and wrinkles by stimulating the production of such materials as collagen, giving the skin a stronger base or foundation. All of these changes in the skin demonstrate an altering of its "structure and function," which according to the 1938 FDA definition, would be considered drug claims. Yet, as mentioned earlier, AHAs have revolutionized the cosmetic industry and are found in many skin care products.

This complexity is also seen in reverse: products once treated as cosmetics might now be classified as drugs. Many people experience severe skin chapping and cracking—sometimes to the point of bleeding—during winter months. This can often be due to a combination of water plus a cold temperature and low humidity outside. In the 1970s a group of estheticians were given a jar of 100 percent Petrolatum (commonly called Vaseline®) and several pairs of cotton gloves; each night before bed they were to apply the Petrolatum to their hands, put on a pair of the gloves, go to sleep, and in the morning remove the gloves and wash their hands with a gentle soap or cleanser. All of them disliked this routine, but within three to five days their skin was once again soft and supple. Technically, this too is altering skin structure and function and therefore given the FDA's definition, Petrolatum should be considered a drug. In fact, today, a jar of Vaseline® carries a "drug fact label" and indeed it is now marketed as an over-the-counter (OTC) drug.

So, what is the difference between the two cases? Both AHAs and Petrolatum change the "structure and function" of skin. Both significantly impact the skin, though their mechanisms of action (how they work) are different. Yet AHAs are sold as cosmetics and 100 percent Petrolatum is sold as an OTC drug. What then permits the 1938 FDA law to classify them differently? Is it the concentration of the ingredient in question? There are no concentration limits set by the FDA for AHA products because they are cosmetics; however, products that contain 30 to 100 percent Petrolatum are generally sold as OTC drug products. Does that mean that any product containing 30 to 100 percent Petrolatum is an OTC drug? These are all very logical questions, but it is difficult to use strict logic to answer the questions as such logic has little to do with how the regulation is applied. What matters when constructing an answer to the question, and thus what forms the basis for the classification, is what the manufacturer claims or says about the product and its activity on the skin. Regardless whether the ingredients actually impact the skin's structure, function, or mechanism of action, and independently of their concentration, regulations only apply if the product or ingredient(s) are discussed in ways that can be interpreted as a drug or pharmaceutical claim. AHA-based products are sold as skin moisturizers, and their packaging and advertising will generally read: "apply this luxuriously rich moisturizing cream day and night for younger more radiant looking skin." This is a cosmetic claim because it refers to "altering the appearance" of the skin—that is, skin looks more youthful and radiant; it is not claiming to make the skin more youthful and radiant. In the case of Petrolatum, products containing 30 to 100 percent Petrolatum usually state "For the temporary relief of chapped skin or lips." This is a drug claim because it refers to "altering the structure" of your skin—that is, chapped skin or lips are relieved of their condition, at least temporarily.

The 1938 FDA law has not kept up with science. Our understanding about what happens in skin when an ingredient or product is applied to it—biochemistry—as well as being able to measure these changes down to the cellular level—analytical chemistry—has become extremely advanced. These capacities did not exist when the FDA developed its law. Today, one can say that almost all ingredients impact the "structure or function" of the skin in one way or another. This being the case, it would appear that the only way the FDA can enforce the 1938 Food, Drug and Cosmetic Act is by either establishing "logical standards," which would require receiving a significant increase in resources (funding, equipment, and personnel); or by continuing to let the cosmetic industry regulate itself. The cost to redefine this almost two hundred billion dollar global industry is more than most governments are willing to do. This is especially the case since the cosmetic industry has caused very minimal problems worldwide.

Any confusion is compounded by differences in regulation between the United States and Europe, for example. It is also a potential problem in light of the vast number of new ingredients and skin care concepts available to chemists, professionals, and consumers. The cosmeceutical revolution that began with AHAs has expanded and become even more sophisticated and effective. Botanically based products are experiencing a renaissance and renewed credibility as chemists and formulators become increasingly precise in their technologies and ability to isolate a botanical's therapeutic components. Carotenoids, for example, as well as flavonoids, peptides, polyphenols, and phytoestrogens all fall into this category. Animal-based ingredients are now replaced with plant-based or synthetically manufactured equivalents, and even botanically derived ingredients have synthetic equivalents that are more frequently used for their purity and predictability. While anti-aging products still represent the lion's share of cosmetic industry sales, there is also growing awareness of the importance of age and damage prevention and thus an emphasis on anti-oxidants, more UVA protection in sunscreens, and new sunscreen labeling requirements in the United States. Nanotechnology is still being researched and developed.

Now in its fourth edition, the aim of this book remains the same: to help skin care professionals and their clients solve the mystery of skin care product performance by helping identify what the ingredient does and why it might be incorporated into a product. Part I is dedicated to understanding the skin—its physiology, its various types and conditions, and how it interacts with cosmetic products. A large number of technical terms often used in cosmetic product development and formulation are introduced and briefly defined here as well. Part II provides a listing of the ingredients that are commonly found in today's skincare cosmetics, both active principles and the ingredients that give a product its texture, color, stability, and acceptance by the skin and consumer. Finally, as ingredient labeling becomes more harmonized and it is increasingly common to find the Latin names of botanicals on an ingredient listing, Part III is a cross index of Latin names with the botanical's "common" name that is generally found in Part II.

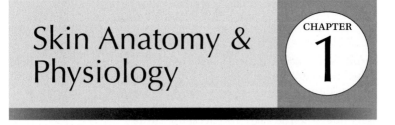

Skin Anatomy & Physiology

CHAPTER 1

INTRODUCTION

The skin is a complex, multipurpose organ that attracts much attention and scientific study. Science is constantly unraveling the intricacies of skin physiology, of the chemical substances present in the skin, and of their interaction. This knowledge, in turn, increases the understanding of how the processes of skin disease and skin aging occur. Scientists are identifying the skin's individual chemical components and the chemical and physiological reactions that accelerate aging. With the aging process better understood, laboratories are developing and incorporating new ingredients into cosmetic products that can reduce or decelerate the effects of aging and other skin problems, as well as counteract and/or correct them. A large number of new cosmetic ingredients are continually being introduced and this trend is expected to continue at a fast pace. Many of the ingredients used in cosmetics are intended to delay the aging process, rejuvenate the skin, improve skin problems, and even reduce the risk of skin cancer. A solid understanding of skin physiology allows for more targeted and effective skin care cosmetic formulations.

THE FUNCTIONS OF THE SKIN

As the body's largest organ, the skin performs a series of key functions resulting from multiple chemical and physical reactions that take place within it. The skin is a barrier, protecting the body from external elements, injury, and oxidation. It helps maintain a constant body temperature through the regulation of moisture loss thereby helping the body adapt to different ambient temperatures and atmospheric conditions. It gathers sensory information and plays an active role in the immune system, protecting the body from disease. In order to perform all of these functions—protective, metabolic, sensory, and immunological—the skin must maintain its own auto-repairing capacities and functional integrity.

Cosmetic products play a major role in the skin's protective function. Sunscreens protect against ultraviolet (UV) radiation and, therefore, against premature skin aging and skin cancer. Creams and lotions with a bactericidal effect reduce and/or control excessive proliferation of bacteria on the skin, a problem particularly associated with oily skin, and one of the main causes of acne formation. By forming an invisible barrier on the skin's surface, specific moisturizing ingredients can help reduce the skin's moisture loss that results in dehydration. The skin also protects the internal organs from exposure to oxygen. Without the skin, the body's organs would rapidly oxidize, much like a peeled banana or apple does when its interior is left exposed to air.

Through the secretion of sweat and sebum, the skin performs an excretory function, eliminating a number of harmful substances resulting from the metabolic activities of the intestine and the liver. The skin also secretes hormones and enzymes. When the skin's chemistry and chemical composition are not compatible with a particular ingredient(s) of a cosmetic product, the result is overall product sensitivity and even allergic reactions.

The large number of nerve endings in the skin makes it sensitive to touch. As a result, the skin is a sensory organ and the point of receptivity for cold, heat, pressure, stretching, pleasure, and pain.

The skin plays an immunological role, primarily through the Langerhans cells, which carry antigens from the skin to the lymphatic system. Excessive UV radiation either destroys or inhibits the performance of Langerhans cells, increasing the risk of skin cancer. The skin tends to be discussed and treated as an entity unto itself, so this close relationship between the skin and the body is often overlooked or forgotten. Although it protects the body in a variety of ways, the skin and its condition are governed by a number of internal body functions. For example, skin oiliness arises from oil gland hyperactivity and pigmentation problems are due to the tyrosinase enzyme; both can be regulated by hormonal functions. Given this relationship between the skin and the body, for the skin to look its best, there is a need to maintain overall health through proper nutrition, exercise, and rest. This connection also highlights the potential problems that ingredients penetrating deep into the dermis may cause if they are systemically absorbed by the capillary system.

When the skin performs in perfect harmony, the result is a beautiful, glowing, healthy complexion. If the skin does not function properly because of deterioration due to age, sun damage, bacterial infection, hyperkeratinization, or simply loss of natural moisture, cosmetic products can be used to assist in restoring its balance and beauty. They must do so, however, by working in conjunction with the skin's very complex structure.

SKIN COMPONENTS AND STRUCTURE

The skin has a very intricate microanatomical structure. In addition to thousands of skin cells, within one square inch of skin, varying from 0.04 inches (1 mm) to 0.16 inches (4 mm) in thickness, there are some

650 sweat glands, 65 hair follicles, 19 yards of capillaries, 78 yards of nerves, thousands of nerve endings, Merkel cells for sensory perception, and Langerhans cells for immunological protection. The skin also contains melanocyte cells responsible for producing the melanin that gives the skin its color and pigmentation spots, or freckles. For a solid visual understanding, draw a one-inch square and attempt to make 650 dots representing the sweat pores in the square. Then take a spool of thread, measure 19 yards, and place it within the square. If you are having a hard time with 650 dots and 19 yards of thread, imagine trying to add 1,300 nerve endings and 78 yards of nerves! All of this is found in one square inch of skin, about as thick as a few stacked sheets of paper.

The skin is home to a variety of glands. These glands are important for their intrinsic functions and also because they represent a route of entry into the skin for certain chemical compounds. Their main function is to synthesize substances that can cool the body, protect the skin, increase skin suppleness, or eliminate impurities such as mineral elements or cholesterol. Among these glands are the sebaceous glands and two sweat glands: the eccrine and apocrine glands.

Sebaceous glands, also known as oil glands, are attached to the same duct that contains the hair follicle (phylosebaceous duct). They are responsible for oil secretion in the skin, and are held within little sacs. The ducts of the oil glands open into the upper portion of the hair follicle. Usually, there is only one oil gland per follicle, but in some locations there may be more, resulting in greater oil (sebum) secretion in that area. Oil glands are found in almost all parts of the body. The face and back contain the highest number per square inch of skin, whereas the palms of the hands and soles of the feet contain none. The sebum secreted by the oil glands lubricates the skin and helps prevent the evaporation of moisture. It also possesses some anti-fungal properties. Excessive oil secretion is associated with the development of acne, while insufficient oil secretion is associated with skin dryness.

Sweat glands are abundant throughout the skin. Eccrine glands are the most numerous. Their secreting duct opens as a pore directly onto the skin surface. Very abundant on the soles of the feet and the palms of the hands, they secrete a transparent fluid composed mainly of water, lactic acid, urea, toxins, and bacteria-fighting substances. The primary function of this secretion is to cool the body and to maintain thermal equilibrium with the environment. The apocrine sweat glands are mainly situated in the axillae (armpit) and the pubic areas. They are inactive until puberty and are stimulated by emotions and stress. The excretion of the apocrine sweat glands is very limited; it does not occur directly onto the skin's surface, but rather into the upper part of the hair follicle, and from there to the skin surface. The perspiration from apocrine sweat glands can smell unpleasant due to a chemical reaction between the excretion, oxygen, and the enzymes produced by the bacteria (microflora) in the hair follicle and on the skin.

It is important to note that impurities and/or congestion seen in the pores occur in the hair follicle. They are the result of a mixture produced by sebum, keratin from stratum corneum cells (corneocytes), and bacteria present in the follicle. Cleansing the skin means eliminating impurities from these pores. Perspiration is not a cleanser. It may help clean the tiny opening of the sweat pores, but perspiration will not cleanse the hair follicle, the pore through which oil is secreted. This is a regular misconception by those who feel that saunas or perspiration cleanse the skin.

The surface of the skin is acidic. Its pH, also known as its protective mantle, is formed by a number of components, including naturally secreted sebum and perspiration (containing small amounts of uric and lactic acids). Chemical reactions occurring in the skin also generate several relatively strong water-soluble acids. At the stratum corneum, the skin's pH level ranges from 4.4 to 5.6, depending where on the body the reading is taken. It also appears to vary by individual and race. As one moves past the stratum corneum through the epidermis and into the dermis, the pH level increases and becomes neutral (pH 7.0).

The skin's acidity helps maintain its strength and cohesiveness, helps ward off infection by preventing the growth of bacteria, and allows for easier and more normal exfoliation of surface dead cells. One of the principal reasons why soaps—especially harsh soaps or cleansers with high pH values—are detrimental to the skin is because the skin needs an acidic environment to function properly. This is why, after using certain skin care cleansers a balancing lotion is needed: when cleansers have a neutral or alkaline pH, the skin's acidic level needs to be restored. Left alone, the skin will regain its acidic value in about 20 minutes (or more) depending on the level of acidic imbalance created.

All of these components and actions are found within the basic building block of skin tissue, treated and discussed as three layers.

LAYERS OF THE SKIN

The skin is a highly specialized and complex set of tissues divided into three layers: the epidermis, dermis, and hypodermis, also known as the subcutaneous layer (Figure 1–1).

There are several different types of cells in the skin, the most important of which are keratinocytes, melanocytes, fibroblasts, and a variety of immune cells (Langerhans, migrating mononuclear

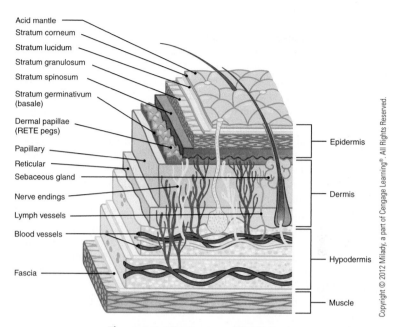

Acid mantle
Stratum corneum
Stratum lucidum
Stratum granulosum
Stratum spinosum
Stratum germinativum (basale)
Dermal papillae (RETE pegs)
Papillary
Reticular
Sebaceous gland
Nerve endings
Lymph vessels
Blood vessels
Fascia

Epidermis
Dermis
Hypodermis
Muscle

Copyright © 2012 Milady, a part of Cengage Learning®. All Rights Reserved.

Figure 1.1 *The Layers of the Skin*

cells and mast cells). In addition to these various cell types, the skin also contains connective tissues that are rich in extra cellular matrix (ECM), the components of which are primarily responsible for the skin's flexibility—its suppleness and elasticity.

Other physiologically important functions such as hydration, temperature regulation, and the regulation of the skin's permeability depend on specific cells and the chemical composition of the ECM. These regulatory functions are closely linked to the interaction between the cells and the chemicals in the skin through special receptors located on the membrane of each cell. These receptors can be thought of as antennae that help cells communicate with each other and with their environment. They are also able to bind with various chemical components that pass between cells. Among these chemical substances are certain ingredients commonly used in cosmetics (such as retinol) that interact with cells and perform a variety of therapeutic functions through cellular receptors. When receptors do not function properly, the skin's physiological performance may be impaired, accelerating damage or deterioration, such as aging. While work with receptors is a concept studied more extensively in medicine and pharmaceuticals, in cosmetics the role of receptors for retinol effectiveness, for example, is well established.

The epidermis is the part of the skin visible to the naked eye. It is a very thin layer approximately 25 to 30 cell layers deep: its thickness varies from 0.063 inches (1.6 mm) on the soles of the feet to 0.002 inches (0.04 mm) on the eyelids. The epidermis contains a variety of cells, including keratinocytes, which are engaged in a constant process of reproduction to replace exfoliated cells; Langerhans cells for immunological protection; melanocytes for skin color; and Merkel cells that are involved in the function of touch. The epidermis is the layer of skin to which products are applied, and the one with which an individual (and cosmetics) comes most in contact when cleansing, exfoliating, healing, and hydrating.

The second skin layer, and dermis, lies below the epidermis and is connected to it by the basement membrane. The dermis also varies in thickness from 0.12 inches (3.0 mm) on the back to 0.012 inches (0.3 mm) on the eyelids. It represents the most important part of the skin. It is made of collagen and elastin (connective tissues), hair follicles, oil (sebaceous) and sweat (eccrine) glands, blood vessels, and nerves that transmit sensations of touch, pressure, pain, itch, and temperature.

The third skin layer, the hypodermis, is the deepest of the three layers. Consisting primarily of fat and connective tissue it houses mostly large blood vessels and nerves. The hypodermis is much thicker than the epidermis and dermis. Its measured thickness, however, depends on the part of the body being evaluated and the fat content of the individual. This layer is important for regulating both skin and body temperature.

A close examination of each layer, including composition and function, is important for further understanding the impact a cosmetic product may have on the skin.

The Epidermis

Understanding the epidermis is extremely important for discussing product penetration, the definition of cosmetic versus pharmaceutical action according to FDA regulation, and product efficacy. The epidermis gives the skin its glow, youthfulness, texture, and good looks. It is responsible for the skin's health, protecting it from moisture loss and the penetration of bacteria. UV rays, acne conditions, visible skin disease, cigarette smoke, pollution, and skin cancer all affect this layer.

The epidermis is a metabolically active tissue that synthesizes lipids and contains all the individual components required to form the protective barrier layer. Since the epidermis represents the outermost layer of the skin, it acts as the initial barrier to oxidant assault. The epidermis has a higher protective and anti-oxidant capacity than the dermis because it houses essential free radical scavengers such as vitamins E and C and superoxide dismutase. This layer also contains large amounts of glycosaminoglycans and ceramides.

The epidermis is divided into five sublayers of cells, all of which play an active role in maintaining healthy skin. From the surface of the skin down to the dermis, these five layers are as follows:

1. Stratum corneum layer
2. Stratum lucidum layer
3. Stratum granulosum layer
4. Spinous layer
5. Germinative (Basal) layer

Epidermal cells are formed in the germinative layer and move upward toward the stratum corneum layer. In their upward migration, epidermal cells undergo a number of chemical modifications, transforming from soft, protoplasmic cells into flat surface "scales" made of keratin that constantly rub off.

The epidermis holds a large amount of water. The layer with the highest water content is the germinative layer, holding about 80 percent. Each subsequent layer has less water as a percentage of its total chemical composition, with the stratum corneum layer containing only 10 to 15 percent water. Water is held in the cell's cytoplasmic gel and in the intercellular channels (spaces between the cells). The younger the body, the more water there is in the skin. The skin's capacity to retain water decreases with age, making the skin more vulnerable to dehydration and wrinkles.

The epidermis is also the first barrier against immunological aggressors, thanks to the Langerhans cells. These dendritic cells are formed in the bone marrow and migrate to the skin's dermal and epidermal layers. Once they complete their migration, Langerhans cells typically are found in the lower layers of the epidermis, comprising about 5 percent of the total epidermal cell population. These cells engulf foreign bodies, carrying the invaders to the lymphatic system to be processed and eliminated. Langerhans cells are sensitive to UV radiation, and are easily damaged by UV rays. Even minor UV exposure will damage the Langerhans cells enough to reduce the skin's immune capacities. With age, these cells also decrease in number. This is one reason why the possibility of skin disease increases with age.

In a young person, it takes approximately 28 days for a cell to travel from the germinative to the corneum layer. With age, the speed of this process drops significantly. It is estimated that after the age of 50, it takes about 37 days to complete the same process.

In terms of skin aging, this indicates that stimulating skin functions, either manually through facial massage or through cosmetic product activity, would improve cellular metabolism. The 28- and 37-day time span is also important when it comes to skin sensitivity and the misuse of facial scrubs. If it takes 28 days or more for a cell to reach the surface of the skin, then we are naturally exfoliating one layer of dead cells a day. Depending on the harshness of the material, the use of scrubs may remove more layers of surface dead cells than appropriate, potentially increasing skin sensitivity. Furthermore, the misuse of scrubs may exacerbate oil gland activity, thereby increasing oil production, the opposite of what one generally wishes to achieve.

Epidermal layers

Understanding the epidermal layers allows us to understand some of the problems of dehydration, sensitivity, aging and pigmentation, which in turn helps associate product and ingredient effectiveness with skin requirements. The cells of the four epidermal layers from the germinative to the stratum lucidum layer are referred to as keratinocytes and are the predominant cell species found in the epidermis. The primary function of the epidermis is to manufacture the uppermost layer, the stratum corneum layer. An improperly functioning keratinocyte formation system cannot generate an esthetically acceptable stratum corneum layer. Therefore, a key factor for beautiful skin appears to be the appropriate metabolism of keratinocytes in order to generate a healthy stratum corneum layer. This is important in order to protect against moisture loss and the penetration of microbes and chemical irritants.

The germinative layer, also referred to as the basal layer, is where the cells reproduce by mitosis (one cell divides into two) creating two cells identical to one another and to the original parent cell. After subdivision, one cell remains in the basal layer and the other is pushed upward toward the upper epidermal layers. In young skin, the germinative layer is the thickest layer of the epidermis. Here, the cells are large and supple, and contain a high percentage of water.

As the cells move upward toward the stratum corneum layer, they begin to fill with a granular substance called keratin (hence the term keratinocyte). The keratinocytes lose water, become flat, and their cellular contents dissolve. As the cells migrate through the layers, they secrete a variety of lipid materials (i.e., cholesterol, fatty acids, and ceramides) into the intercellular spaces, increasing cohesion between the cells, thus helping make the epidermis an effective barrier.

In their last stage of migration, the cells reach the stratum corneum layer. This layer is considered so important to product penetration, skin hydration, and the reduction of skin sensitivity that it is often studied separately from the other epidermal layers. The stratum corneum layer is what we see as our skin. In healthy, young skin, it is composed of 18 to 23 layers of flattened, dead cells (also called corneocytes) firmly cemented together. The actual number of layers depends on a variety of factors, including oil secretion and exfoliation rate. The stratum corneum is thickest on the palms of the hands and soles of the feet and thinnest on the eyelids. Scientists divide the stratum corneum into two distinct layers: the compact layer, where the corneocytes are linked one to another and act as a barrier, and the outer sloughing layer. In this second layer, the breakdown of cellular union provokes exfoliation, allowing for the continuous elimination of cells. Here, as the corneocytes gradually detach, numerous spaces are formed between the cells where the bacteria living on the skin find refuge and thrive, feeding on the remaining corneocytes and lipids. These bacteria are adapted to the acid environment of the stratum corneum. Other bacteria, known as transients, may be present on the surface of the skin, but the pH conditions are unfavorable for their development and proliferation.

The natural cellular exfoliation process is enzymatically controlled. Specific enzymes dissolve the bonds holding the corneocytes together, enabling them to slough off. If this process is not functioning properly, too many dead cells will accumulate on the skin surface causing hyperkeratosis (too much keratin), and leaving the skin looking thick, rough, and esthetically unpleasing. The stratum corneum layer retains only about 10 to 15 percent of its original moisture. Its principal activities are to prevent skin dehydration by stopping water from evaporating through the skin (transepidermal water loss) and inhibiting foreign matter from penetrating the skin. The cells are held together and surrounded by lipids and ceramides, as well as glycoproteins, desmosomes, peptide breakdown products, sebaceous products, and active enzymes. The intercellular lipids play a crucial role in the skin's water-retention properties by acting as a barrier, trapping water, and preventing excessive water loss. Ceramides account for up to 40 percent of the total intercellular lipids and also play a vital role in the skin's water-retaining capacity.

The stratum corneum layer includes a natural moisturizing factor (NMF) made of hydrosoluable (able to dissolve in water) and hygroscopic (able to retain water) substances that regulate the stratum corneum's selective permeability. The NMF is composed of about 40 percent free amino acids, some 12 percent PCA, 12 percent lactose, 7 percent urea, and approximately 30 percent of a large variety of other materials. Exposure to harsh detergents and climatic conditions can result in decreased NMF levels, rendering the skin fragile and dry.

The thickness of the stratum corneum layer, the appropriate arrangement of its surface cells, and the strength of the cellular cement greatly determine a product or ingredient's ability to penetrate. A well-formed stratum corneum tends to be thin and compact with an orderly cellular structure mimicking a basket-weave and yielding a strong barrier function. When the stratum corneum layer is thick and its cells are arranged in a compact, uneven pattern, the natural barrier function of the skin is reduced, allowing for potential irritants to penetrate. This is one reason why products may produce an irritation or a burning sensation. When the skin is excessively moist, sensitivity may also occur because the barrier has been disrupted, making it easier for certain irritants to penetrate. Ingredients such as alpha hydroxy acids (AHAs) restructure or "normalize" an abnormal stratum corneum, giving it a healthier structure and restoring its protective capacities.

Skin pigment or melanin is formed at the deepest layer of the epidermis by the melanocyte cells. This pigment is later transferred to the keratinocytes, giving the skin its color. Excessive melanin production can be induced by sun or UV light exposure (e.g., sunbathing, tanning beds) and/or hormonal imbalances. In the first case, the melanocytes produce additional melanin in an attempt to protect the skin from free radical damage. Once UV light exposure is stopped, cellular migration and normal exfoliation allow the skin to slowly eliminate the pigmented cells and recover its normal color. For example, a few months after summer vacation, the skin returns to its normal color. In the second case, hormonal imbalances cause shifts that trigger greater melanocyte activity, producing an overabundance of pigment in the skin. This is most commonly observed during pregnancy (melasma). Additionally, severe irritation reactions can also stimulate excessive melanin production in a similar manner as hormones, resulting in post-inflammatory hyperpigmentation (PIH).

Immunological protection is provided in the epidermis by the Langerhans cells. Their function is to detect foreign bodies that have penetrated the epidermis, capture them, and carry them to lymphocytes in the lymphatic system. An immune response is then triggered, neutralizing and finally eliminating the foreign element.

Touch is sensed by the Merkel cells that are situated between the keratinocytes. Merkel cells are a modified epidermal cell associated with a receptor. As a nerve ending in glabrous (hairless) skin approaches the base of the epidermis, it expands into a flattened leaf or "ivy" shape and lies close to specialized cells near the epidermal/dermal junction. These are sometimes referred to as hederiform or "ivy-shaped" nerve endings or Merkel disks, after the scientist, Friedrish Sigmund Merkel, who first described them. However, not a great deal is known about these endings.

These three types of specialized epidermal cells—the melanocytes, the Langerhans cells, and the Merkel cells—account for 13 to 20 percent of total epidermal cells.

The complexity of the epidermal layer is astonishing, especially when considering its thinness. In addition to the different cells present, their individual functions, and their relationship to one another, there is constant activity in the skin: cellular receptors are communicating, and a host of physiological and chemical interactions are ongoing. All of these elements need to remain in proper equilibrium in order to ensure the appropriate keratinocyte metabolism and functioning. Without such balance, the beauty and the health of the skin are impaired. Thus, caring for the skin and avoiding unnecessary harshness become critical for the skin's health and beauty.

The Dermis

The dermis is the second layer of the skin. It is 10 to 40 times thicker than the epidermis. Within the dermis are the appendages of the skin, the hair follicles, sebaceous glands, the two types of sweat glands (eccrine and apocrine), plus a complex capillary and nerve network. The dermis is made of 80 percent moisture, elastin fibers that supply elastic properties, and collagen fibers that provide a structural framework Collagen represents about 70 percent of the dermal proteins and provides resistance, resilience, and traction. About 20 different types of collagen fibers have been identified with collagen I and III being most common to the skin. Optimum wound healing is achieved when the repair process begins with the production of very thin collagen fibers and continues with collagen fibers of increasing thickness. Keloids are formed when wound healing begins with thicker forms of collagen. In addition to collagen and elastin, the dermis has a variety of other fibers, grouped together as structural glycoproteins, and a set of chemicals grouped under the term glycosaminoglycans. These are responsible for hydration, suppleness, and water retention. They also regulate permeability, provide resistance to pressure, and are responsible for the orientation of proteins.

By means of its vast network of capillaries and blood vessels, the dermis provides energy and nutrition to the viable epidermis, and plays a critical role in healing and thermoregulation. It is responsible for the supporting framework and elasticity of the skin, which also depends on well-balanced water content in the dermis and other skin layers. To facilitate this essential hydration, the dermis acts as a water storage site. It also protects the body from mechanical injury, and plays an important role in sensory perception and as an internal regulator. Langerhans cells, responsible for immunoprotection, are also present in the dermis.

The dermis consists of a thick connective membrane crisscrossed by blood vessels, lymphatic vessels, nerve fibers, and many sensory nerve endings. Collagen and elastin protein fibers, the two main components of the dermis, act as a structural support system for the nerve fibers, hair follicles, blood vessels, and oil and sweat glands located in this layer, and also provide the skin with strength and elasticity.

Collagen is the dermis' principal component and is basically a chain of amino acids including alanine, arginine, lysine, glycine, proline, and hydroxyproline. Its production begins with the elaboration of procollagen, which later undergoes a series of modifications and is transformed into regular collagen. Procollagen is very hygroscopic and binds many times its weight in water. A decreasing procollagen content over time may be related to the increased dryness, wrinkles, and lack of elasticity associated with mature skin.

In undamaged or normal skin, different types of elastin fibers account for 2 to 4 percent of the dermis. They form an interconnected structure that provides skin elasticity and resilience. Under a microscope, elastin looks like short, overlapping fibers that form an irregular network within the dermis, primarily concentrated in the layer's lower segments. The importance of elastin is disproportionate to the relatively small quantity found in the dermis.

Filling the space between collagen and elastin are various types of glycoproteins and glycosaminoglycans. These form a significant part of the ECM and provide structural support for the dermis. Glycoproteins are large molecules that combine a protein with a carbohydrate. The most common glycoprotein is fibronectin. This molecule plays a major role in cell adhesion, growth, migration, and differentiation and is important for wound healing. Glycosaminoglycans are large carbohydrates that can bind to proteins creating what are called proteoglycans (a type of glycoprotein) or can be found as independent molecules in both the epidermis and dermis. Glycosaminoglycans are fundamental dermal materials that provide support, lubrication, and the proper environment for the development of dermal cells. They also have a great water-binding capacity and are, therefore, crucial for the skin's turgor, water content, and elasticity. The most common glycosaminoglycan is hyaluronic acid. With age, the skin's glycosaminoglycan content diminishes, thus decreasing the skin's capacity to retain water and increasing the propensity for skin dryness.

The proper functioning of the dermal layer, as well as its water content, accounts for the skin's hue, smoothness, and elasticity. A properly functioning dermis is key for a youthful appearance and beautiful skin.

The Hypodermis

The hypodermis or subcutaneous fascia (fat) is the third and last layer of the skin. It lies just below the dermis and the deeper tissues known as fascia and muscle. This layer gives the skin its shape and works as a thermal insulator, shock absorber, and nutritional depot where nutrients can be stored until needed. The layer is firmly attached to the lower surface of the dermis but loosely bound to its underlying structures, giving the skin mobility over the deeper fascia. The fat lobules of the tissue are surrounded by collagen fibers, which support vascular networks, lymph vessels, and nerves from the underlining tissues to the dermis. It is not present where the skin is especially thin such as the eyelids, nipples, genitals, and shins.

Generally speaking, this layer is not normally considered when formulating cosmetic products, except when trying to minimize cellulite and/or reduce the overall thickness of various body parts, for example the thighs and belly in the case of slimming products. Additionally, recent research has shown that nutrients taken orally may be stored in this tissue, such as fat soluble anti-oxidants, that can later be transferred to the dermis and/or epidermis to minimize damage from free radicals. Lastly, it should be noted that working with this layer of skin can be important in other therapeutic areas like Rolfing.

SUMMARY

The skin, with its many tiny components and multilayered structure, is astonishingly complex. For the skin to be healthy and beautiful, the balance and the proper working of all interrelated elements are essential. As more light is shed on how the skin works, cosmetic chemists have new elements to consider when exploring improvements in the functioning of different skin mechanisms and the formulation of appropriate skin care products.

As more is known about the skin and its complexity, its chemical composition, and how it functions and why, there are greater opportunities to identify ingredients or compounds that can provide significant benefit to the skin. This includes maintaining the beauty and health of the skin, and delaying the damage caused by the passage of time—assuming, of course, that these ingredients remain unchanged when they reach their targeted destination within the skin.

Skin Types, Conditions, & Problems

INTRODUCTION

In today's world it is essential to know as much as possible about the skin before treating it or applying products to it. Understanding the skin's anatomy and physiology, and the basic skin types (normal, oily, and dry) is important. Paramount to providing appropriate and effective skin care, however, is collecting information about specific conditions and/or problems that the skin may be experiencing or has experienced in the past. This chapter is intended to provide a better understanding of the skin's different types, conditions, and problems, as well as the tools to best work with them.

THE FIVE BASIC QUESTIONS

The biological variation between people is vast, and the days of guessing a person's skin type or sensitivity level are long gone: mothers will react differently than their daughters; women of color may be more sensitive than the red hair, fair complexion, green-eyed individual. Therefore, one needs to do much more than just guess a person's skin or photo-skin type. In a professional skin care context, five minutes of time to gather as much information as possible can save several hours of problems later. This can help build a positive, long-lasting relationship between skin care professionals and their clients. The following five basic questions provide a significant amount of important information that can help determine the most appropriate course of skin care:

1. Are you planning a pregnancy, pregnant, or nursing?
2. Are you currently taking any medications?
3. Have you ever experienced a skin irritation, rash, or acne?
4. Have you ever had a reaction to medicine, food, clothing, flowers, cosmetics, hair dye, perfumes, or jewelry?
5. Do you consider yourself to have sensitive skin or eyes?

Cosmetics, and skincare products in particular, are no longer designed as discussed in this volume's introduction. In 1938, the FDA defined cosmetics as "any product, except soap, intended to be applied to the human body for cleansing, beautifying, promoting at-tractiveness, or altering appearances." Many products are now avail-able that contain biologically active ingredients (vitamins, peptides, anti-oxidants, etc.), and can interact with the body's biochemical mechanisms, going far beyond the 1938 definition in their action. Such products are called *cosmeceuticals*, a term combining the words *"**cosme**tics"* and *"pharma**ceuticals"*** to imply that the product will do more than the 1938 FDA definition. (They are also sometimes re-ferred to as "active cosmetics.") Therefore, if products can do more, it is important to understand more about the products in order to avoid causing unintentional problems.

Why the pregnancy question? Some vitamin A (retinol) products could contain one to four times the Recommended Dietary Allow-ance (RDA) for this vitamin. There is some concern over too much Vitamin A during pregnancy. Could there be a problem or risk if a woman is pregnant and using one, two, three, or even four products all containing high levels of Vitamin A? This is question best left to a medical doctor. However, if it is discovered that a client is or is try-ing to become pregnant she should speak to her doctor to make sure there are no concerns with using the product(s) being recommended.

Taking medications into account is also important. For instance, if someone is using a topical steroid for a skin condition it may cause another product to penetrate too deeply into the skin, resulting in an adverse reaction. People taking a drug for herpes should be aware that some skin care treatments (e.g., chemical peels, dermabrasion, etc.) could cause an outbreak. An individual with a minor outbreak of herpes should suspend all treatment regimes until the skin lesions are gone. Skin care professionals are not medical professionals, and if there are any doubts, a medical doctor should be consulted to make sure there are no concerns.

The final three questions all focus on a person's past history of skin reactions. Many people have had some type of adverse reaction but have never thought of it as such. Thus it is important to ask, "Have you ever experienced a skin irritation, rash, or acne?" Additionally, it is important to ask about more than just a problem with cosmetics. Many similar ingredients are used in different types of products and are found in nature. A person who cannot wear fake jewelry may not tolerate a product that contains iron oxides, titanium dioxide, zinc oxide, or any type of metal as they can all contain nickel—a metal to which about 10 percent of the women in the United States are aller-gic. People who have a problem with certain flowers such as primrose may also have problems with hair dyes containing para-phenylene-diamine (PPD), or with hydroquinone-based skin bleaching agents. Why? Because all three can contain 1,4-benzoquinone. Lastly, at least

25 percent of the population believes they have sensitive skin or eyes. This means they may be *atopic* or "not typical" and have reactions that are not visible, such as itching or burning. In the face of uncertainty a simple patch test can help identify allergies or intolerance, and this can be done before beginning product use:

> To an area about the size of a quarter on the skin of the inner arm where the elbow folds, apply and rub-in a small amount of the product in question. If after several hours or overnight no reactions are seen (no redness, no swelling, no itching, or no burning) there is a 95 percent chance that the person will be able to use the product. If at any time the person experiences a reaction (i.e., redness, swelling, itching or burning) the person should wash the area where the product was applied and not use it.

There are many interactions that one would not expect, and which are still not understood. Taking a few minutes to talk to a client before performing a treatment procedure or recommending a product can make a world of difference in the outcome. When in doubt consult with a doctor or call the product manufacturer and ask any specific question(s) regarding use or compatibility. In a professional setting, when speaking with clients sometimes changing the way the question is asked, or asking fewer or more questions works better. Ultimately, we are all continually learning, and adding to one's knowledge base can help get the maximum benefit from cosmetic products.

SKIN TYPES

Skin types are a combined expression of our genes (hereditary) and the climate in which we live (environment). This combination of heredity and environmental attributes produces three basic categories: normal, oily, and dry. These skin types can occur to varying degrees, ranging from slightly oily or slightly dry, all the way to very oily or very dry. Additionally, it is not unusual to observe a combination of these skin types, which is generally referred to as "combination skin," with normal to oily and normal to dry being most common. These conditions or combinations usually occur in the "T-zone"—the area across the forehead, down the nose and to the chin.

Most people will fall into one of these three categories, but there are always exceptions to any rule. People often identify their skin type incorrectly and are usually off by one or two categories. The best example is among those who exhibit slight oiliness in the T-zone area. When asked, some will say that their skin is very oily and that they are using an exfoliating cleanser followed by a strong oily skin cleanser every day. Such a cleansing regime is far too aggressive for this skin type and often the person will have red, irritated skin that is dehydrated (i.e., lacking moisture but not oil) from damage to the stratum corneum layer. Thus, it is important to appropriately evaluate the skin, and recommend or use products based on what is seen not just on what is perceived or said.

Normal Skin

Normal skin has good hydration, tone, and resilience produced by a properly functioning epidermis and dermis that is well hydrated and adequately supported by adipose tissues. There is strong biological activity at the basal layer, blood circulation is active, and the metabolism is balanced. Normal skin looks soft, moist, plump, and dewy, and has a healthy glow and color. The stratum corneum layer is translucent, showing a fine texture, and there are no visible lines from dehydration or large pores associated with oiliness. The best example of normal skin is that of children, from birth usually until puberty.

Aging due to the passage of time, sun exposure, and other external elements such as harsh climate, dehydration, and poor skin care, is the primary factor behind the deterioration of normal skin. Other factors include insufficient water intake and an inadequate diet. Food devoid of vitamins, enzymes, and amino acids does not provide the cells with the nourishment necessary for proper cellular reproduction and growth. Improper skin care, such as lack of cleansing, is quite prevalent in children and teenagers due to the lack of skin care awareness. Yet, in these cases, keeping the skin clean is essential. Cleansing twice a day (morning and evening) with an appropriate cleansing product can reduce acne by up to 25 percent. The use of harsh soaps and scrubs as well as the environment contribute to the deterioration of normal skin. Exposure to sun and the elements without protection dries, dehydrates, and prematurely ages the skin.

Normal skin requires proper morning and evening cleansing, plus protection from oxidation caused by free radicals and the sun. The consistent use of protective moisturizers containing anti-oxidants and a sunscreen during the day to prevent moisture loss and free radical damage, along with hydrating creams at night is essential. It is important that these moisturizers contain anti-oxidants such as vitamins E and C, idebenone, or coenzyme Q10. Occasional exfoliation is also beneficial. Sun protection is extremely important, even for children. Children should not be allowed on the beach without a proper sunscreen or in the snow without a good protective cream that includes UV and anti-oxidant protection. For normal skin the key is damage prevention and control.

Oily Skin

Oily skin is a condition that develops due to overactive sebaceous (oil) glands producing an abundance of sebum (oil). This activity is mainly controlled by androgens or the masculine hormone. Oily skin can be recognized by its shiny, thick, and firm appearance. Pores look enlarged, usually due to oil, stratum corneum cells and bacteria trapped in the philosebaceous follicle. An oily complexion tends to look dirty and uncared for—with occasional blemishes on the chin, cheeks, and/or the forehead area—and feels oily to the touch.

Hot and humid climates tend to exacerbate oil gland secretion, making the skin oilier. Additionally, oily skin problems can be aggravated by the misuse of skin care products. There is a tendency to dry the skin either through the use of harsh soaps or through the excessive use of astringents or scrubs disrupting the barrier function of the skin and allowing water to evaporate. Overstimulation of skin functions through scrubbing or stimulating massage should be avoided.

Oily skin can be classified into two subcategories: oily (*without* water deficiency) and oily dehydrated (*with* water deficiency). In the first case, the skin has proper hydration; while it feels and looks oily, it does not have the sensation of "dryness." In the second subcategory, the skin lacks moisture. All the characteristics of oily skin are present but the individual tends to complain of "dry skin." Often those with oily skin tend to use drying, dehydrating ingredients in an effort to feel "less oily." The end result is skin that feels flaky, rough, and scaly. The usual thought when this type of condition develops is to "self-diagnose" as a dry skin type and purchase products rich in oils. As the skin already has enough oil, these products only aggravate the oily condition and result in blemishes, blackheads, etc. It is not unusual for individuals with oily skin to conclude that they do not need a moisturizer because they have oily skin. Thus, it is important to remember that oiliness comes from the oil glands, and moisture from the intercellular channels.

Care of oily skin requires thorough yet gentle cleansing morning and evening. Oil-free moisturizing gels or lotions will help the skin maintain its suppleness and moisture. Other products such as those that claim to help regulate oil gland secretion can be used; however, the effectiveness of these products is questionable and will be discussed in the next chapter. It is essential to keep oily skin clean and hydrated with appropriate cleansing and moisturizing. Exfoliators that also provide moisture to the skin, such as alpha hydroxy acids (AHAs) or beta hydroxy acids (BHAs), or the weekly use of enzyme peels designed for oily skin are highly recommended. These products help improve the look and texture of oily skin by reducing oiliness, and pore size, and by normalizing exfoliation rates. When properly cared for, this is the preferred skin type since the wrinkle process appears to be delayed.

Dry Skin

Dry skin develops mainly as a result of under-active sebaceous glands, abnormal exfoliation of surface cells (hyperkeratosis), and environmental insults. As all body activities slow down with time, oil gland activity and exfoliation slow down as well. In fact, many women may find that their skin has gone from oily to dry after menopause. The lack of oil in dry skin reduces its ability to retain moisture, since oil on the surface of the skin acts as a natural barrier against moisture loss. Thus, dry skin is usually dehydrated and often feels scaly, rough, and itchy. Dry skin can frequently be characterized as very fine, overly delicate, and thin, with almost invisible pores. As a result, dry skin can have fewer cells in the stratum corneum layer than oily skin. The skin also tends to wrinkle easily and is often filled with tiny superficial lines. However, a dry skin type that is associated with abnormal exfoliation, sun damage, or general premature aging can appear thick and flaky.

Dry skin problems are aggravated by exposure to the sun, wind, and heat. Improper skin care, especially the lack of protection against moisture loss, further exacerbates this problem. Care for dry skin should include products that will add emollients or oils to the skin surface as well as those that add to or stimulate the skin's natural production of humectants (water binding ingredients). Adding emollients or oils to the surface of the skin helps form a "sealing" film, minimizing moisture loss. These products could also include high molecular weight ingredients, such as collagen, hyaluronic acid, and dimethicone. Moisturizing ingredients such as glycolic and lactic acids, glycerin, urea, ceramides, and cholesterol help boost the skin's natural water-retention ability and maintain moisture in the skin. Such multifunction moisturizers are essential for dry skin and are highly recommended. As with every skin type, the use of products with anti-oxidant ingredients is essential to delay cellular damage. The use of nourishing, hydrating masks is also advisable for dry skin.

Combination Skin

Combination skin occurs when oily, dry, or normal skin types are present simultaneously. It is unclear why this happens; however, the most common forms of combination skin tend to be either normal cheeks with an oily T-zone or dry cheeks with a normal T-zone. The skin generally is not dry and oily at the same time. Oily skin, however, can have areas that are dehydrated and require moisture. For normal to oily or oily skin with normal/dry-dehydrated patches, oil-free products that contain water-based humectants such as glycerin or sodium PCA are recommended. Products that contain ingredients that stimulate and/or repair the skin's moisture retention capacity, for example glycolic or lactic acids, essential fatty acids, ceramides and/or cholesterol, are better suited for normal to dry skin types.

Skin Phototype

There are several skin typing systems that are based on how a person reacts to sun or ultraviolet light. One that is commonly used was developed by Dr. Thomas Fitzpatrick in 1975. It is a scale that classifies six different skin types using Roman numerals 1(I) through 6(VI). Table 2–1 has been slightly modified by separating out the

Table 2–1 *Modified Fitzpatrick Classification Scale*

Skin Type	Characteristics	
	Appearance/General Characteristics	Reaction to UV Sun Exposure and Laser Treatment Damage Risks
I	Very Fair; Blond or red hair; light-colored eyes; freckles common.	Always burns, never tans. High risk for skin cancer, vascular damage.
II	Fair-skinned; light eyes; light hair	Burns easily; tans with difficulty. High risk for skin cancer, vascular damage.
III	Very common skin type; fair; eye and hair color vary	Sometimes burns, gradually tans. Risk of hyper/hypopigmentation. Moderate risk of skin cancer and vascular damage.
IV	Mediterranean Caucasian skin; dark brown hair; medium to heavy pigmentation.	Rarely burns, tans easily. High risk of hyper/hypopigmentation High risk for scarring. Moderate risk for vascular damage.
V	Middle Eastern skin; dark and black hair; brown eyes; rarely sun sensitive	Skin darkens; may never burn. High risk of hyper/hypopigmentation. High risk of scarring from treatments and trauma. Moderate risk for vascular damage. Lower risk for solar-pigmented conditions and actinic aging (from sun exposure).
VI	Black skin, brown eyes; rarely sun sensitive.	Tans easily; may never burn. Very high risk of hyper/hypopigmentation. Very high risk for scarring from treatments and trauma. Moderate risk for vascular damage. Lower risk for solar-pigmented conditions and actinic aging.

Copyright © 2015 Milady, a part of Cengage Learning®. All Rights Reserved.

characteristics of how a person "burns" and "tans" after sun exposure. As mentioned earlier in the "Five Basic Questions," biological variation between people is common and stereotyping how people react to anything based on skin, hair, or eye color can be a large mistake. Yet, when asked how they react to sun exposure using the characteristics in this scale, it is possible to get an idea of how sensitive a person is to the sun. As much as 90 percent of premature aging is from sun exposure, therefore, it is essential to gauge how susceptible someone is to the sun in order to properly prevent and/or treat premature aging.

Another identification system commonly used to evaluate photoaging was developed by Dr. Richard Glogau in 1996 and is outlined in Table 2–2. The table has been modified, removing the category of "Typical Age" since lifestyle and not age plays the major role behind the skin damage that appears. For example, Group I, Mild with No Wrinkles had a Typical Age of 28 to 35. This may be true if as a child the person frequently used sunscreens and avoided sun exposure. On the other hand, if the person started surfing or playing tennis as a teenager they would more than likely be classified as Group II, Moderate with Wrinkles in Motion by the age of 21. Therefore, regardless of what technique used to evaluate sun damage, taking lifestyle into account when considering appropriate skin care products can make a significant difference.

Table 2–2 *Modified Glogau Classification Scale*

Group	Classification	Description	Skin Characteristics
I	Mild	No wrinkles	**Early Photoaging:** mild pigment changes, no keratosis, minimal wrinkles, minimal or no makeup
II	Moderate	Wrinkles in motion	**Early to Moderate Photoaging:** early brown spots visible, keratosis palpable but not visible, parallel smile lines begin to appear, wears some foundation
III	Advanced	Wrinkles at rest	**Advanced Photoaging:** obvious discolorations, visible capillaries (telangiectasias), visible keratosis, wears heavier foundation always
IV	Severe	Only wrinkles	**Severe Photoaging:** yellow-gray skin color, prior skin malignancies, wrinkles throughout; no normal skin, cannot wear makeup because it cakes and cracks

Copyright © 2015 Milady, a part of Cengage Learning®. All Rights Reserved.

SKIN CONDITIONS

Skin conditions develop over time and apply to all skin types, leading to the many combinations that make everyone's skin unique. The most common skin conditions are acne, aging, couperose, dehydration, pigmentation, and rosacea. Skin conditions can develop for a variety of reasons, including hormonal imbalances, lack of environmental protection, over exposure to the sun, use of tanning beds, free radical damage, inflammation, low water content in the skin, unbalanced or excessive melanin production, the use of products containing ingredients that can trigger vasodilatation or allergic reactions, or improper daily skin care.

Acne

There are various forms of acne, which is the combination of non-inflammatory lesions called comedones (whiteheads and blackheads) and inflammatory lesions called papules and pustules (small red and white bumps, respectively, that are usually filled with fluid). Acne becomes prevalent at puberty when androgen hormones (e.g., testosterone) start to develop. Androgens stimulate the sebaceous glands to produce sebum (oil), which is then deposited into the follicle. Only follicles that have sebaceous glands attached to them (sebaceous follicles) are involved with acne. These follicles are located on the face, chest, upper back, and upper arms.

The production of acne involves more than just the stimulation of the sebaceous glands; bacteria (*Propionibacterium acnes* or *P. acnes* for short) must also be present, along with sloughed stratum corneum cells that line the follicle. Together, these various materials can provoke an acne response. When all of these elements combine, a plug is formed inside of the follicle, causing the follicle to expand in the middle, thereby reducing the size of the follicle's orifice (follicle opening) and trapping the materials inside. If the orifice remains open, the material that is contained in the follicle remains visible, becomes oxidized, and appears black in color, hence called a blackhead. If the orifice completely closes up, the comedone will appear white and thus the term *whitehead* is used. When one tries to remove the plug from the follicle by physically pushing it out with a device or fingers (extraction) it very often causes the follicle to rupture, leaking the contents (sebum, bacteria, and stratum corneum cells) into the dermis, provoking an inflammatory reaction (papules and/or pustules). This is the reason why many people complain about breaking out with clusters of papules or pustules following extractions. It is important to understand that this reaction is not related to the product(s) used, but it is a direct result of rupturing the follicle and causing an inflammatory reaction. Lastly, whether a lesion becomes a small papule/pustule or a large nodule depends on the severity or depth of inflammatory response provoked by rupturing the follicle.

There are many different ways to work with slight to moderate acne. Severe acne should not be treated with just basic cosmetics, cosmeceutical products, or procedures. This condition can be somewhat disfiguring and requires prescription medication such as oral retinoids or antibiotics. Individuals with slight to moderate acne respond well to a basic skin care regime appropriately designed for their skin type, i.e., a cleanser, toner or astringent, and a moisturizer used morning and evening. Additionally, one can incorporate a salicylic acid-, sulfur-, or benzoyl peroxide-based product into the regime to fight off more persistent acne or to accelerate healing. Botanical ingredients that have shown some benefits in subjects with acne are tea tree oil for its antibacterial benefits and willow bark for its salicylic acid content. Women of color that suffer from acne will often feel that acne lesions are not removed by some of these treatments. Unfortunately, the acne lesion is removed but often the inflammation associated with acne causes a slight depigmentation of the skin, making it look like the lesion is still there because of the uneven skin tone. One last note: acne often improves with sun exposure. A chemical called porphyrin is a byproduct of the *P. acnes* bacteria. When exposed to sunlight porphyrin produces a free radical that kills the bacteria, thus reducing acne. This is why acne usually improves from spring to summer and can worsen from fall to winter. However, since sunlight is the major cause of premature aging, one must balance out the risk of too much sun exposure and minimizing acne lesions.

Aging

Skin aging is a complex, biological process affecting various layers of the skin—most significantly the dermis—and includes a modification of genetic material. Among the events that occur in the aging process are deficiencies in the nutritional components within the different tissues, cellular destruction through excessive sun exposure, the effect of free radicals on the cellular membrane, deterioration in the genetic programming of the DNA, and a decrease in cellular proliferation. The impact on skin tissue is a loss of elasticity, a reduced ability to regulate water, and a less efficient replication or renewal process. The consequences are skin atrophy and a general process of degeneration.

Aging skin is characterized by a thick stratum corneum with a thin epidermis and dermis. It exhibits an accentuation of lines and wrinkles as a result of increased dryness and dehydration caused by skin thinning and reduced oil gland activity. The complexion looks withered, and assumes a lackluster hue as melanin production diminishes. Aging skin can be recognized by its poor elasticity, lack of normal firmness, and sagging due to the breakdown of collagen and elastin in the dermis. Aging is accompanied by a slowing down of cell proliferation. Skin thickness decreases with age. On average, the skin loses about 6 percent of its thickness every 10 years. This means that someone who is 100 years old will have lost approximately 60 percent of their initial skin volume. This impacts both the epidermis and dermis.

Skin aging can be grouped into two categories. The first is intrinsic or chronological aging, which results from the passage of time, and is the slow irreversible process of tissue degeneration. Intrinsic aging is linked to the transformation of connective tissue and the decrease of cellular regeneration. The second category is extrinsic aging. It is often referred to as photoaging since it is primarily due to sun (UV) exposure, which damages or destroys cellular reproductive abilities and degenerates collagen and elastin. Its clinical characteristics include fine lines and wrinkles, roughness, pigmentation, couperose, actinic keratosis, and skin cancer. Other factors that can cause or accelerate extrinsic aging are exposure to outdoor elements, stress, and lifestyle choices. In addition, skin aging is compounded by health problems, hormonal imbalances, improper care while young, and improper nutrition, which robs the skin of appropriate nourishment for cellular reproduction and growth. Recent research in the field of aging has linked both intrinsic and extrinsic aging to free radical damage. In the case of intrinsic aging, such damage is associated with the improper neutralization of free radicals that are produced in and by the cells when using oxygen to make energy. With respect to extrinsic aging, free radical damage arises from environmental insults such as excessive sun exposure. In reality, we are not aging we are oxidizing, and therefore, anti-oxidants are key in reducing the appearance of aging.

Anti-aging treatments emphasize the return to a smoother, more youthful appearance by softening and normalizing the look and feel of sun-damaged or otherwise extrinsically aged skin. With today's skin care technology, however, it is increasingly possible to emphasize the prevention of skin aging as well as the correction or improvement of its visible signs. It is well established that premature skin aging is mediated by free radical damage. One of the primary factors behind such damage is UV light, followed by cigarette smoke. Thus, the first step in an anti-aging treatment is to protect the skin from free radical formation and damage by using sunscreens and by increasing the skin's anti-oxidant levels through antioxidant-rich products. Furthermore, a diet rich in anti-oxidants will help both intrinsic aging from oxidative damage as well as help the skin prevent damage from the inside out. If correction is attempted without prevention, what is corrected at night can easily be re-damaged during the day.

Highly effective ingredients are available for correction in many cosmeceutical products. Among the most sophisticated ingredients currently available are idebenone and coffee-berry, powerful anti-oxidants that reduce collagen destruction and appear to affect intrinsic aging from oxidative damage. Various forms of vitamin A, especially retinol or retinoic acid, glycolic and lactic acids, numerous peptides and amino acids are among the many ingredients that appear to be effective when working with aging skin. Among the beneficial botanical ingredients for anti-aging treatment are apricot, for its vitamins A, B, C, and D and anti-oxidant content; carrot, for its vitamin A and mineral salts; and horseradish, for its ability to improve skin connective tissues, regulate skin functions, increase the skin's defense mechanisms, and prevent and/or counteract wrinkle formation.

When treating aging skin, it is important that the active principles be revitalizing, normalizing, stimulating, and hydrating, as well as protective. No single ingredient or product can accomplish all of this. A complete skin care regime should include daily sunscreen applications for protection; properly hydrating and anti-oxidant moisturizers; and corrective creams, lotions, gels, or emulsions with active principles that stimulate and revitalize skin function, nourish the skin, neutralize damaging chemicals formed in the skin, and activate intercellular activity and communications.

Couperose

Couperose can be a temporary or chronic redness appearing on the face. It shows up as small, dilated, winding, bright red blood vessels on the cheeks, around the nose, and sometimes on the chin. Couperose occurs primarily as a result of poor elasticity in the capillary wall. When there is a sudden rush of blood because of blushing, excessive heat, or other stimuli, the capillaries expand, making room for the increase of blood. When the amount of blood recedes, the capillaries contract to their normal size. If the capillary wall is not sufficiently elastic, it will expand but not contract again to its original shape or size. The result is a distended capillary that will hold blood cells within its structure, thus giving the appearance of diffuse or local redness.

Couperose is aggravated by atmospheric conditions such as hot or cold climates, by the use of excessively cold or hot water, nervous disorders, digestive disorders, saunas, exercise that causes the face to turn very red, drinking alcohol and very hot liquids, eating spicy foods, blushing, and excessive sun exposure. Individuals with couperose that are also using topical retinoids should consult with a physician, as this product may aggravate the condition as well. Care should be taken that couperose skin is not exposed to excessively hot or cold water. Night creams or lotions that help strengthen the capillary walls are helpful. Products with vasoconstrictive ingredients are also beneficial. Botanical ingredients of benefit for couperose include plantain; grape; horse chestnut; St. John's wort, for anti-inflammatory activity; and acacia, for its soothing capacities.

Dehydration

Dehydration—a lack of sufficient moisture in the cellular system and intercellular channels—is one of the most common skin conditions. Dehydration is caused by the compromised permeability of the lipid barrier; cracks in the skin due to a decrease in the suppleness, softness, and flexibility of the stratum corneum; a reduction in size of the flattened corneocytes; and a lower capacity by the skin to retain moisture, usually resulting from decreased glycosaminoglycan levels due to skin aging or damage.

Dehydration is aggravated by atmospheric conditions that include too much sun and wind as well as not using sunscreens and/or daytime protective moisturizers containing anti-oxidants. Other factors such as an overuse of inappropriate skin care products including cleansers containing harsh soaps or detergents, caffeinated products, diuretics and not drinking enough water also contribute to skin dehydration. Dehydrated skin looks dry, scaly, flaky, and it can feel tight. When gently pulled, the skin "crinkles" in a way that is similar to pulling a corner of very thin tissue paper. Sometimes the skin appears as if it had an additional thin layer of skin placed on top. This is particularly evident on the nose and forehead.

Dehydration is one of the most difficult skin conditions to diagnose. It is usually confused with dryness, which is technically a lack of oil. Unfortunately, dehydration and dryness have many similarities. Both dry and oily skin types may be dehydrated. Dry skin can be dehydrated because thin skin has difficulty retaining inner moisture. Oily skin becomes dehydrated through the use of harsh soaps and the excessive use of astringents. When oily skin becomes dehydrated, the surface layers of cells harden up and block oil secretion. The result is an entrapment of the oils under the stratum corneum layer. This is particularly detrimental in the case of someone with acne because it also results in the entrapment of the infection. To end the confusion between dehydration and dryness, the best approach is to first diagnose the skin type and then the skin condition.

Care for dehydrated skin requires the use of moisturizers containing ingredients that will protect the skin from moisture loss as well as restore internal skin hydration. Moisturizing ingredients that can help the skin retain inner moisture by reducing transepidermal water loss are generally high molecular weight ingredients that form a protective barrier on top of skin, for example silicones, polymers, and natural oils. The use of glycolic and lactic acids can activate the water-retention capability of glycosaminoglycans and could be complemented with ingredients that add moisture to the skin, such as glycerin, urea, and hyaluronic acid. In order to restore or improve the skin's intracellular matrix (and thereby reduce transepidermal water loss), ingredients such as ceramides, cholesterol, and essential fatty acids are key. In addition to moisturizers with these ingredients, proper care can include the application of hydrating masks on a weekly or biweekly basis, depending on the level of dehydration.

Pigmentation

Melanin production is a normal process in the skin's cellular activity, and gives rise to skin color or pigmentation. Melanin is produced and stored in organelles called melanosomes, which are found in melanocyte cells, located in the basal layer of the epidermis. Melanin is disbursed through the skin by a chemical process that allows the melanosomes to pass into the keratinocytes or skin cells. Once in the keratinocyte, the melanosome loses its membrane and releases the melanin, giving the skin its natural color. Melanin production is a very complicated biochemical reaction that is driven by the tyrosine protein, which is activated by the tyrosine's enzyme in an oxidative chain reaction. Exposure to UV light and the consequent increase in the oxidative process that can occur from such exposure causes an increase in melanin production. This reaction can also be hormonally controlled, which explains why melasma (also known as the mask of pregnancy) can result from pregnancy as well as be associated with the use of contraceptives. Menopause and prolonged periods of intense stress are also believed to cause melasma in susceptible individuals.

Hyperpigmentation results from an uneven distribution of melanin over the skin surface, either due to pigment accumulation, as in the case of age spots or lentigo, or because of uneven melanin production/absorption by the melanocytes, as in the case of melasma. The rate of melanin production varies from person to person and from race to race, being greater in darker-skinned individuals. Melanin acts as a filter, protecting the skin and body against the harmful effects of the sun's radiation. Therefore, a suntan is the body's protective response against internal skin damage from over exposure to the sun. Surface irritation, caused by irritants or allergic reactions, can also trigger either an increase in melanin production augmenting the amount of pigment in the skin (called Post-inflammatory *Hyper*pigmentation), or a decrease in the amount of pigmentation in the skin (Post-inflammatory *Hypo*pigmentation). Additionally, dark spots in lightly pigmented skin or light spots in heavily pigmented skin can also be the result of surface irritation caused by acne conditions.

The best treatment for pigmentation is based on bleaching agents and ingredients that can help regulate melanocyte activity. Bleaching and skin-lightening agents, both botanical and synthetically manufactured, can include all citruses, idebenone, kojic acid, linden, and yarrow. Hydroquinone, a very effective bleaching ingredient, has been removed from the cosmetic ingredient category in a number of countries due to a potential melanocyte-damaging effect. Some bleaching agents should only be applied at night, as some of the ingredients tend to react with sunlight and further aggravate the problem.

Other ingredients that can minimize melanin production are arbutin (a hydroquinone derivative which is banned in several countries), niacinamide, methyl gentisate, and anti-oxidants that can inhibit the oxidation reactions needed to produce pigment in the melanocyte. Such ingredients include idebenone, super oxide dismutase, alpha lipoic acid, green tea, and vitamins E and C. In addition, anti-inflammatory and soothing ingredients, for example licorice or bisabolol, are essential to reduce potential skin irritation, which can also stimulate melanin production. Ingredients such as glycolic or lactic acids and/or salicylic acid can help ferry pigment out of the skin via exfoliation.

Hyperpigmentation is one of the most challenging skin conditions to treat and, regardless of its cause, it is essential to use a broad spectrum sunscreen with a high SPF and UVA rating at *all times* during the day, no matter if it is sunny or cloudy, summer or winter. Direct sun exposure in the summer should be avoided, as UV light increases the process of oxidation responsible for pigmentation. The use of tanning beds should be avoided, of course. Failure to use a sunscreen could neutralize whatever result the treating product may give.

Rosacea

Rosacea is a chronic inflammatory skin condition of the face that impacts approximately 16 million people in the United States alone. Although the exact cause of rosacea is still unknown, various theories about its origin have evolved. These include facial blood vessels that dilate too easily, whereby the increased blood near the skin surface makes the skin appear red and flushed; certain bacteria present on otherwise harmless Demodex mites that could prompt an inflammatory response; overproduction of two inflammatory proteins that increase the levels of a third protein that leads to rosacea symptoms; a high level of stratum corneumtryptic enzymes (SCTE), the precursor of a rosacea-causing peptide. Many of these potential mechanisms have been studied, but none have yielded a cure for the condition.

People with rosacea will experience inappropriate flushing that is not usually associated with sweating and/or persistent facial redness. They commonly have broken blood vessels (telangiectasias or couperose) and experience bouts of inflammation that cause papules or pustules. However, comedones (blackheads and whiteheads) are not part of rosacea. Clinically, rosacea may resemble acne vulgaris and is often confused with couperose and/or sensitive skin; however, these are separate conditions requiring different solutions. Rosacea seems to be linked to the vascular network of the central facial skin and causes redness, bumps, pustules, and other symptoms that rarely appear anywhere other than on the face. The presence of rosacea is independent of skin type, as it can affect dry, flaky skin as well as normal or oily skin. The key is to identify the skin type and use the skincare products most suitable for it.

Skin with a rosacea condition may be sensitive and easily irritated. It is important to avoid ingredients and products that burn, sting, or irritate the skin, including those with alcohol, witch hazel distillate, fragrance, menthol, peppermint, eucalyptus oil, clove oil, salicylic acid, as well as scrubs, toners, astringents, and exfoliants. Products containing sulfur or azelaic acid may be medically prescribed as an alternative to antibiotic therapy and some success has been made with the use of anti-oxidants in order to suppress the inflammatory reactions associated with rosacea.

Sunscreens containing zinc oxide or titanium dioxide that are effective against the full spectrum of UVA and UVB can be especially important for rosacea skin, as this condition may be particularly susceptible to sun damage resulting in rosacea flare-ups. The U.S. National Rosacea Society (www.rosacea.org) is the world's largest support organization for rosacea, offering information and educational services to hundreds of thousands of rosacea patients and health professionals each year. Rosacea cannot be cured.

ADVERSE REACTIONS

By now, the complexity of the skin should be apparent. Not only are there several different ways to evaluate and categorize skin types, there are also a variety of conditions that need to be identified prior to selecting a product in order to truly help a skin condition rather than aggravate it. Additionally, obtaining a brief individual history (the "Five Basic Questions") to avoid an adverse reaction is very important. However, being able to understand the type of reaction is equally if not more important as it can help a skincare professional to (*i*) reassure a client that everything will be fine and (*ii*) direct them to a dermatologist or medical professional to have the reaction treated quickly, thereby minimizing its severity. This section, dedicated to skin reactions, is intended to give a clear, general understanding of the type of reactions that can be experienced when using cosmetics and an ability to assess if a particular ingredient or product is appropriate for a specific individual. It is not intended to replace the knowledge of a physician.

In skin care, an adverse reaction can be defined as "any unwanted effect associated with a treatment." Adverse reactions are not always bad, just unwanted. (In fact, some adverse reactions have led to interesting discoveries. For example, researchers developed a high blood pressure medication that, during the course of testing, caused hair to grow in unwanted places. Needless to say, many women participating in the study were not very pleased with this reaction, but men and women with premature hair loss were. The active principle was then changed from being administered as a pill to being applied in liquid form directly on the scalp.) Two of the more frequent types of reactions observed in skin care are irritation and allergy.

Basic or Simple Irritation

It is probable that everyone has either seen or experienced some form of skin irritation. In Caucasian, European, and Hispanic skin (light to medium pigmentation), irritation can range from a simple, small, pale-red patch of skin to a large area that is intense crimson red in color. Asian skin can react more intensely to irritation, demonstrating deeper red colorations. In contrast, women of color (medium to dark pigmentation) may not exhibit redness at all. Instead they will often demonstrate a decrease in color at the site of irritation, causing an imbalance in overall skin coloration.

Skin irritation only appears in the area where a product has been applied and usually develops within 6 to 24 hours after product use. In the event a person develops this type of reaction they should (*i*) wash the product off the skin as soon as possible and (*ii*) discontinue product use until the reaction completely disappears, usually within 72 to 96 hours. It is recommended that those who are very upset about the reaction, contact their doctor or dermatologist. Usually this type of reaction can be suppressed with a topical anti-itch and/or anti-inflammatory cream. This said, it is important that skin care professionals not give medical advice, including counseling on how to treat an adverse skin reaction, and that they refer clients to a physician.

Cumulative Irritation

Cumulative irritation is something that occurs after continued product use. There will be no signs of irritation for three or more days and suddenly a reaction will occur. The skin will react in the same manner as basic or simple irritation described earlier and the product should be washed off and discontinued until the reaction has subsided. These types of reactions are more common when one or more products are being used at the same time, for example in regime skin care. Often the skin can tolerate one or more products for a few days, but over time it becomes less tolerant and an irritation reaction occurs. For this reason, skin care professionals should consider contacting a client three to seven days after beginning a new skin care regime to ensure that the products are being tolerated and used correctly.

Chemical Folliculitis

Chemical folliculitis is a form of irritation that is commonly confused with acne, and leads people to say "I'm breaking out" from the product(s). Like cumulative irritation, these reactions usually arise when clients use multiple products. However, instead of getting a rash or redness they develop small bumps. The reaction usually entails a cluster (10 to 20 small blemish-like lesions) that can appear red or white in color and can be filled with fluid. These lesions are inflammatory in nature and are not white or blackheads (non-inflammatory lesions or comedones). In cases of chemical folliculitis, stop all product use until the reaction is gone and then start using one product at a time. For example, the skin care regime can be resumed using the cleanser morning and night for the first week. If no reactions occur, the next product can be added the following week, for example a moisturizer after cleansing. If still no problems are observed when using two products, a third product can be reintroduced, and so on, leaving about a week in between each additional product. The schedule of product introduction can be adjusted according to the individual. If a person is very sensitive, the cleanser can be used once a day for the first week and twice a day the second, and in the third a moisturizer can be added to the mix, and so on.

Subjective Irritation Reactions: Burning/Stinging/Itching

Burning, stinging, and itching are subjective irritation reactions that are considered sub-clinical in nature, i.e., not visible to the eye. It is not clear why people experience this type of reaction; however, there is a direct correlation between subjective irritation reactions and a drop in temperature and humidity in the air. More specifically, when the climate goes from warm to cold and there is less humidity or moisture is in the air—in winter, for example—there is an increase in the amount of skin burning, stinging, and itching complaints. For these types of reactions, minimizing the number of products used, as described for chemical folliculitis, and/or using a simple cleanser with a heavy moisturizer such as a barrier cream can be helpful until the skin acclimates to the changes in the environment.

Allergic Reactions

Allergic reactions are often very complex and can be difficult to determine. Therefore, it is always best to leave it up to experts—for instance allergists or dermatologists—who are familiar with "Contact Dermatitis Patch Testing." There are several types of allergic reactions with many different mechanisms of action. Three of the most common forms are immediate hypersensitivity, delayed hypersensitivity or allergic reactions, and utricaria. Ingredients that can most often cause such sensitivity are fragrances, preservatives, and some chemical sunscreens.

Immediate hypersensitivity is exactly what its name implies: the reaction typically occurs within 30 minutes of being exposed to a product or ingredient to which one is allergic. These reactions can often be very severe, producing significant swelling and redness, and potentially causing a person to go into anaphylactic shock and stop breathing. In the event of a severe reaction, medical treatment should be obtained immediately at a nearby hospital emergency room. In reactions not involving difficulty in breathing, clients should see their physician as soon as possible to minimize the length and severity of the reaction. Treatment usually consists of either injectable or oral steroids, as topical treatment with creams or gels is too slow and usually avoided.

Delayed hypersensitivity is a reaction that normally occurs within 24 to 96 hours after a person comes in contact with a product or ingredient to which they are allergic. The reactions observed can range from mild to severe redness and swelling, and the skin can be itchy and somewhat uncomfortable. Normally, there is little potential for anaphylactic shock; however, medical treatment should be obtained as soon as possible to avoid the reaction from getting worse and lasting longer than 7 to 10 days.

Utricaria relates to breaking out in hives which are raised red, itchy welts on the surface of the skin. While this type of reaction is more commonly reported as a result of excessive stress, certain foods, medicines, and topical skin care products can also be a cause. Most of the time, these reactions relate to histamine circulating in the blood. They occur within 30 to 60 minutes of coming in contact with a product, and normally go away by themselves within several hours (or faster with an oral anti-histamine).

There are a several points worth mentioning about the difference between irritation and allergy. First, irritation is normally less severe and shorter in duration. It usually lasts only a few days compared to allergic reactions, which can require immediate medical care and last up to 10 days. Second, irritation is usually confined to the area to which the product was applied. Allergic reactions can spread to areas near the application site, and in cases where histamine is involved, reactions can occur anywhere on the body. Third, the major difference between irritation and allergy is that once an irritation reaction clears, the product can be reintroduced into a skin treatment regime. If there is an allergy to the product, a person will be allergic to it forever and should never use it again.

Post-inflammatory Hyper- or Hypopigmentation (PIH)

Post-inflammatory hyperpigmentation (too much) or hypopigmentation (too little) reactions are either irritant or allergic in nature, and can be caused by the inflammation associated with either adverse reaction. A *hyper*pigmentation reaction causes an overproduction of melanin in the skin, resulting in a darker and uneven skin tone where the adverse reaction occurred. A *hypo*pigmentation reaction causes the opposite to occur leaving the area with less pigment than the surrounding skin. The latter reaction is more common in darker skin tones. Both types of pigmentation reactions are uncommon but can occur after an adverse event, and are very difficult and time-consuming to treat.

SUMMARY

The best way to avoid an adverse reaction is to first take account of a person's experience with their skin through a brief history (the Five Basic Questions). Then, identify the basic skin type (normal, oily, and dry), know how they react to the sun (skin phototype), and be aware of any skin conditions that may impact the course of skin treatment. If there is any uncertainty as to how a person may react to a product, a good rule of thumb is to start low (maybe using one or two products) and go slow (add additional products after the first or second week). Lastly, in a professional context it is always best to call the client a few days to a week after they begin a new treatment regime to make sure the products are being correctly used, and no problems are being experienced. Following these suggestions will permit an effective skin treatment, minimize any possibility of adverse reaction, and build positive relationships.

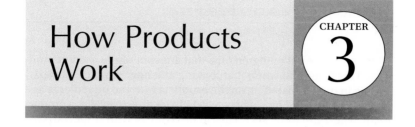

How Products Work

INTRODUCTION

With the advent of cosmeceuticals and skin care products that can cost between US$400 to US$750 an ounce, "Does this product work?" is an important question to answer. Understanding the types of ingredients used, product safety and efficacy, clinical testing conducted (if any), and the claims being made by the manufacturer is critical to guiding product selection and obtaining results that meet expectations.

Do not be impressed by large words, pretty brochures, or complicated science. Be aware of what makes a product safe and effective. Ask questions. You will quickly see a change in how sales people treat you, which will save you time and money by avoiding products that do not live up to their claims. Remember, that the majority of sales people will not have the answers to some, or most, questions. When possible, allow them to research the answers by asking the manufacturer and the product researchers. People who appear to have all the answers are often making it up as they go along. Any reputable cosmetic company should be willing to share data, explain why their product is worth using, and why it can lead to the results claimed.

COSMETIC INGREDIENTS

There are roughly 69 million individual chemicals and/or chemical combinations used in the world today. This is the number published by the Chemical Abstract Society (CAS) that assigns the unique Chemical Abstract Numbers used to track each substance. Additionally, approximately 15,000 new chemical substances are submitted for CAS numbers every day. The fact that there are that many chemicals substances is worrisome, but more alarming is that less than 1 percent of them have been tested for safety.

According to one of the largest trade association groups, The Personal Care Product Council (formerly known as the Cosmetic, Toiletries and Fragrance Association, CTFA), there are approximately 17,500 different ingredients and ingredient mixtures that can be used in cosmetic products. Part II of this book, "Product Ingredients," is a comprehensive list of ingredients that are commonly used in products. This is helpful when first looking at a new product. Comparing the ingredient labeling on the products with the ingredients and functions described in this book will help identify the value a product holds. There are three key issues to be aware of with respect to cosmetic ingredients and mixtures:

1. Ingredients can be multi-functional.
2. Paired ingredients can work synergistically so that one plus one equals more than two.
3. The order in which cosmetic ingredients are listed on a label.

Most ingredients can be multi-functional. For example, salicylic acid is commonly used as an acne active in over-the-counter (OTC) products, but it is also considered an effective preservative, a pH buffer, and an anti-aging ingredient because it is a beta hydroxy acid (BHA) and thus capable of reversing the signs of premature aging. Lactic acid, an alpha hydroxy acid (AHA), is an exfoliating agent, but it can also normalize epidermal structure, and stimulate the production of hyaluronic acid, collagen, and elastin. When evaluating a product it is important to understand what an ingredient can be expected to do in the product, i.e., is it serving primarily as a preservative, as an anti-aging ingredient, a solvent, etc.

Pairing ingredients with specific functions is also an important dimension with respect to cosmetic ingredients. For example, salicylic acid can be a more effective anti-acne agent when paired with glycolic acid; vitamin A-based products may offer better results when formulated in conjunction with an AHA, such as glycolic or lactic acids. Often when combining ingredients one plus one equals much more than two.

The final issue can be called the "ingredient label game." Based on the Fair Packaging and Labeling Act, consumer products must list their ingredients in order of concentration starting with the highest and ending with the lowest up to 1 percent. (Note that only cosmetic products packaged for professional use are exempt from the requirement to list ingredients.) This is why water is usually the first ingredient listed on most labels. Ingredients used in concentrations below 1 percent can be listed in any order. Listings can be followed by a "may contain" section, which is used mainly for color cosmetics as a short cut to avoid producing hundreds of ingredient labels for individual shades. When looking at an ingredient label and the first ingredient is not water, but perhaps "aloe gel," the manufacturer is not indicating that the ingredient is in a water-based solution. While the product label may claim it contains 80 percent "aloe gel" it is highly probable that it contains approximately 0.5 percent (or less) of Aloe and

79.5 percent (or more) water. Some products are formulated so that only four or five ingredients are above 1 percent and the sixth ingredient listed in the formula is present at infinitesimally small concentrations, for example 0.0001 percent vitamin C. Yet, the product's label and marketing materials can state "contains Vitamin C." Both of these practices are misleading. They imply that because a product contains an ingredient it is effective. Products are effective because they contain many ingredients that are designed to work together in the formula. Just because a product contains a trendy ingredient, does not mean it works. When possible, ask for the clinical data or look at a company's website to see if results are displayed and then determine if the product is of value.

PRODUCT AND INGREDIENT PENETRATION

Product and ingredient penetration are tricky subjects when it comes to skin care because many companies do not test whether or not a product penetrates the skin or how deeply it can penetrate. Some companies conduct clinical testing on a product, and based on the results will determine the level of penetration. For example, if a skin biopsy is taken before and after a product has been used for a period of time and there is an increase in collagen deposition, it can be concluded that the product penetrates to the fibroblast cells in the dermis and causes more collagen to be present. Skin penetration studies are very expensive and are more commonly performed by pharmaceutical companies evaluating the absorption, distribution, metabolism, and excretion (ADME) of a drug. Additionally, product penetration into the lower levels of the skin is not always desired. Sunscreen products need to stay on top of the skin in order to effectively absorb and/or reflect UV radiation from the sun.

Regardless of the complexities of ADME studies, there are a number of factors that can promote or inhibit ingredient penetration into the skin. The skin acts like a mesh or a screen, allowing small molecules to pass freely, but generally screening out larger substances. Depending on the source of information, a substance with a molecular weight or size less than 1,000 can penetrate the skin. To enter the cell, it must be even smaller, approximately around 400 in terms of molecular weight. Substances below 100 may enter the blood stream. To put molecular weight in context and as an easy point of reference, water has a molecular weight of approximately 18 and hyaluronic acid can range from 5,000 to 20,000. Beyond molecular weight or size, there are many other factors that determine and impact ingredient penetration, including water or lipid solubility, and the charge of a molecule (i.e., its polarity). The fact that a given molecule is incorporated into a formula with many other ingredients only complicates matters. For instance, an ingredient may bind to other ingredients in the formula making it larger. This is why conducting a clinical study and observing what changes occur in the skin gives a clearer picture of penetration. It is not possible to simply say that the molecular size of an ingredient will enable it to or prevent it from penetrating the skin.

Increasingly, nanotechnology is featured when discussing ingredient size and penetration capacity. This is an exciting topic in skin care, and it is a logical source of concern for regulators worldwide. Nanotechnology is the science of making ingredients very small in order to boost their penetration capacity. As noted earlier, materials below a molecular weight of a 100 can enter the blood stream. Nanoparticles can be 25 to 95 percent smaller than that, meaning that not only can these particles pass through the skin, enter the blood stream, and circulate in the body, but they can also easily pass through membranes, enter into DNA, and alter a variety of biochemical functions that we may not be able to control. At the same time, there are a number of benefits associated with this technology. Most benefits are related to making things stronger and/or lighter. For example, the resins used for eyeglasses and/or ceramic coatings can be made thinner and stronger with the use of nanotechnology. Additionally, there have been some clinical trials showing promising results for people with certain types of lung disease. It is important, however, that where the particles go is controlled, which can be accomplished through controlled delivery systems. (*See also* Chapter 4.)

Peptides are also commonly said to penetrate the skin based on their size. Peptides are generally a linked grouping of a few amino acids (which are very small) linked and bound to a carrier molecule, such as palmitic acid, for stability reasons. Peptides can incite a cell to produce collagen and other proteins that enhance the skin's appearance. When evaluating products containing peptides, it is important to review clinical studies or data on the finished product and not just on the peptide itself. In this way it is easier to determine if the benefits claimed are associated with the peptide or with the whole formulation.

There are other factors, not related to an ingredient's size, that affect product penetration. Many people are uncertain as to why a toner containing alcohol or other solvents would be used in a skin care regime or as a skin-prepping agent, especially since solvents can be drying. The reason is that solvents change the solubility of the skin, allowing more water-soluble (hydrophilic and polar) ingredients like lactic acid to penetrate the skin. Tape stripping, dermabrasion, and chemical peels work because they remove part or most of the stratum corneum barrier, thereby allowing materials to penetrate the skin much more easily. Ultrasound, mild electrical currents, or occlusion (covering the skin with cellophane, tape, or a patch) enhance product penetration into the skin because they change the skin's absorption properties.

Most recently, light therapy is being explored for its ability to promote skin penetration and the therapeutic benefits of a skin care regime. Like nanotechnology, this is an emerging field that requires a better understanding of how to control it in order to reap its possible value. In the discussion on acne in Chapter 2, porphyrin was mentioned: when exposed to light, porphyrin improves the acne condition by killing the bacteria in the follicle. Researchers have found the specific wavelength that is responsible for this reaction and a variety of products are now currently available that permit the therapeutic benefits to be realized without exposure to damaging sunlight. Other wavelengths have been identified that may stimulate cells to produce collagen and other materials needed for healthy skin. This technology is still at its inception. A significant amount of research needs to be completed in this area and thus caution should be exercised when investigating light-based devices or treatments.

Below is a summary of the factors that can influence an ingredient's ability to penetrate the skin:

- Ingredient size (molecular weights of under a 1,000 penetrate more easily)
- Absorption channels (e.g., follicles, pores, sweat glands, and sebaceous glands)
- Solubility—either lipophilic or hydrophilic (i.e., fat soluble or water soluble)
- Polarity—polar or non-polar (i.e., positive- or negative-charged molecules)
- Solvents (e.g., ethanol, acetone, DiMethylSurfOxide—DMSO)
- Tape stripping or dermabrasion (i.e., physically removing the stratum corneum barrier)
- Sound waves (i.e., ultrasound)
- Mild electric currents (i.e., iontophoresis)
- Occlusion (transdermal delivery systems)

SAFETY TESTING

The introduction to this book mentioned the 1938 Food, Drug and Cosmetic Act in which the FDA defined the difference between a cosmetic and a drug product. The other significant point in this law, still in effect today, is that the FDA shifted the responsibility of ensuring that a product was safe for consumer use away from the government to the product's manufacturer. The law states that if the manufacturer does not test the product for safety, the product label must include the following notice in a legible manner for consumers to read:

Warning–The safety of this product has not been determined.

No company has ever been willing to place such a statement on a product label, and thus all manufacturers test their products for safety prior to consumer use. There are some nuances however, which are important to be aware of. Unfortunately, there is no FDA guidance on the specific types of testing that should be conducted in order to determine consumer safety. Thus, individual companies decide for themselves the battery of tests and testing procedures that are adequate to determine product safety. This has led to some very large discrepancies in the amount and type of testing undertaken. Some companies never test a product formulation, instead they look at the tests conducted on the ingredients used in the product and determined that the product is safe for use. Other companies spend an extraordinary amount of time, money, and effort testing the product on several hundred people prior to marketing. The average cosmetic product manufacturer will generally undertake some combination of the tests to determine safety.

Eye Irritation

Up until the mid-1980s the cosmetic industry routinely conducted a Draize Rabbit Eye Irritation Test to evaluate the ocular irritation potential of products. This test, as well as all animal testing, was suspended by the cosmetic industry due to a variety of social pressures. Since then, many *in vitro* tests (testing in part or in cells, not the whole animal) have been used to determine eye irritation. The Draize Skin Irritation Test has also been replaced by *in vitro* testing although most companies will do the *in vitro* ocular test first and if the product does not produce clinically relevant irritation they will start testing on human skin.

Human Patch Testing

This could be a simple patch, similar to a Band-Aid, which is applied with a product and placed on the upper back or upper arm of 25 to 100 people for one to two days and removed to see if any irritation was produced. Most companies use a Repeat Insult Patch Test (RIPT), which requires applying a product to a patch in a similar manner as in the simple patch test described above, but tested on as many as 200 people several times over a five- to six-week period. The RIPT is preferred over a simple patch test because it measures not only basic irritation potential, but also cumulative irritation and several types of allergic reactions.

Photo Patch Testing

This test is similar to the Human Patch Test, except it adds an additional step that includes applying the product to the skin and then exposing it to ultraviolet (UV) light. In this way, the manufacturer simulates what might happen to the skin when a product is applied and then exposed to sunlight. This test is used mainly for products that have had a history of phototoxic or photo allergic reactions, such as those containing fragrance, as well as perfumes, colognes, and sunscreen actives.

Clinical Use Test

This test evaluates the finished product (i.e., the actual formulation that will be marketed and its packaging) according to the use directions that will be written on the package. Subjects are normally allowed to use the product at home and then come back to the clinic to be evaluated by a clinician at various, predetermined points. Testing can be as short as one week but it can also last several months. It can include as few as five people or as many as several hundred. It might involve a dermatologist and/or ophthalmologist, depending on the type of product being evaluated. Additionally, subjects are usually asked to fill out questionnaires during and/or at the conclusion of testing in order to compare what they tested to other products they used. They are also asked a variety of questions about how the product worked. This test indicates if the product can be used safely as directed. It can also be used to substantiate or validate product claims from the consumer's perspective, for example, "do you feel the product reduces lines and wrinkles?"

Comedogenicity Testing

This test is conducted to determine if a product can cause comedones (i.e., whiteheads, blackheads, and non-inflammatory lesions). The reasoning behind this test was that heavy oils, waxes, and other ingredients could clog pores, allowing a comedone to develop. This was more of an issue in the mid-1970s when the diagnosis or term *Acne Cosmetica* was given to women in their 30s and 40s who developed comedones after using certain skin care and makeup products. The problem of *Acne Cosmetica* has dropped significantly over the years; however, with the introduction of so many new cosmetic ingredients many companies still undertake this test. The method most commonly used entails applying patches containing a product to the upper back of people with large pores over a period of three to six weeks, and then evaluating the skin for micro-comedones. There are other tests that allow people to use the product for several weeks (similar to the clinical use test) and count acne lesions before and after product use. *In vitro* tests are also an option, measuring water evaporation through a membrane (artificial skin) coated with the product to see if the membrane/skin can still breathe.

Microbiological Testing

Most companies differentiate microbiological testing from safety testing; however, they are the same. Over the past few years, the FDA has become more active, requiring that manufacturers recall all types of products—including foods—because consumers have gotten sick or died after using a product due to contamination by microorganisms, such as *E. coli*. Prior to introduction into the market place, it is essential to test every product in order to ensure it is not contaminated. More importantly, however, the product should be able to withstand repeated exposure to microorganisms. This is particularly critical with respect to products packaged in jars that can be contaminated by the microorganisms on our fingers on a daily basis. On average, the cosmetic industry very rarely experiences problems relating to microbiological contamination because it has set a very high standard in this respect—in most cases higher than that for food products—thereby keeping such problems to a minimum. This type of testing is extremely important in products marketed as "preservative free" because products without a preservative system usually have a very short shelf-life (six months or less).

Product Shelf-life

Nothing is more problematic then buying a product that begins to separate, significantly change color, and/or smell badly shortly after its purchase. Unlike over-the-counter (OTC) drugs (e.g., sunscreens, acne medications, antiperspirants, etc.), cosmetic products are not required to have expiration dates. In the cases of products that do provide a date, these can still change over time. It is important that cosmetic users be aware if a product contains an ingredient like an anti-oxidant or vitamin, which may change the product's attributes over the course of use. This is information that a skin care professional can easily communicate. All cosmetic product manufacturers should conduct shelf-life stability studies and be able to disclose whether the product remains effective over time, even though it may change slightly. This said, products may no longer be appropriate to use if they are badly separated or smell rancid.

Analytical Testing

In some cases, ingredients can react with each other once incorporated into a formulation, yielding ingredients that are not listed on the ingredient label. In other cases, ingredients may contain an unexpected contaminant. For instance DMDM hydantoin, a product preservative, can cause formaldehyde to form in the product; and at one time asbestos was a common contaminant in talc—a significant issue for the baby powder industry. It is impossible to know the likelihood of either of these cases without being told by the manufacturer or the press. They are, however, good questions for skin care professionals to ask product manufacturers in the event of an adverse reaction.

A final note with respect to the press and "alarmist" interest groups that publicize the potential health hazards of cosmetics: please remember that these groups function in their own interest. Their objective is to sell something, be it a newspaper, magazine, or subscription, and provocative headlines tend to attract more attention and boost sales. When in doubt contact the manufacturer, ask about the issue, and make an informed decision based on the facts. Remember there are more than 69 million chemicals in the world and very little is known about most of them.

EFFICACY TESTING

All products making a claim should be clinically tested in order to substantiate that the product will do what is being claimed. Many product manufacturers will use testing conducted on an ingredient contained in the product and not test the actual formulation. Others will use data that was generated or published by another source, for example on the benefit or effectiveness of certain vitamins or antioxidants. However, these studies were likely to be conducted under conditions dissimilar to the product being sold. Relying on this type of information to substantiate a claim is not always dependable. Many cosmetic products are highly complex, with their formulations containing dozens of ingredients. In general, it is very difficult to determine what is happening chemically in a formula when it contains more than six ingredients. Therefore, claiming product efficacy because it contains one particular ingredient among dozens can be misleading or inaccurate for a number of reasons, including:

- the ingredient in question can bind to another chemical in the formulation and become inactive;
- the ingredient may only be effective at higher concentrations than what is used in the product;
- the ingredient may only be effective under certain conditions, for example, a specific pH, if no water is present in the formula.

When evaluating a cosmetic's efficacy, caution should be taken when relying on claims based on a specific ingredient within the product. Such a claim should always be substantiated based on the actual formulation. In addition, regardless of whether or not a clinical study was conducted on the product, there is no guarantee that it will provide the same results for 100 percent of the people that use it. The biological variability and diversity among individuals is vast, and what works well or very well for some, may not work at all for others. Monitoring product use in order to ensure the product works is what matters. Following is a brief description of the main types of claim-substantiation or efficacy tests that are conducted. (More in-depth information on these tests can be found on the Internet or by reading books specific to the subject found in a nearby library or medical library.)

Claims Testing

Companies will normally conduct a clinical use test (as described in the discussion on safety testing earlier) and add expert grader evaluations and/or instrumentation analysis to demonstrate specific claims. Expert grader evaluations are normally conducted by a dermatologist, nurse, or a lab technician with years of experience measuring specific testing parameters such as lines and wrinkles, skin roughness, dryness, elasticity, pigmentation, and global or overall improvement. Instrumentation analysis utilizes a variety of highly specific machines that measure skin hydration (electrical conductance or impedance), the depth of lines and wrinkles (image analysis or profilometer), pigmentation (chromometer), skin elasticity (cutometer or twistometer), and transepidermal water loss (evaporimeter). Normally, some form of mathematical statistical analysis is conducted on the data generated from these tests to determine if the product produced a change that can be considered statistically significant and reproducible. If the result is statistically significant then efficacy can be more easily claimed for the product.

FDA OTC Monograph Testing

Many cosmetic manufacturers also produce OTC drugs that are regulated by the FDA and some require testing to prove that they are efficacious prior to sale, for instance sunscreens and anti-perspirant products. However, some categories, like acne products and skin-bleaching products, only need to contain a certain concentration of an FDA-approved active ingredient in order to make a specific claim. For example, if a product contains between 0.5 and 2 percent salicylic acid it can be considered safe and effective as an acne treatment product. As long as the product still contains the correct amount of salicylic acid during product shelf-life testing, and this can be clinically demonstrated, no acne testing is required.

Many types of OTC products are available on the market. The product categories discussed here represent only a few. In the United States all OTC product packaging has a "Drug Facts Labeling." This is a grid or series of boxes on the back of the package that identifies the "active ingredient(s)" along with concentration and function in the formula, plus directions for use, warnings, expiration dates, etc.

The FDA also publishes testing guidelines for a product's Sun Protection Factor (SPF), which measures only UVB protection, and for Broad Spectrum Testing, which relates only to UVA protection. When considering sunscreen products, it is important to remember that most people do not know the difference between UVB and UVA; there is significant controversy surrounding how to test for UVB and UVA efficacy and people are not truly aware of the potential damage caused by UV light regardless of its source, be it from natural sunlight or the artificial sunlight associated with tanning beds.

First, UVB is a short UV wavelength (280–320 nm) that does not penetrate very deeply into the skin. However, it is responsible for sunburn and free radical damage that can cause cell death. UVA is a longer wavelength (320–410 nm) that can penetrate deeply into the skin, reaching the dermis and damaging collagen and elastin, the skin's main support structures. Unlike UVB, it does not cause sunburn, but like UVB it does produce free radicals. Free radical damage is associated with both UVB and UVA exposure. A point to stress is that sunscreen actives do not stop free radicals from being produced, regardless of the wavelengths they reflect or absorb. This is because sunscreens are not anti-oxidants; rather they are UV absorbers and/or reflectors. Using a sunscreen without anti-oxidants will not fully protect against premature aging. Sunscreens and anti-oxidants must be used together, either as two individual products or as a two-in-one product. This is why sun exposure is responsible for the majority of premature aging today.

Second, regulatory agencies in the United States, Europe, Asia, Australia, and other countries around the world disagree on the best way to test for UVB and UVA efficacy. They also disagree on how this information should be communicated to the consumer. While the technical points to this debate are many, two of the finer points are creating consumer confusion. The main issue is that the same formula when tested in the United States may demonstrate an SPF 30, but when tested in Australia or elsewhere the demonstrated protective value is an SPF 20. This has led manufacturers to label the same product differently depending on the country where it is sold. The second issue has to do with how UVA protection is indicated. Some countries would like UVA protection expressed numerically, for example UVA10, while others want it expressed symbolically using a "star rating," whereby five stars are better than three stars, and so on. This can again result in the same product sold with different labels around the world, or worse, that the same product is expressing UV protection differently, causing consumer confusion depending on where they purchase the sunscreen.

Finally, most people do not understand the consequences associated with UV exposure, regardless of whether it is from natural UV light (i.e., from the sun) or artificial UV light (i.e., from tanning beds). A number of facts relating to this issue are listed below. More information is also available on the Skin Cancer Foundation's website (http://www.skincancer.org/).

- One or more blistering sunburns in childhood more than doubles an individual's chances of developing melanoma later in life. A person's risk for melanoma doubles if he or she has had more than five sunburns at any age.
- One in five Americans will develop skin cancer and 1 in 55 will be diagnosed with melanoma in the course of a lifetime.
- About 90 percent of non-melanoma skin cancers and about 65 percent of melanoma are associated with sun exposure.
- Indoor UV tanners (i.e., people using tanning beds) are 74 percent more likely to develop melanoma than those who never tan indoors.
- People who use tanning beds are 2.5 times more likely to develop a non-melanoma skin cancer.

There is no such thing as a "safe tan" or a tan free from UV exposure. The only way to tan is via UV light, and UV light damages the skin.

CLAIM SUBSTANTIATION

The majority of safety and efficacy tests are also used to substantiate product claims. For example, the RIPT is used to support "Dermatologist Tested and/or Clinically Tested and/or Allergy Tested"; SPF testing demonstrates UVB sunscreen efficacy and SPF claims

(SPF 15, SPF 30, etc.). There is a basic rational behind many of the common phrases used to support product claims. Some of these are listed below, together with general comments regarding their meaning. Hopefully this will provide a better idea of how claims are made and what they mean, and will make it easier to sort through the marketing terms and catch phrases commonly seen or heard on television, the press, radio, product packaging, and marketing materials.

In the United States there are several agencies that watch over what is said and done in the cosmetics industry. These include the national television networks (e.g., ABC, NBC, and CBS) through the Network TV Broadcast Standards; the Federal Trade Commission (FTC) has a National Advertising Division (NAD), which is part of the Better Business Bureau and the FDA; some cable shopping channels such as QVC and Home Shopping Networks follow claim substantiation guidelines. At the same time, the Internet, local print media, and local TV and radio are not as easily regulated often due to the sheer volume of information available, the incredible speed at which things come and go, and the lack of agency resources to enforce regulations relating to inappropriate or misleading claims. Given this, it is important to understand that boundaries are often overstepped. Skin care professionals, their clients, and cosmetic users generally have a right to request that manufacturers substantiate their claims. In the United States, if a product does not give the results promised, the NAD can be notified. If other complaints have been filed, they will go to the manufacturer in order to evaluate the testing and conclude whether the claim is substantiated or not. If the conclusion is negative, the manufacturer will be requested to remove the claim from their advertising. If a product has caused any injury, the manufacturer should be contacted in order to report the adverse event. At a minimum, most manufacturers should be willing to refund the product cost and/or any other out-of-pocket expenses associated with an adverse event, such as unpaid medical expenses, medications, etc. If this is not the case, the FDA can be contacted, the incident reported, and again if other complaints have been logged for that product or manufacturer an official investigation into the problem should be initiated by FDA.

Dermatologist or Ophthalmologist Tested

"Dermatologist Tested" or "Ophthalmologist Tested" simply means that a dermatologist or ophthalmologist—usually board certified or licensed—has had some part in testing the product. Generally, this claim is substantiated by a RIPT. The claim can also be substantiated by a dermatologist or ophthalmologist that conducts a clinical use/efficacy study on the product. In either case, a report with the dermatologist or ophthalmologist's signature should be on file with the manufacturer. Additionally, on "Ophthalmologist Tested" eye area formulations the phrase "suitable for contact lenses" may be noted. This claim is substantiated by including subjects who wear contact lenses as part of the clinical use test. It should indicate that the product has been evaluated in some manner by a trained professional, and that it is safe/effective when used according to directions.

Fragrance-free

This claim refers to the fact that a "complex fragrance oil" (often listed as simply "fragrance" on an ingredient label), usually containing a few hundred ingredients, has not been used in the formula. An essential oil, such as lavender or sage, can give the same results as a complex fragrance oil and the product can be considered "Fragrance Free."Every raw material used in a product has an odor, some pleasant, some not so pleasant, thus even products that are not fragranced can have a smell. No product is odor free, but as long as a complex fragrance oil has not been used, the "Fragrance Free" claim can be substantiated. Fragrances are still the number one cause associated with adverse reactions, primarily allergic reactions. Therefore, if the formula is without a complex fragrance oil the implication is that it is safer to use. Fragrances or essential oils are generally added to cosmetic products in order to mask or cover up the odors associated with certain raw materials that can be unpleasant or not esthetically pleasing.

Hypoallergenic

There are ingredients or categories of ingredients, such as fragrance oils and preservatives, which can cause allergic reactions. "Hypoallergenic" products should be less likely to cause an allergic reaction. There are no guidelines for what makes a product hypoallergenic, but most manufacturers minimize the use of ingredients that have a greater potential to cause an allergic reaction and/or they perform additional testing on groups of people with sensitive skin.

In general terms hypoallergenic products are less likely to cause a reaction. More specifically however, it means: less likely to be allergenic or to cause an allergic reaction. *Hypo* means "less" and allergic refers to allergic reaction.

Non-comodogenic

A comedone is a non-inflammatory lesion (a whitehead, blackhead, or blemish). This claim is substantiated via product testing on subjects prone to developing non-inflammatory lesions in order to ensure none are produced through the product's use. The term non-comedogenic has also been used to substantiate such claims as "allows skin to breathe" and "will not clog pores."

The claim is aimed at anyone who is prone to whiteheads, blackheads, or inflammatory lesions, or wants to use a product to cover up any such blemishes.

Oil Free

Depending on how the term oil free is defined, it is possible to determine if a product is truly "oil free." If it refers to "no animal, mineral, or plant oils" (e.g., fish liver oil, mineral oil, corn oil, etc.) then, yes, most products are "oil free." If the term oil is replaced with synthetic oils or esters then most products contain oils. If a more rigid stance is taken and esters are excluded from the definition, then generally a water-soluble solution or suspension or a gel is oil free. These formulations, however, are not as esthetically pleasing as emulsions (creams or lotions) containing esters. Oils have been suggested to clog pores and aggravate such conditions as oily skin, non-inflammatory lesions, and acne.

Alcohol Free

"Alcohol free" refers to products that do not contain fermented alcohol and specifically SD Alcohol 40 (B) is a fermented alcohol or ethyl alcohol (drinking alcohol) that has been denatured. There were concerns that if the ingredient was identified as ethyl alcohol, people would drink the products. SD Alcohol is not commonly used in skin care products, but can be found in perfumes/colognes and in products that are intended to "de-fat" skin or to enhance product penetration. Companies using emulsifying ingredients such as cetyl alcohol or stearyl alcohol can make an alcohol-free claim because these ingredients are not derived from fermented alcohol and do not de-fat the skin.

Alcohol is a solvent that removes dirt and oil from skin and can change the water solubility of the skin for a brief period, thereby allowing more water-soluble ingredients to penetrate. Alcohol is a very good prepping solution for skin peels, acne medications, or acne treatments.

There are a few alternatives to alcohol but they are less popular, such as acetone, or not as effective, "alcohol free Witch Hazel extract," for example.

Natural

This is a very popular claim that can mean different things. Strictly speaking, "natural" should mean that ingredients are sourced from nature, are usually plant-based, and have been purified to some extent for health and safety reasons. (A manufacturer cannot responsibly use ingredients straight from a plant source without cleaning or purifying the material.) Some examples of natural materials that are commonly purified according to government requirements are colorants and vitamins. Petroleum and/or animal by-products can also be considered natural; however, most people avoid using these materials for a variety of reasons.

For consumers, the difficulty comes with determining which ingredients are purified and not chemically altered to such an extent that the final product is no longer natural. There are a few ingredients, polysorbate and sodium lauryl sulfate for instance, that are very hard to consider natural even if they are initially derived from a plant source because they undergo numerous chemical reactions to arrive at their final form. Additionally, there is no agreement on how many times a material can be purified and still be natural. A more straightforward approach is for the manufacturer to state what percentage of the product is "natural." This means subtracting out those ingredients that are not natural and identifying the percentage of the formula that is natural, thus stating "98.4 percent natural" rather than simply "natural." Such an approach can indicate the degree to which a specific formulation is truly "natural." Many regulatory groups are trying to determine possible guidelines for "natural" that would be acceptable for consumers and applicable to the cosmetic industry. (Ironically many of these groups are also questioning whether or not water is natural since all manufacturers use some form of distilled or purified water, and water comprises 60 to 95 percent of a skincare product.) Unfortunately, most people would need to become chemists to understand if a product is truly natural. At the moment the best way to identify what is meant by "natural" in any given product is to speak with the manufacturer and ask how the term is being defined and determined.

Is "natural" any better than "synthetic"? Until recently natural products were considered problematic by cosmetic chemists. Naturally occurring ingredients can be inconsistent: active ingredients vary from year to year based on rainfall, sun exposure, and other environmental issues, and they can contain materials that cause adverse reactions. Furthermore, consideration is given to the vast number of fruits and vegetables containing chemicals that are listed on some government agency sites as causing cancer. Natural ingredients are chemicals, too, and today it is easier to separate out the fractions or chemicals that provide the therapeutic benefit being sought. Everything that exists, be it natural or not, is made of chemicals. There is no such thing as "chemical free"; the only possible question is whether or not the 69 million chemicals in the world are derived from a natural or synthetic source. Using synthetic ingredients can be a way to remove unsafe impurities from natural materials while also purifying and/or concentrating active ingredients, thereby improving quality control and yielding more effective products. There is little to nothing indicating "natural products" are more effective than those that are "synthetically based." In fact, they can often be less effective. Therefore, natural versus synthetic is not really a claim relating to efficacy; it is a statement relating to lifestyle choice.

Preservative Free

"Natural" and "preservative free" are very similar claims. Preservative-free primarily indicates that a conventional preservative such as methylparaben or imidazolidinyl urea has not been used in the formula. Earlier in this chapter the multi-functionality nature of ingredients was discussed and specifically such chemicals as salicylic acid that can be used as an anti-acne agent, anti-aging active, a pH adjustor, and a preservative. Additionally, fragrances/essential oils, alcohols, various glycols, and even alpha hydroxy acids (AHAs) can kill micro-organisms. Ultimately, if a product does not have to be refrigerated or discarded after a few months there is something in the formula "acting like" a preservative. Therefore, can or should it really be considered "preservative free"? It is possible to create a preservative-free product; however, these products have an extremely short shelf-life compared to products that are adequately preserved, an average of a few months compared to three to four years.

The only benefit of a preservative-free product is that/it suits an individual who is sensitive or allergic to preservatives. In such cases, preservative-free products must be used. However, in the United States the number of people sensitive or allergic to preservatives is estimated to be approximately 2 percent. The 69 million or more chemicals available and for which there is no safety information should be of greater concern than whether or not a product contains preservatives, since most cosmetic products—and their preservatives—are tested to be safe.

Subjective Claims

A claim is like a guarantee; it is a promise. Why pay US$750 for a set of new tires that claim to last 100,000 miles, if in reality they will only last 25,000 miles and should have cost only US$250. If a tire company did that they would be sued and lose the case once it was proven that the tires only lasted 25,000 miles. Stating that a skin care product will make anyone 10 years younger (or look 10 years younger) is not just a claim; it is also a guarantee: a promise that the product will do that. If it does not a consumer should be at least able to get their money back.

Product labels and marketing information is full of subjective or "puffery" phrases. For example, words like luxurious or rich lather etc., are considered subjective. They are terms that mean different things to different people. What is luxurious to one person may not be so luxurious to someone else.

Appearance claims, for example, look, feel, etc., are also subjective. Statements such as "leaves skin looking and feeling younger" beg the question "looking and feeling younger than what?" "Helps" is another term requiring some caution. The claim "helps reduce the appearance of lines and wrinkles" does not mean that the product will eliminate lines and wrinkles; it means exactly what it is saying, it will help reduce their appearance, which will depend on individuals and their perception. Such phrases are often used in magazines, advertising, or other marketing materials.

Using claims such as these can reduce stringent testing requirements and minimize legal or regulatory issues. Unfortunately many manufacturers have to use subjective or vague words (e.g., look, feel, and helps). If they clearly stated that the product "removes" or even simply "reduces" wrinkles, the FDA would perceive the product as a drug since the claim indicates the product "alters the structure and/or function of the skin." In turn, the product would require FDA approval, something that can take up to 10 years and cost millions of dollars to obtain. The only way to know for sure if a product truly works is to try it. Do not be misled by claims; seeing how a product works on an individual's skin is the only real proof.

SUMMARY

The information provided in this chapter is a reflection of what should be involved in getting a product into the marketplace. It takes into account everything from the ingredients used, considerations relating to delivering key ingredients to the right place (penetration), the types of testing required to ensure a product is safe and efficacious, and the claims or catch phrases used to entice people into buying, selling, and using a product. It is important that cosmetic users be prudent, ask questions, do their homework, and not take things at face value or believe everything that is said—delve past big words and the science manufacturers produce. Understanding how and why a cosmetic works, and how to evaluate what is being claimed, makes for a smarter cosmetic consumer.

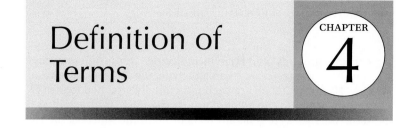

Definition of Terms

CHAPTER 4

INTRODUCTION

This chapter provides a listing of commonly used terms in cosmetic chemistry and cosmetic formulations. Many of these terms are used throughout the individual ingredient listing in Part II of this volume. It is intended to give a general understanding of what the terms mean and their function in a formulation, as many of these terms are fields of study unto themselves.

COMMONLY USED TERMS DEFINED

acid—refers to the pH level of a substance, ranging from 0 for the most acidic to 6.9 for the least acidic. Acids are used in cosmetic formulations for a variety of reasons: to neutralize substances that otherwise would be too alkaline for the skin; as active principles that perform a specific function based on their own particular properties (e.g., hyaluronic acid, essential fatty acids); and as exfoliating and peeling agents (e.g., alpha hydroxy acids). Only those acid ingredients with a very low pH will be irritating to the skin because the skin itself is acidic.

active principle (active ingredient)—an ingredient with "treatment" value. When placed on the skin, it performs a therapeutic or beneficial function, such as healing, hydrating, soothing, toning, etc.

alcohols—widely used in cosmetics as solvents, carriers, and astringents. When incorporated as active ingredients, it is for antiseptic, anti-viral, and bactericidal purposes. Alcohols are organic compounds containing a hydroxyl group (OH) in their molecule. They are recognized by the suffix -ol, such as ethanol for ethyl alcohol and isopropanol for isopropyl alcohol. Compounds listed with an -ol ending should be recognized as alcohols, even if the word alcohol does not follow. Alcohols are also present in essential oils. Geraniol, nerol, and linalool are examples.

aldehyde—can be used as a chemical reagent, solvent, fragrance, or, when used as an active ingredient, as a soothing or antiseptic compound. An aldehyde is an organic compound containing a carboxyl group (O and H) in its molecule. This is different from the OH of the alcohols. In an aldehyde, the "O" for oxygen and the "H" for hydrogen are each individually attached to the "C" carbon atom. In the alcohol group, the "OH" is attached as a unit. Aldehydes are generally recognized by the suffix -al, such as citral, geranial, or ethanal for ethyl aldehyde.

alkali—a pH level measurement: a substance of 7.1 is the least alkaline and a substance of 14 is the most alkaline. Alkalis are used in cosmetics to balance formulas that have an undesired acid level: they raise the pH of formulas with a low acid level that might be irritating to the skin. For example, if a formulation has a pH below 4, an alkali may be added to raise the pH to 4.4 or 5.6, which is closer to the pH value of the skin. At the same time, cosmetics with a high alkaline level will be irritating to the skin.

anti-oxidant—refers to the ability of an ingredient to slow down, prevent, or block oxidation caused by the damaging effects of free radical activity.

The skin's own anti-oxidant defense system of enzymatic and non-enzymatic components protects it from free radical damage. However, when the amount of free radicals formed is greater than the capacity of the skin's natural defense system, cellular damage immediately occurs. Thus, as part of a "damage prevention process," anti-oxidants are added to cosmetics to increase the natural anti-oxidant reservoir of the skin. Some of the most common anti-oxidants used in cosmetics are beta carotene, coenzyme Q10, glutathione, green tea, idebenone, superoxide dismutase, and vitamins E and C. It is well established that a mixture, or "cocktail," of anti-oxidants may enhance the photoprotective effects of a formulation. A single anti-oxidant exposed to free radicals may become a free radical itself, albeit a less active one. When used in conjunction with other anti-oxidants, there is often a chain reaction that occurs among the various anti-oxidants, where each "takes a turn" in a process of continual neutralization of a free radical until it is totally neutralized. Anti-oxidants are key to age prevention and their daily use in cosmetic products helps reduce UV-induced skin damage. The term anti-oxidant can also apply to a compound that prevents other compounds from oxidizing or becoming rancid (in the case of fats and oils). Thus, some ingredients with anti-oxidant properties are also used in preservative systems. *See also* free radicals; free radical scavengers.

aromatherapy—refers to the use of essential oils for therapeutic purposes and perfumery. Its use in skin care ranges from a marketing tool to the fragrance of cosmetics to the therapeutic value associated with the topical applications of essential oils. The therapeutic value is derived both from topical use as well as more subtle psychological changes that result from scent inhalation. These can include an overall feeling of well-being, mood changes, and even an increase and/or decrease in productivity levels. *See also* botanicals.

astringent—refers to the constriction of tissues. It is considered to improve the appearance of large, open pores. An astringent is also used to reduce the oil content on the skin's surface, and rebalance the skin's acid level after the use of certain cleansers. This is particularly the case with cleansers that have a pH that is higher than the pH of the skin. Excessive use of astringents may result in surface dryness.

atom—the smallest component of an element that still retains the element's properties. An atom is made up of positive and negative charges called protons and electrons, respectively. The protons are in the nucleus of the atom and the electrons are found in layers around the nucleus. Each atom has the same number of electrons and protons. A combination of atoms forms a larger substance called a molecule.

bioavailable (bioactive; bioavailability)—refers to the amount of ingredient(s) absorbed and made available at the action site in the skin after its application.

bioflavonoid—a category of plant constituent with therapeutic attributes. Bioflavonoids have anti-oxidant properties, allowing them to absorb oxygen radicals that may cause skin oxidation. They are also anti-microbial, which may aid in anti-inflammatory activity against microbially caused skin irritations.

Bioflavonoids can be grouped into four categories: proanthocyanidins, quercetin, citrus bioflavonoids, and green tea polyphenols. Proanthocyanidins (PCOs) are found in red wine and many plants, with most commercially available sources being derived from grape seeds and maritime pine bark. The quercetin group represents the most active of the various flavonoids. Citrus bioflavonoids (e.g., rutin, quercitrin, hesperidin, and naringin) have clinically demonstrated results for treating capillarian permeability, easy bruising, and varicose veins. Green tea polyphenols are derived from *camellia sinensis*, and obtained by steaming the fresh cut leaf. Green tea polyphenols—i.e., catechin, epicatechin, epicatechin gallate, epiallocatechin gallate, and proanthocyanidin—are a form of bioflavonoid.

botanical—a plant element containing active plant constituents that can elicit certain biological responses when applied on the skin. Botanicals provide a wide range of benefits depending on the specific constituents of the plant. Efficacy is often associated with the concentration level of the active constituents present in the formulation, the skin's capability to absorb these, the effect that other ingredients present in the formulation might have on the active constituent, and the constituent's degree of penetration. Although botanicals were traditionally used as remedies for any number of external and internal disorders, their value was nearly reduced to folklore and hearsay when compared to the identified, measured, and tested effectiveness of synthetic ingredients. As research unravels the different molecular components of botanical extracts, it is being established that all botanicals have biologically active molecules. These molecules are responsible for the plant's attributed therapeutic properties. For example, bisabolol has been isolated and identified as one of the calming constituents in chamomile, and flavonoids, present in a large variety of plants, are now recognized as powerful anti-oxidants with anti-inflammatory, anti-allergenic, anti-viral, anti-aging, and anti-carcinogenic activity.

Botanicals can be incorporated into a product in several forms: as the whole phytocomplex (e.g., macerated rose petals or macerated carrots), as an extract (e.g., licorice root extract); as fractions or particular elements of the extract (e.g., flavonoids or terpenes); and as individual constituents or active chemical components of the extract (e.g., glycyrrhetinic acid which is naturally occurring in licorice root). The therapeutic activity associated with a botanical can also vary based on the part of the plant used. A plant's fruit extract may have therapeutic values not found in an extract from the plant's leaf, for example. Regardless of the form in which the botanical is incorporated (whole, fraction, or individual constituent), the proper concentration of an active chemical component incorporated into cosmetic formulations is crucial to determine the benefit provided by that particular plant extract. Merely adding an extract into a cosmetic product does not guarantee treatment benefits. Awareness of botanical performance and the part of the plant incorporated into the formulation is important in order to differentiate actual benefits from marketing techniques.

Research continues to identify the active constituents that give botanical compounds their therapeutic value. As more becomes known about how the biologically active constituents of botanicals work, the use of botanicals in skin care preparations will continue to rise. Currently, cosmetics based on botanical ingredients represent one of the fastest growing market segments.

Not all botanicals are appropriate for skin care, however. Depending on the ingredient, the skin type and condition, or amount of product used, some botanicals can cause severe irritation and/or react with other chemical ingredients on the skin, resulting in allergic reactions. As botanicals and their therapeutic properties are increasingly understood, knowledge of their proper use and management in cosmetics will increase as well.

buffered—refers to a chemical process by which a compound (or compounds) is added to a formulation in order to keep the formulation's pH unchanged, regardless of the other ingredients added. The compound permitting such a process is called a buffer.

carbomers—a group of high molecular-weight polymers widely used as thickeners, suspending agents, and emulsion stabilizers in a variety of skin care products. The high clarity and unique texture they impart have led the way in the evolution of gel products. The benefits associated with carbomers include specific texture and formulation flow control, highly effective oil/water emulsion stabilization, and permanent suspension of insoluble or immiscible ingredients.

carrier (vehicle)—a formulation component that can affect a product's ease of application and depth of penetration. Carriers may also impact an active ingredient's efficacy, stability, and time release, as well as skin tolerance and final location in the different skin layers.

chemical reaction—refers to the transformation of one or more substances into one or more different substances.

color—can be found listed as FD&C, D&C, and Ext. D&C. FD&C colors are FDA approved for use in food, drugs, and cosmetics. D&C colors may be used only in drugs and cosmetics, including those that come in contact with mucous membranes and those that are ingested. An Ext. D&C listing indicates the use of a color certified for use in drugs and cosmetics that do not come in contact with mucous membranes and that are not ingested. (Note: these definitions should be used only as guidelines, as some FD&C colors are no longer approved for cosmetic use.)

A color listing can be broken down into three parts. For example, with FD&C Red No. 4, the first part indicates under which category of FDA certification the pigment falls, the second gives the color, and the number indicates which red is being used. If listed as FD&C Yellow No. 6 Al Lake, the Al Lake refers to "aluminum lake," and indicates the use of an organic pigment of the lake group, a water-soluble dye absorbed on alumina.

Three types of coloring matter are used in cosmetic products: inorganic, organic, and dyestuffs. Inorganic pigments are insoluble compounds based on metal ions. They tend to have good stability, and are widely used in eye and face makeup. Organic pigments tend to be bright but offer less variety in shades. This type of pigment is further divided into three subsets: lakes (water-soluble dyes absorbed on alumina), toners (organic barium or calcium salts), and true pigments. Although the true pigments are the least popular for use in cosmetics, they are the most stable of the three. The lakes are the least stable, and toners fall in between. Dyestuffs are used primarily in toiletry products such as shampoos and lotions. There are six classes of water-soluble dyestuffs commonly used in cosmetics and whose stability is dependent on chemical structure. These include azo, indigoid, and xanthene. Dyestuffs are also naturally occurring in some plants.

The colors listed on an ingredient label fall under FDA jurisdiction. Currently there are 65 different ingredients that are approved by the FDA for use as color additives in cosmetics. These can range from naturally derived ingredients such as beta-carotene, to minerals such as mica and zinc oxide, to the FD&C, D&C, and ext. D&C colors previously discussed. Most of these were approved prior to 1988.

comedogenic—describes an ingredient that tends to increase keratinocyte agglomeration in the philosebaceous follicle, thus creating a blockage of the follicle and causing the formation of comedones.

controlled release—describes a gradual and systematic release of an active ingredient into the skin, thereby avoiding the "peaks and valleys" of availability characteristically associated with regular topical applications. It includes encapsulating technologies such as liposomes or polymer entrapment. Encapsulated or entrapped actives can have a more controlled evaporation and greater skin compatibility, cause less irritation, and maximize the amount of time an active ingredient is present on the skin surface or within the epidermis. When required, such a system will reduce potential penetration. These systems can release their content, usually at once, by breakage due to pressure, abrasion, or dissolution of their shell. *See also* encapsulation.

cosmeceutical—a combination of the words cosmetic and pharmaceutical. This term is applied by the cosmetic industry and in marketing to a type of ingredient and a category of cosmetics. There is no legal or official definition of a "cosmeceutical." It is used to describe a range of products that promote attractiveness and affect the structure of the skin. With increased knowledge of skin physiology and chemistry, many more of these types of ingredients are being incorporated into products marketed as cosmetics. These are positioned primarily as "correctors" that influence the biological function of the skin for anti-aging, anti-wrinkle, and skin rejuvenation purposes. Some of the mechanisms of action attributed to cosmeceutical ingredients include activating cellular receptors (retinoids); enhancing barrier function (most moisturizers); increasing exfoliation (AHAs and BHAs); normalizing cellular repair (copper peptides) inhibiting oxidation (anti-oxidants); and regulating cellular communication (peptides). As knowledge increases, it is expected that the cosmeceutical category will continue to grow and increase its use of sophisticated ingredients. From the commercial standpoint, the term cosmeceuticals is being used to indicate that a given product may have greater efficacy than whatever can be said under cosmetic claims.

cytokines—a generic name used to describe a group of soluble peptides and proteins that act as regulators modulating the functional activities of individual cells and tissues.

delivery system—a chemical system that delivers the active principle to the targeted site of action in the skin in order to optimize performance. Delivery systems can affect skin reaction, ingredient penetration, and ingredient efficacy. Unless the active ingredient is delivered to the right place within the skin and at the appropriate concentration, the efficacy of the product can come into question.

dispersing agent—an ingredient that is able to coat solid particles, like clays or pigments, to stop them from clumping or sticking together in a formula.

emollient—a fatty substance with lubricating action that makes the skin feel softer and more pliable. Emollients also have a hydrating effect by reducing moisture evaporation from the skin surface through water diffusion into the corneum layer and underlying tissues. Although virtually any fatty material can make the skin feel softer, different emollients produce different results and skin feel. There are over 600 emollients, providing a variety of characteristics to a formulation, such as oily, dry, draggy, slippery, penetrating, non-penetrating, shiny, dull, or any combination the formulator wishes to achieve. The selection of an emollient is a formulator's choice based on desired product performance and the other ingredients present in the formulation.

emulsifier—in a homogenized system, an emulsifier holds the oil-based and water-based ingredients together, helping stabilize the interaction between both phases, and thereby avoiding their separation in the cosmetic formulation.

emulsion—oil and water blended together as one substance, such as a cream or lotion, by use of an emulsifier. When oil is dispersed in water, the emulsion is called an oil-in-water emulsion, abbreviated as o/w. The oily phase of such emulsions can include oils, fats, and waxes. Oil-in-water emulsions provide a number of benefits: they can act as emollients imparting a pleasant skin feel by filling in the crevices between dead cells; or soften and improve the skin's moisture-retention properties by leaving a water-repellent film. The contrary emulsion form is a water-in-oil or w/o emulsion where water is dispersed into oil. Depending on the ingredients and product purpose, this can facilitate ingredient penetration to a desired target site. When emulsions destabilize, it may be due to any one or combination of factors such as high temperature, water evaporation, microbial contamination, or undesired chemical reactions. Emulsions are the most common delivery system used in cosmetic products because they enable the quick and convenient delivery of a wide variety of ingredients.

encapsulation (microencapsulation)—the process of enveloping microscopic amounts of substance in a thin film of polymer or in a vesicle. Liposomes are an example of encapsulation. Some of the many reasons for the use of encapsulation in cosmetic formulations are controlled release in order to reduce irritation, reduce evaporation, and facilitate ingredient delivery through the lipid barrier. *See also* controlled release.

enzyme—a highly specific and complex biological protein present in cosmetic formulations for at least three reasons: as a catalyst, an exfoliant, and an anti-oxidant. As a catalyst it can accelerate or produce a chemical reaction. Without enzymes, given the temperature and pH usually found in cells, most chemical reactions would not proceed fast enough to maintain the cell's life. Enzymes are specific to the type of reaction they catalyze, and they can increase a reaction rate anywhere from 100 to 1,000 times.

As exfoliants, the most common enzymes are of vegetable origin, such as papain from papaya. They tend to be used for boosting the activity of naturally occurring enzymes in the skin that are responsible for the surface exfoliation of dead cells by breaking intercellular bonds. As anti-oxidants, enzymes such as superoxide dismutase (SOD) work to convert dangerous and highly reactive oxygen free radicals into a less reactive form. Enzymes have also been used in cosmetics to reduce the preservative content since some of them can protect cosmetic formulations from bacterial attack.

The correct concentration of any enzyme in a product is very important: too little will not be effective and too much might cause adverse reactions or be toxic.

essential fatty acid (EFA)—the basic building blocks of body fats and cellular membranes. If the skin's EFA content declines, so will its elasticity. Meanwhile, transepidermal water loss will increase, together with skin roughness and scaliness. Because cell membranes are largely made of phospholipids, topically applied EFAs may be metabolized in the skin, normalizing the cell lipid layer and improving the water-retention capability of the corneum layer. Examples of EFAs are Omegas 3, 6, and 9.

essential oil—a volatile oily substance obtained from plants. Essential oils contain vitamins, hormones, antibiotics, and/or anti-septics. These oils are present as tiny droplets between the plant's cells. They play an important role in the plant's biochemistry, and are also responsible for its fragrance. Essential oils have many established and attributed properties, including antiseptic, antibiotic, soothing, and calming and can also act as preservatives. These oils are extracted by a variety of methods that allow the integrity of the oil to be maintained, distillation being the most common. The yield of essential oils varies between 0.005 and 10 percent of the plant, depending on the type of plant. The lower the yield, the more expensive the oil. The quality and chemistry of essential oils may vary according to the methods of cultivation, the time of day and/or year in which the source plant was picked, the location where the plant grows (lowlands, highlands), and the part of the plant from which the oil was extracted (root, bark, flowers, leaf).

esters—products resulting from the combination of organic acids and alcohols. They can be natural or synthetic, liquid or solid, depending on properties of the reacting substances. Insoluble in water, they replace oils and fats to provide a more uniform composition and preservation. They have good skin tolerance and a lubricating and emollient action. Esters are also found in essential oils. Often even small amounts of esters are crucial for the finer notes in the fragrance of an essential oil.

fatty acid—*see* essential fatty acid.

flavonoids—also known as bioflavonoids. The term refers to a type of plant extract classified as flavonoids, isoflavonoids, and neo-flavonoids. There are approximately 3,000 identified flavonoid substances. In addition to an anti-oxidant effect, flavonoids have also demonstrated anti-inflammatory, anti-allergenic, anti-viral, anti-aging and anti-carcinogenic activity. They are used for treating skin aging, as they appear to improve collagen and, to a lesser degree, elasticity, roughness, and skin hydration. In addition, they seem to regulate oil gland secretion.

Flavonoids are widely distributed in plants and fulfill many functions. They provide flowers with their yellow or red/blue pigment and protect the plant from attack by microbes and insects. The beneficial effects of fruit, vegetables, tea and even red wine have been attributed to their flavonoid components rather than to known nutrients and vitamins. Flavonoids are found in berries, citrus fruits, cocoa, green tea, parsley, red wine, and soybean.

The most important flavonoids are quercetin, which is considered the most active of flavonoids and found in many medicinal plants, and epicatechin, which is found in cocoa. Studies show that these flavonoids, together with those from grape leaf, citrus fruits, and green tea, can penetrate the skin.

fragrance—natural and synthetic compounds added to a cosmetic formulation to give an aroma, mask chemical odors, or to achieve subtly communicated messages such as image and market positioning. Studies conducted on consumer perception of product efficacy demonstrated that, using the same product base, consumers gave the product a different performance rating depending on the fragrance used.

Fragrances have also been the source of cosmetic allergies. An FDA study determined that more than 1 percent of all cosmetic contact dermatitis cases were due to fragrances. Observations indicate that 7 to 18 percent of all individuals may have some form of sensitivity or intolerance to fragrances. Thus, products positioned as hypoallergenic are fragrance-free.

On an ingredient label, it is very difficult to determine if the fragrance used is natural or synthetic, a known fragrance, or a proprietary blend. Terminology such as plant extracts indicates extracts used for therapeutic purposes and/or for adding fragrance. There is no definite way of knowing the origin of a fragrance by just looking at the label.

With the increased popularity of aromatherapy, many skin care products depend on already incorporated botanicals for fragrance. The dual function of aromatherapy is appealing: the formulator achieves potential therapeutic value and fragrance without offending a consumer's sense of "green" or creating a fear of increasing skin sensitivity.

free radicals (reactive oxygen species)—electrically charged, highly unstable, and very reactive oxygen atoms or molecules. Free radicals are formed when an oxygen atom loses an electron. The loss of the electron makes the atom or molecule electrically unstable. To regain stability, free radicals tend to capture electrons from other substances in order to neutralize. This reaction can give rise to two different processes: (a) the neutralization effect of one free radical can cause the formation of another, causing a chain reaction of free radical formation where innumerable free radical reactions occur within seconds of the initial reaction; or (b) it can attach itself to the cellular membrane, allowing the free radical to restabilize, but in the process a new oxidation compound is formed that damages the cellular membrane, the DNA, the cellular repair mechanisms, etc. This is why it is important that the skin has a reservoir of anti-oxidants.

The instability and high reactivity of free radicals is corrected when they give or take an electron from another molecule. Oxygen is necessary for an organism's survival and is a primary producer of free radicals in the body. Internally, free radicals are produced by metabolic reactions. Externally, they are a result of UV radiation, pesticides, air pollution, drugs, cigarette smoke, stress, and unhealthy lifestyles. The body has its own natural mechanism of protection against free radical-induced damage. This protective ability diminishes with age and when the body is exposed to situations where the quantity of free radicals formed is greater than the body's natural ability to neutralize them. In addition, the production of free radicals over and above that from which the body can protect itself is responsible for numerous undesired problems. Free radicals are considered the number one factor behind skin aging. They damage DNA, cellular membranes, and the dermal connective tissue, particularly collagen, by stimulating collagenase enzyme production. The overall result is cellular damage, alterations in the structure of the cellular membrane, and decreased skin elasticity and pliability. Free radicals also harm the Langerhans cells, diminishing the efficacy of the skin's immune system. In addition, free radicals favor the production of secondary chemicals in the skin. These cause negative chemical reactions and cellular damage that further accentuates skin aging. It is important to note that a certain amount of free radicals are necessary for proper skin functioning. It is the excessive amount that causes serious and often irreversible damage.

free radical scavengers (anti-free radicals, anti-oxidants)— components that counteract the destructive effect of free radical activity. Compounds such as vitamin E (the different tocopherol forms), vitamin C (ascorbic acid form), and flavonoids are examples of ingredients currently considered free radical scavengers. They can be systemically or topically incorporated to help reduce the free radical effect by decomposing the free radicals into compounds against which the body can defend itself.

humectant—used in cosmetic formulations to increase the skin's moisture content. Humectants can bind moisture and are considered moisturizers.

hydrogenate—a process of combing a substance with hydrogen. Most often added to unsaturated oils in order to produce a solid fat.

hydrolysis—a chemical process by which complex proteins are degraded to smaller molecules of lower molecular weight, including into their individual amino acid components. Hydrolysis can be performed by means of acid reactions or enzymatic action. Hydrolyzed proteins are proteins of lower molecular weight than their source and have greater skin affinity, enabling them to be more easily incorporated into cosmetic formulations. Generally, the term hydrolyzed, commonly found on cosmetic labels, does not identify the amino acids involved or the process of hydrolysis used.

hygroscopic—describes an ingredient that readily absorbs and retains moisture.

hypoallergenic—describes a cosmetic product as one that is not likely to produce allergic reactions. Usually, this term is applied to products that are fragrance-free and have a select type of preservative. The causes and varieties of allergies are so broad and widespread that it is very difficult to state that a product is truly hypoallergenic. Allergenicity is not a matter of the product but rather the sensitivity of the individual.

in vitro—relates to biological studies conducted on part of an organism, for example, a cell culture study.

in vivo—relates to biological studies conducted on a whole organism, for example, a human clinical trial.

lipid—refers to fat or fat-like substances (oils, waxes), and encompasses diverse compounds, including triglycerides, phospholipids, and sterols such as cholesterol. Lipids are an important element for the corneum layer's healthy structure and function. They account for a significant volume of the stratum corneum, constituting 6 to 10 percent of the normal corneum layer by weight. They are primarily found in the intercellular spaces. Intercellular lipids serve as a barrier against the passage of a variety of substances through the skin.

Lipids incorporated into cosmetics help moisturize the skin by renewing its barrier function, either by replacing lipids that have been removed with washing, by allowing epidermal lipids to remain despite adverse environments, or by renewing the skin's ability to bind moisture. The skin's barrier function against moisture loss is proportional to the corneum layer's lipid content.

liquid crystal—defined as a substance that flows like a liquid but maintains some of the ordered structure characteristics of crystals. In cosmetics, it applies primarily to compounds that can encapsulate active substances and allow for a time-release pattern. They are considered intermediates between solids and liquids.

masking—refers to an ingredient that can help "hide" any unpleasant odor that may naturally arise from the combination of chemicals that are used to formulate a cosmetic. A masking ingredient may be very different from a fragrance. While a fragrance may impart a pleasant odor, a masking ingredient may simply help neutralize unpleasant ones.

molecule—a substance made from a combination of similar or different atoms held together by chemical bonds. Molecules have their own characteristic set of properties. For example, a water molecule is composed of two hydrogen atoms and one oxygen atom. The size of a molecule is established by its number of atoms and will determine its ability to penetrate the skin layers.

nanotechnology—a rapidly developing technology based on extremely small (nano) particles (one nanometer is to a meter like a marble is to the size of the Earth), with multiple applications. At nanoscale, molecules tend to change many of their characteristics. For example, zinc oxide and titanium dioxide change from white to being colorless. The cosmetic industry also classifies nanotechnology into insoluble and soluble nanoparticles, nanoemulsions, and nanodelivery systems.

Insoluble nanoparticles of titanium dioxide and zinc oxide have been used for many years as UV filters in order to provide a broad spectrum of UVA and UVB protection. These two molecules are transparent at nanoscale rather than their characteristic white color, and thus they do not leave a white film on the skin. It has been established that the insoluble nanoparticles, titanium dioxide, and zinc oxide do not penetrate further than the stratum corneum.

Nanotechnology utilizing organic ingredients is now being used in formulating anti-aging products with the belief that smaller particles are more rapidly absorbed into the skin and will repair damage more easily and more efficiently. However, at a nano size, organic compounds have deeper penetration capabilities and different toxicity characteristics than the same compound or chemical at its "regular" size. Thus, organic nanoparticles that do penetrate risk provoking secondary reactions, the nature of which is not yet established. Nanoemulsions and nanodelivery systems are being used for the efficient delivery and rapid penetration of active principles through the skin.

Given expressed concerns over the potential unintended effects of nanotechnology, a comprehensive regulatory system is seen as key to ensure the safe implementation of this technology. Both the U.S. FDA and the European Commission are looking into nanomaterials because of uncertainties surrounding the rapid and unknown level of penetration. The FDA and the Scientific Committee for Cosmetic Products of the European Union concluded that titanium dioxide and zinc oxide nanoparticles are safe for use in sunscreens. For other nanoelements, the FDA is seeking feedback from the cosmetic industry to develop the recommendations that its Nanotechnology Task Force will utilize to establish guidelines for this field.

Capitalizing on the nano concept, some companies are renaming a variation of this technology as "mega-small" ingredients. Therefore, consumers need to be aware of the manipulation of nano concepts.

Nanotechnology can either become a revolutionary concept in skin care or become a government-regulated area that requires special approval for use. The relative newness of the technology and its potential controversy have not been sufficiently developed to foresee its future in cosmetics.

natural cosmetics—strictly speaking, natural cosmetics should refer only to cosmetics made of all natural ingredients. However, this terminology is applied to a variety of concepts that range from products made using mostly organically grown plants to chemically manufactured products that contain some plant extracts.

The term natural in cosmetics can be misleading, since everything that comes from nature is considered natural, including plants, minerals, animals, and insects. From this very strict perspective, mineral oil and petrolatum should be considered natural, as they are found in nature.

This classification also covers products formulated with "ingredients of natural origin." These products include those with natural ingredients that have been, or might have been, chemically processed.

In almost all instances, chemical products are present in "natural cosmetics." In almost all instances, except in the case of essential oils, preservatives are added to these products. The more organic compounds a product has, the greater its chance to perish in a short period of time if not properly preserved. A consumer needs just to consider how long an apple or a container of milk lasts even when refrigerated.

While consumers increasingly insist on "natural" and/or "organic" products, it is important to examine manufacturers' claims with a level of skepticism. The term natural is not regulated by any government agency and therefore guidelines and standards have not been set as to what can and cannot be considered a "natural cosmetic." It is thus left open to interpretation by manufacturers and consumers. *See also* organic cosmetics.

natural moisturizing factor (NMF)—found in the corneum layer, the NMF is comprised of hygroscopic, water-soluble substances that regulate the layer's selective permeability. The NMF is composed of about 40 percent free amino acids, 12 percent PCA, 12 percent lactose, 7 percent urea, and approximately 30 percent of a large variety of other materials. Exposure to harsh detergents and climatic conditions can result in decreased NMF levels, rendering the skin fragile and dry.

The design of modern moisturizers has depended on selecting various hygroscopic ingredients with properties and effects similar to the NMF and combining them with effective vehicles.

neutralized—when a chemical product has been added to bring the formulation's pH to near 7, or neutral. Partially neutralized is when a chemical product is added to move the compound up or down the pH scale toward 7 or a more neutral value.

occlusive ingredients—used to decrease the level of moisture loss by the skin. Occlusive ingredients tend to be film-formers because of their large molecular size.

oligoelement—refers to trace elements with important catalytic action in enzymatic reactions to ensure normal cell metabolism. These elements include copper, magnesium, selenium, and zinc. Some sources indicate that indiscriminate application of these oligoelements, whether alone or in combination with one another, may be ineffective and even harmful to the skin. Others cite experimental tests showing that the presence of selected oligoelements in a formulation may improve the ability of a protein derivative to increase skin moisturization.

organic cosmetics—tend to refer to cosmetics that incorporate either extracts or macerations of organically grown plants. The latter are usually more active than the former, may have a greater tendency to cause sensitivity or allergic reactions, and have a shorter shelf-life.

Unlike the case with organic food products, the term organic in cosmetics is not government regulated or even defined. The standards have been given by laboratory or manufacturer associations in individual countries and follow no uniform pattern from one country to the next. In Europe, the European Cosmetics Standards Working Group, comprising seven organizations, is working to harmonize organic personal care standards. In 2005, the U.S. Department of Agriculture stated that agricultural products, including personal care products, that have an organic agricultural content may meet the National Organic Program (NOP) standards and be labeled as "100 percent organic," "organic," or "made with organic [ingredients]" pursuant to the NOP regulations. Prior to the use of this statement, companies could receive organic certification for the agriculturally produced ingredients but not for the finished product. However, cosmetics that do not conform to the NOP's organic standards still can use the word organic in their products because the word organic is an unregulated marketing claim.

Lack of regulation and a consumer perception that "organic" is better have resulted in a significant level of marketing manipulation with respect to the concept of "organic" cosmetics. Under the best self-imposed guidelines, organic cosmetics are made with certified organically grown vegetal materials, do not use genetically modified ingredients, use only selected preservatives (usually a significant amount of natural alcohols and salicylic acid), follow a list of restricted raw materials used for processing, do not use radioactive radiation for disinfection, and do not use synthetic dyes and fragrances. Often, a small amount of chemical ingredients, about 5 percent of a formulation's total, is allowed.

However, even the best guidelines can be manipulated and lead to misinterpretations. For example, a product can cite a percentage value of organic material as if it represented the total value of organic ingredients. More careful reading would indicate that in reality, the percentage listed represents the amount of organic materials in the total quantity of the product's vegetal material. Since the label does not indicate the total percentage of vegetal material present in the formula, the true amount of organic materials cannot be calculated. For example, the product may have 20 percent of vegetal material, and 80 percent of that may be of organic agriculture. The label and the advertising can be written in a way that the consumer can interpret that 80 percent of the product to be "organic," when in truth only 16 percent (80 percent of the 20 percent) of the total formulation is.

Regretfully, given present regulatory practices, consumers have no easy way of distinguishing which organic cosmetics are most "truthfully" organic.

pH—refers to the level of acidity or alkalinity of a given chemical ingredient or product. As the hydrogen in a substance determines the ingredient or product's level of acidity or alkalinity, the symbol pH stands for the power (p) of the hydrogen molecule (H). The pH of acids ranges between 0 and 6.9 and of alkalis between 7.1 and 14. A pH of 7.0 is considered neutral. The importance of a product's pH is based on its correlation to the skin's pH. Human skin has a pH in the acidic range, varying from 4.4 to 5.6 depending on the individual and the area of skin tested. The value of the surface pH is due to acids present in the stratum corneum. External factors, such as perspiration, tend to make the skin more acidic. The higher the skin's pH number the less acidic it is, and the greater its sensitivity reaction to very acidic compounds, often experienced as burning or redness. The lower the skin's numeric pH the more acidic it is, and thus it will be less sensitive to acid compounds such as peelings and other exfoliants. As a practical example, skin with a pH of 5 will be more sensitive to an AHA product with a pH of 3.8 than will skin with a pH of 4.4.

parabens—a family of synthetic preservatives widely used in cosmetics worldwide since the 1920s because of their efficacy, low risk of irritation, and stability. This family includes butylparaben, ethylparaben, methylparaben, and propylparaben, with the last two being the most commonly used. All of these parabens are effective against a broad spectrum of micro-organisms, including most fungi and most bacteria, and prevent the growth of other possible contaminants such as yeast and mold. They are used in quantities of 0.1 to 0.5 percent of total formulation, and it is estimated that 30 percent or less of the total amount of paraben used (0.03 to 0.15 percent) may penetrate the skin.

In 2004, the safety of parabens as preservatives became an issue. This was the result of a UK study that focused on the use of paraben-containing deodorants. It evaluated if long-term use of parabens was biocumulative and thus somehow related to breast cancer. Since then, cosmetic chemists who are familiar with the skin-penetration activity of parabens maintain that an accumulation of parabens from topical application is not possible because once parabens enter the skin, they form metabolites that are incapable of mimicking estrogen. Other studies indicate that after entering the skin, parabens are metabolized to para-hydroxy-benzoic acid with only a small percentage remaining as the original paraben.

The most recently conducted studies seem to invalidate the claim of potential breast cancer risk when using cosmetics with parabens. Studies have shown that parabens are 1,000 to 1,000,000 times less estrogenic than estradiol, the major estrogenic compound in the body. Methylparaben has the weakest estogenic effect, approximately 2.5 million times less potent than 17-B estradiol, followed by ethylparaben. Phytoestrogens, substances from plants that have estrogen-like qualities including soybeans, clover, strawberries, sage, dong quai, red clover, pumpkin, and rosehips (among others), are considered to have natural estrogenic effects 1,000 to 1,000,000 times stronger than parabens.

The U.S. Food and Drug Administration (FDA) has stated: The "FDA is aware that estrogenic activity in the body is associated with certain forms of breast cancer. Although parabens can act similarly to estrogen, they have been shown to have much less estrogenic activity than the body's naturally occurring estrogen." Despite this statement, the use of parabens in cosmetics remains controversial. More comprehensive studies are needed to conclusively determine the true scope of the potential harm caused by prolonged exposure to parabens resulting from daily use of cosmetics.

While the parabens used in cosmetics and toiletries are synthetically manufactured, parabens are naturally formed by an acid (p-hydroxy-benzoic acid) reportedly found in raspberries and blackberries.

peptides—short polymers formed by linking alpha amino acids. When such an amino acid chain is small, the molecule is called a peptide. When it is larger, it is called a polypeptide. Proteins are polypeptide molecules. While proteins cannot penetrate the skin, smaller peptides can be absorbed.

The ability to link different numbers of amino acids, thereby forming different peptides and polypeptides, gives these ingredients a variety of beneficial properties when incorporated into cosmetic products. These benefits range from increased skin elasticity and smoothness to improvements in the appearance of wrinkles, a reduction of inflammation, and tissue repair. There are also claims that peptides can activate regenerative skin functions, increase collagen, and synthesize other epidermal components.

For cosmetic application, natural peptides are derived from cotton, rice, wheat, casein, and whey. They have various applications in hair and skin care formulations based on their molecular weight distributions, amino acid content, solubility, and odor profiles. Peptides can be natural or synthetic.

phytotherapy—refers to the use of plants or plant extracts for their therapeutic value in a cosmetic product. It includes the use of plant extracts, distilled waters, and essential oils.

phytoestrogen—a plant constituent that has estrogenic efficacy. Estrogen stimulates the fibroblast to produce collagen and hyaluronic acid and thus, phytoestrogen-containing plants are claimed to improve collagen formation and hyaluronic acid content. Blackberry, lily extract, spinach, red clover, and soy isoflavones have estrogenic efficacy.

polymers—large molecules constructed of smaller molecules of the same substance. In cosmetics, polymers are part of the encapsulation concept used for a sustained and controlled release of active ingredients. Polymers improve the delivery of lubricants and skin protectants and the duration of skin hydration. They also act as emulsifiers. *See also* controlled release.

polyphenols—a family of very powerful botanical anti-oxidants. Polyphenols also reinforce collagen and elastin while preventing the degradation of fundamental tissue elements required for healthy skin. The polyphenols present in green tea include catechins, such as epigallocatechin gallate (EGCG), epigallocatechin (EGC), epicatechin 3-gallate (ECG), and epicatechin (EC). These are naturally occurring anti-oxidants that also act as anti-inflammatory and anti-carcinogenic agents. The stabilized grape seed polyphenol works with essential fatty acids to protect cells against free-radicals. Polyphenols are claimed to treat and/or prevent skin conditions, including fine lines and wrinkles, acne rosacea, surface irregularities of the skin, and hyperpigmentation.

precipitate—small particles (above 1 micron) that have settled out of a suspension due to gravity or as a result of electrical discharge.

precursors—intermediate compounds of high biological potential that, when activated, are converted to another specific substance. This is the case, for example, of ergosterol (provitamin D_2), which is changed by ultraviolet radiation to vitamin D. Carotene (provitamin A) is a precursor that can be transformed into vitamin A.

Biological precursors are also defined as small molecules capable of penetrating the skin and, once in the skin—through a chemical reaction with skin's own chemicals and/or enzymes—convert into another, related compound that could have not penetrated the skin in its original state because of molecular size or affinity problems. One example is retinyl palmitate. When applied to the skin, a percentage of it converts to retinol through an enzymatic process. Some substances labeled as biological precursors are said to stimulate the synthesis of collagen, elastin, proteoglycans, and structural glycoproteins.

preservative—added to a formulation to ensure its micro-biological safety and stability. Preservatives guard products during consumer use from undesirable micro-organisms (usually seen as mold growth) that can be introduced into an open container and become a possible health hazard. This is especially true for products that contain plant extracts. Without preservatives, these everyday items would become overloaded with bacteria, mold, and fungus.

An ideal preservative system should include a broad anti-bacterial/anti-fungal spectrum; be non-toxic, non-irritating, and free of other sensitizing effects; be compatible with other products in the formulation; and be compatible with the product's packaging. While only some preservatives may cause irritation and sensitization, people tend to believe this is the case with most or all preservatives. This has led to "preservative-free" cosmetics. In reality, "preservative-free" products do not lack a preservative system. They are considered "self-preserving" based on a low pH value, the surfactants and anti-oxidants incorporated, aroma chemicals, alcohols, and some essential oils and other ingredients used to make the growth and survival of microorganisms difficult. The idea that preservative-free cosmetics are safer than those with preservatives is not necessarily true. The use of preservatives in cosmetics is a regulatory requirement.

protein—a chain of amino acids joined by peptide bonds. Incorporating proteins into skin care preparations can provide such benefits as film-forming and moisturizing, regenerating, stimulating cell proliferation, and reducing the irritation potential of certain surfactants. Originally, most of the proteins used were animal derived. These are now generally replaced with those of vegetable origin. Common and suitable sources for vegetable proteins include almond, oat, rice, soybean, and wheat.

reactive oxygen species—*see* free radicals.

retinoids—refers to a family of ingredients derived from vitamin A, including retinol, retinyl esters, and retinyl palmitate. Retinoids play an important role in repairing damaged and photodamaged skin. Retinoid treatment can result in the regeneration of the dermal collagen tissue by inhibiting excessive formation of the collagenase enzyme responsible for the breakdown of dermal collagen and by also promoting collagen synthesis. The ability of retinoids to increase collagen types I and II makes them helpful in the prevention of bruising, tearing, and ulceration in mature skin. Retinol has become the preferred retinoid for cosmetic use.

sensitizer—refers to an ingredient(s) that can provoke a sensitivity reaction such as skin redness, swelling, itching, or any other adverse reaction.

skin conditioner—a general term referring to an ingredient's ability to help keep the skin in an optimal state. A skin conditioner might help improve skin tone, texture, softness, smoothness, and overall appearance.

solubilizer—helps dissolve normally insoluble materials such as fragrances and oils.

sun protection factor (SPF)—a measurement of the time that it takes the skin to turn red when exposed to ultraviolet energy. It refers only to UVB protection. It does not apply to UVA protection. A sunscreen's SPF number identifies the exposure time required to produce a minimal redness or minimal erythema dose (MED) on unprotected skin. Therefore, SPF 15 means that the sunscreen offers 15 times greater protection against redness from exposure to UVB rays than if no sunscreen were applied. Because MED response varies by individual, the SPF value time varies accordingly.

In 2011, the U.S. FDA issued a Final Rule on Sunscreen Labeling and Effectiveness testing. This ruling classifies sunscreens as Broad Spectrum SPF and SPF. Broad Spectrum SPF indicates that the product provides both UVB and UVA protection. In order to be categorized as Broad Spectrum, the formulation will have had to pass a test indicating that it protects from wavelengths equal to or greater than 370 nm. In addition the UVA protection provided will need to be proportional to the SPF value. Thus the higher the SPF value, the higher the UVA protection will need to be. A sunscreen labeled Broad Spectrum SPF 30 will be offering greater UVA protection than a sunscreen labeled Broad Spectrum SPF 15. Note that the SPF remains strictly related to protection against UVB. Products that do not provide UVA protection or that fail the Broad Spectrum test will be labeled with an SPF value only, as is the current practice.

In 2012, the FDA revised definitions for establishing product performance categories for SPF: any product with an SPF of at least 2 and no more than 12 is considered to be a minimal sunburn protection product. Products with an SPF between 12 and 30 are considered to be a moderate sunburn protection product. Products with an SPF above 30 are considered a high sunburn protection product.

sunblock—a term not incorporated into the FDA's May 1999 final monograph, rendering it "non-monograph." This means that the term sunblock cannot appear anywhere on product labeling or promotional materials. *See also* sunscreen.

sunscreen—as a technical term it refers to specific chemicals or compounds designed to protect the skin from harmful ultraviolet (UV) rays. Sunscreens can absorb, reflect, and/or scatter UV radiation, shielding skin from the sun's damaging effects. More loosely, however, the term is used to name a special class of personal-care products containing sunscreen ingredients. Unlike regular skin care or other cosmetics, in the United States, these products are classified as drugs and are therefore regulated by the Food and Drug Administration (FDA).

Sunscreens should absorb and/or reflect both UVB and UVA rays. This is very important because while UV light is responsible for tanning and UVB causes sunburn, both UVA and UVB damage the skin and increase the risk of skin cancer. The formulation of an effective UVA/UVB sunscreen requires the use of several sunscreen chemicals since those that are most effective against UVB rays are not necessarily effective against UVA. Daily protection against UVA is very important, as UVA radiation is a constant, year-round phenomenon.

Sunscreens should be reapplied every few hours or after 40 to 80 minutes of swimming or outdoor activity (e.g., tennis, golf, hiking). If exposure is incidental, for example when driving a car it is best to follow the directions for product use as it is rare that people will reapply the sunscreen, even though this would provide the best protection.

Category I ingredients are those which the FDA classified as Generally Recognized as Safe and Effective. In the case of sunscreen chemicals, the following Category I table was approved by the FDA and implemented in 2012.

Achieving a higher sun protection factor (SPF) product is not necessarily a question of adding in more sunscreen chemicals, as this may increase the irritation potential and cost of the finished product. Alternatives are necessary. Several of the chemicals listed above are generally used together in a sunscreen formulation in order to provide wide spectrum protection.

Table 4–1 *Active Sunscreen Ingredients and Maximum Concentrations*

Drug Name	UV filter, drug, or chemical name	Maximum Concentration
Aminobenzoic acid (PABA)	Aminobenzoic acid	15%
Avobenzone	Butyl methoxydibenzolmethane	3%
Cinoxate	Cinoxate	3%
Dioxybenzone	Dioxybenzone	3%
Homoslate	Homosalate; Benzoic acid	15%
Menthyl anthranilate	Meradimate	5%
Octocrylene	Octocrylene	10%
Octyl methoxycinnamate	Octinoxate	7.5%
Octyl salicylate	Octisalate	5%
Oxybenzone	Oxybenzone	6%
Padimate O	Padimate O	8%
Phenylbenzimidazole sulfonic acid	Ensulizole	4%
Sulisobenzone	Sulisobenzone	10%
Titanium dioxide	Titanium dioxide	25%
Trolamine	Trolamine salicylate	12%
Zinc oxide	Zinc oxide	25%

Adapted from the FDA-CFR Code of Federal Regulations Title 21, 2012.

There is also the need for consumer education. Sunscreen efficacy is not only dependent on the ingredients used. It also depends on the adequacy of sunscreen application by the user. Sunscreen products must be applied evenly and in sufficient amounts to achieve adequate protection. A sunscreen's stated SPF is based on regulated laboratory testing of the product when it is applied with an even thickness of 2 mg/cm^2. Compare this to 0.5 mg/cm^2, the average thickness of sunscreen applied by the average person. Note that in the case of typical use, the average thickness of sunscreen application on individual sites can vary—ranging from 0 to 1.2 mg/cm^2. Also, sunscreens are a category of product that must remain on the surface of the skin for optimal protection. Thus, it is not correct to massage the sunscreen during application to ensure "penetration." Sunscreen application should be evenly spread on the skin's surface with gentle tapping motions. *See also* UV absorbers.

surfactant (surface active agent)—ingredients that lower the surface tension of cosmetics and aid in the spreadability of products when applied on the skin. Surfactants are often found in cleansing agents, emulsifiers, foaming agents, solubilizers, and wetting agents. There are almost 2,000 different surfactants available to the cosmetic formulator. The current focus among ingredient manufacturers is to develop low-irritation surfactants that achieve a maximum emulsifying, solubilizing, and dispersing effect while causing minimal reaction with epidermal cells. The damaging effects of surfactants on the skin include dryness, roughness, scaling, and redness.

Irritation by surfactants accounts for a large number of adverse skin reactions. The level of irritation depends on the type of surfactant used, its concentration, and the duration of contact with the skin. Exaggerated use of surfactants coupled with preexisting sensitivity, extremes of temperature or pH, low humidity, or the combined use of other potential irritants such as abrasives, bleaches, or lipid solvents can bring about reactions such as skin irritation, inflammation, chapping, and roughness.

thickening/gelling agent—gives "body" to cosmetics, increases their stability, improves suspending action, and contributes to product feel and ease of application. Some thickening/gelling agents have film-forming characteristics, and can act as carriers/releasers for active ingredients. Most thickeners are synthetic, with only approximately 10 percent being of natural origin.

ultraviolet radiation—a form of energy from the sun traveling through space in the form of visible light. Sunlight is composed of many wavelengths spread across the electromagnetic spectrum. As these solar rays pass through the Earth's atmosphere, some of the wavelengths are filtered out. The remaining wavelengths reach Earth as UV and infrared light, and are grouped into three categories: UVA, UVB, and UVC. The atmosphere filters almost all light in the UVC range, but not in the UVA or UVB ranges. UVA penetrates deeply into the skin and can cause a phototoxic effect at the dermal level. UVB, with a shorter wavelength, is primarily responsible for causing skin redness, as its penetration and concentration is almost exclusively in the epidermis. Overall, UV light can cause a wide range of reactions including mild skin burn, edema and hyperpigmentation, premature aging, DNA damage, and skin cancer. In addition, UV light can trigger the production in the skin of secondary chemicals (e.g., collagenase enzyme) with capabilities to accelerate aging and damage normal skin function. *See also* UVA; UVB; UVC.

UVA—light composed of wavelengths ranging between 410 and 320 nm. UVA has the lowest energy potential but penetrates deeply into the skin, interacting with more skin structures and damaging collagen and elastin through the production of secondary chemicals that digest the elastin and collagen, leading to wrinkles. UVA may also damage cellular structure, cause DNA mutations or deletions, and inactivate some DNA repair mechanisms. UVA is a particularly potent carcinogenesis promoter, and it also promotes immunosuppression. UVA damage is cumulative, and is evidenced in wrinkles, sagging skin, and other visible signs of aging. UVA light accounts for about 95 percent of all UV radiation that penetrates the skin. UVA rays also come from sunlamps and sunbeds and thus is just as damaging as those rays that come directly from the sun.

UVB—light composed of wavelengths ranging between 320 and 280 nm. This is called the burning or erythemal region because it can penetrate through the stratum corneum and epidermis, causing skin redness and sunburn. Directly absorbed by DNA molecules, UVB is a complete carcinogen in the skin and, in conjunction with certain chemical agents, can act as both a tumor initiator and tumor promoter.

UVC—light composed of wavelengths ranging between 280 and 200 nm. UVC has the lowest wavelength and the highest energy since wavelength and energy are inversely related. Almost all of the light in this range is filtered out by Earth's atmosphere.

UV absorbers (UV filters)—another term for chemical compounds able to absorb UV light, remitting or reabsorbing it in a harmless

form, and thus defusing its damaging energy. When UV light
strikes a molecule of a UV absorber, the molecule is stimulated
to a higher energy level. When it returns to its original energy
state, the excess energy that was absorbed is emitted as light with
a different energy state. Each sunscreen molecule can repeat this
absorption–emission cycle multiple times before it decays. Common UV absorbers include organic compounds. Inorganic sunscreens are insoluble particles that lie on the skin surface and are
not absorbed by the skin layers. Common UV absorbers include
the following families of chemicals:

- *benzophenones*—these absorb UV light that goes beyond
  the 320 nm range. Unfortunately, as materials, they are solids, which make them difficult to handle and hard to incorporate into cosmetic products.
- *cinnamates*—early sunscreen compounds, particularly
  benzyl cinnamate. They have good UV absorption in the
  305 nm range. Currently, ethylhexyl methoxycinnamate
  (formerly octyl methoxycinnamate) is preferred because
  it is insoluble in water, making it ideal for waterproof
  products.
- *physical blockers*—compounds able to reflect UV light,
  thereby preventing it from reaching the skin. Titanium dioxide and zinc oxide are the two most common and popular physical blockers. Innovations in the manufacturing
  technology of zinc oxide and titanium dioxide have created
  micronized versions where UV light is not reflected but
  rather scattered, not leaving a noticeable film on the skin.
- *salicylates*—the first sunscreen chemicals to be widely used
  in commercial preparations. Benzyl salicylate, ethylhexyl
  salicylate (formerly octyl salicylate), and homomethyl salicylate are among the most popular. Salicylates are ideal
  for use in UVB sunscreens because they absorb UV rays
  falling between the 310 and 300 nm range. They also have
  an excellent safety profile.

See also sunscreen.

UV filters—*see* UV absorbers.

vehicle (carrier)—a cosmetic compound used to dilute an active
ingredient, regulate its penetration into the skin, and/or help its
surface application. It has been observed that the degree of ingredient effectiveness varies according to the vehicle used. This
is called the "vehicle effect." In sunscreens, for example, the
same amount of an active material in an oil or alcohol vehicle

is less effective than the same material in a lotion vehicle, and this in turn is less effective than using a cream vehicle. The term vehicle also refers to components used in a cosmetic that provide the formulation with stability or consistency. A formulation can have one or more vehicles. Many times, a vehicle may also be an active principle (for example, alcohol).

vitamins—a group of substances essential for normal cell function, growth, and development. Vitamins are grouped into two categories: fat-soluble, which are stored in the body's fatty tissues; and water-soluble, which are used by the body right away. Chemical and cosmetic research into the impact of vitamins in skin care has resulted in validating and increasing the role that certain vitamins play in cosmetic products. Vitamin A and its derivatives are key among the anti-aging ingredients; vitamins E and C are superb anti-oxidants with synergistic effects; and other vitamins such as B, F, H, and P have been used as cosmetic ingredients at different times. Presently, vitamins A, C, and E are scientifically established as having greatest cosmetic value.

Though most consumers consider vitamins to be natural materials, in cosmetics they can be either naturally derived or synthetically produced. Most of the vitamin ingredients currently used in cosmetic formulations are synthetic versions of vitamins, vitamin derivatives, or some specific vitamin element.

PART II

Product Ingredients

A

acacia (*Acacia senegal*) (**acacia gum; black catechu; gum acacia; gum Arabic**)—commonly used in traditional remedies as a soothing and anti-inflammatory agent. It is also used as a vegetable gum for product thickening. In extract form, acacia is recommended for dry, sensitive, or delicate skin. Acacia is the dried gummy sap from the stems and branches of various species of the African acacia tree. It may cause skin rashes in cases of allergy.

acacia gum—*see* acacia.

açaí (*Euterpe oleracea*) **pulp oil**—appears to have powerful antioxidant properties and an ability to help regulate skin lipids, thereby promoting skin repair activities. Derived from açaí tree berries, its constituents include essential fatty acids (omega-6 and omega-9), vitamin C, polyphenols, and phytosterols. It is recommended for use in moisturizers, after-sun products, and cosmetic preparations destined to improve skin softness. The açaí tree is part of the palm family.

acerola extract—credited with anti-oxidant and free-radical scavenging properties because of its high ascorbic acid content. It is also hydrating and said to enhance capillary strength. Acerola is derived from the ripe fruit of the West Indies or Barbados cherry variety.

acetamide MEA—a humectant recommended for use in emulsions. According to manufacturers, it has counterirritant properties. It is also referred to as ethanol acetamide.

acetate—a salt of acetic acid. Although listed on labels as acetate, to determine its appropriate action, it needs to be preceded or followed by another name (for example, tocopherol acetate), as this other name will indicate the compound's function.

acetone—a solvent considered to be non-comedogenic and occasionally used in skin toners. It is primarily used in nail polish remover. It could be drying and very irritating to the skin depending on the concentration and frequency of use.

acetyl glucosamine—an amino monosaccharide that is naturally occurring in the body as part of other chemicals such as glycoproteins. Studies indicate that acetyl glucosamine promotes keratinocyte and fibroblast production, and acts as a precursor for glycosaminoglycan biosynthesis, thus stimulating hyaluronic acid production. It is considered to be wound healing and moisturizing, as well as able to improve skin suppleness and reduce the appearance of fine lines and wrinkles. It also appears to normalize stratum corneum exfoliation, and some formulations may use it instead of alpha hydroxy acids (AHAs). In other studies, acetyl glucosamine has demonstrated anti-inflammatory properties, and anti-hyperpigmentation activity by inhibiting tyrosinase production. Given this variety of attributes, cosmetic formulators may select acetyl glucosamine for moisturizing, anti-aging, skin lightening and brightening, treating post-inflammatory hyperpigmentation, stimulating hyaluronic acid production, and as an anti-inflammatory (for example after sun exposure). In cosmetics, it can be synthetically produced or enzymatically derived, and is reported to have a good safety profile.

acetyl hexapeptide-1—a melanin-regulating peptide that appears to stimulate the skin's production of melanin. It is said to mimic the skin's own natural defense mechanism against UVB. Found in sun-protection products and products that treat age or sun spots.

acetyl hexapeptide-3—a peptide claimed to intercept and stop the transmission of the chemical signal responsible for muscle contractions that can lead to fine lines and wrinkles formation, while also helping reduce the appearance of existing wrinkles. Found primarily in anti-aging and anti-wrinkle creams, as well as in eye creams.

acetyl hexapeptide-8—an anti-wrinkle peptide. Synthetically produced and considered to be highly effective, clinical studies indicate it can reduce the depth of existing wrinkles. May be incorporated into products marketed as having a topical-BOTOX® or "wrinkle-erasing" effect.

n-acetyl-l-cysteine—a skin conditioner. It may also be used as an anti-aging ingredient given a demonstrated ability to regulate skin atrophy and reduce the appearance of fine lines and wrinkles. *See also* cysteine.

acetylated lanolin—an emollient that helps form water-repellent films on the skin.

acetylated lanolin alcohol—exhibits skin-softening and anti-allergenic properties. This is an ester that resembles steroids generally found on the skin. It is considered highly comedogenic by some sources, with only a mild irritancy potential.

achillea extract—*see* yarrow extract.

acrylamide/sodium acryloyldimethyl taurate copolymer—used as a thickener and/or stabilizer. It is considered non-irritating. *See also* polymer.

acrylates—*see* acrylates copolymer.

acrylates/acrylamide copolymer—a film former similar to acrylates copolymer.

acrylates copolymer—able to absorb skin secretions, thereby reducing skin shine and providing an improved skin surface for makeup application. Acrylates copolymer also imparts a pleasant feel to a cosmetic preparation and helps reduce any feeling of oiliness the product may have. It is incorporated into numerous types of cosmetic formulations including skin cleansers, oil control treatments, makeup, and loose and compressed powders. When used in conjunction with a variety of other ingredients, including glycerine, cyclomethicone, retinyl palmitate, and vegetable oils, acrylates copolymer prolongs the availability of these other ingredients to the skin through a form of time-release activity. It also helps counteract some negative properties when applied to the skin, or further enhance positive ones. For example, acrylates copolymer reduces the tackiness and greasiness of glycerine while prolonging its availability in the interstitial network of the skin. When present with retinyl palmitate, acrylates copolymer improves the stability of the formulation and increases its skin contact time.

acrylates/C$_{10-30}$ alkyl acrylate crosspolymer—an emulsifier for oil-in-water emulsions. It has thickening and formula-stabilizing properties, similar to a carbomer, but with better waterproofing capabilities. It permits a formulation's oil phase component to be released immediately upon rubbing the product into the skin. It is used in moisturizer emulsions and creams, waterproof sunscreens, and fragrance emulsions. *See also* carbomer.

acrylates/dimethicone methacrylate copolymer—an emollient with film-forming capacities. It also prevents caking in cosmetic preparations.

acrylates/t-octylpropenaide copolymer—provides a barrier to moisture loss as well as waterproofing/water-repelling properties. It is commonly found in skin care products requiring a film-forming component, including waterproof sunscreens, smudge-proof eye products, and hand and body moisturizers. Studies indicate that it allows for the gradual release of active principles over a period of time. Other properties include rub-off resistance and fragrance retention.

acrylic acid/acrylonitrogens copolymer—used as a primary emulsifier given its binding and viscosity controlling capacities. It can also contribute to a product's moisturizing properties by acting as a film former on the surface of the skin. It is often found in preparations requiring waterproofing properties.

A

acrylic acid polymers—can be employed as thickeners, dispersion stabilizers, and viscosity modifiers. Clinical studies indicate no dermal reactions or irritations.

adansonia digitata—*see* baoab.

adenosine—an amino acid. Studies indicate anti-wrinkle and skin-smoothing capacities. Although little is written about its direct skin benefit, adenosine plays an important role in biochemical processes. As adenosine triphosphate (ATP) and adenosine diphosphate (ADP), it is involved in energy transfer, and as cyclic adenosine monophosphate (cAMP) in signal transduction.

adenosine phosphate—a nucleotide (building blocks of nucleic acid) added to skin care products to bind water and moisture.

agrimony extract (*Agrimonia eupatoria*)—astringent. This botanical ingredient would be primarily used in toners.

AHA—*see* alpha hydroxy acid.

Ajidew A-100—*see* PCA.

Ajidew N-50—the trade name for sodium PCA. *See* sodium PCA.

alanine—an amino acid that can act as a skin-conditioning agent. It is usually used in combination with other amino acids.

albumen—*see* egg protein.

albumen extract—*see* egg extract.

alchemilla extract (*Alchemilla vulgaris*) (lady's mantle)—according to contemporary phytotherapy, alchemilla is an astringent, and beneficial for wound healing and to stop bleeding. It is anti-inflammatory and soothing. In addition, it is credited with anti-free radical and UV-filtering properties. Its constituents include tannins, saponins, salicylic acid, fatty acids, sterols, and amino acids. The root, flowering stems, and leaves are the parts used. *See also* lady's mantle extract.

alcohol (alcohol SD-40; alcohol SDA-40; ethanol; ethyl alcohol)—widely used in the cosmetic industry as an antiseptic as well as a solvent given its strong grease-dissolving abilities. It is often used in a variety of concentrations in skin toners for acne skin, aftershave lotions, perfumes, suntan lotions, and toilet waters. Alcohol dries the skin when used in high concentrations. It is manufactured through the fermentation of starch, sugar, and other carbohydrates.

alcohol, C_{12-16}—a mixture of fatty alcohols with an attached carbon series (12 to 16 carbons in length). Such modifications are used to either facilitate the penetration of another ingredient into the skin or simply create a larger molecule when needed for formulatory reasons. *See also* alkyl benzoate, C_{12-13}.

alcohol, C$_{14-22}$/C$_{12-20}$ alkylglucoside—an emulsifier suitable for spray-on preparations.

alcohol benzoate, C$_{12-15}$—*see* alkyl benzoate, C$_{12-15}$.

alcohol SD-40 (alcohol 40)—a high-grade version of ethyl alcohol designed especially for cosmetic use. It evaporates almost immediately, leaving the active ingredients on the surface of the skin. Anti-bacterial properties are ascribed to it. "SD" is the acronym for "specially denatured" and the number 40 does not relate to the percentage of alcohol in the formulation but rather to the alcohol's grade. *See also* alcohol.

alcohol SDA-40—another way of describing alcohol SD-40. This could be read as "alcohol, special denatured alcohol." *See also* alcohol SD-40.

aleppo gall extract—a botanically based extract derived from the gall that forms on Valonia oak trees (formerly Aleppo oaks). Aleppo gall can help combat the harmful effects of UVA rays and protect the skin, thanks to its UVB-filtering abilities. It also has astringent and antiseptic properties, making it useful for treating burns and healing wounds. Traditionally, aleppo gall was also used in the treatment of eczema and other dry skin disorders. Minor constituents of this botanical include mucilage, sugar, and resin. It contains a significant percentage of gallotannic acid, a polyphenol and form of tannic acid found in oak galls. Gallic acid, a phenol with anti-oxidant, astringent and anti-fungal properties is another primary constituent. A gall is a hard growth that is formed in response to the presence of insect larvae.

alfalfa extract (*Medicago sativa*)—a botanical considered to have tonic and decongestant properties. Alfalfa is a widely cultivated perennial plant that can also be found growing wild on the borders of fields and in low valleys. The extract is obtained from the leaves.

algae extract (seaweed extract)—an active substance used to normalize the skin's moisture content and provide suppleness and firmness to the epidermis. There are many types of algae and they exhibit different properties. Depending on the variety used, benefits to the skin can include immunological, anti-free radical activity, an improved dermal condition, restructuring, wrinkle reduction, and tissue renewal. Algae can also act as a film former, moisturizer, hydrator, and emollient. Cosmetic manufacturers may choose not to disclose the specific strain of algae employed. This often remains as a part of the formulation's "secret."

algae extract and pullulan—used as a skin tightener. Manufacturers claim an immediate and long-term skin tightening effect thanks to an ability to stimulate and strengthen the skin's collagen fibers. This algae-based polysaccharide (pullulan is a natural sugar with film-forming and moisture-retention capacities) can also have some anti-oxidant activity. Manufacturers indicate it as beneficial for anti-aging and anti-wrinkle formulations and cosmetics wishing to claim a "lifting" effect. Constituents include vitamins B_{12} and C.

algae oil—*see* algae extract; seaweed extract.

algae protein—studies note that some specific varieties are good substitutes for animal-derived collagen. Researchers are also finding that algae protein has potentially better moisturizing benefits at lower levels of use, and a reduced feeling of tackiness often associated with the higher-use levels of animal-derived collagen. *See also* algae extract; seaweed extract.

algin (alginic acid; potassium alginate; sodium alginate)—used in cosmetic formulations as a thickener, stabilizer, and gelling agent. It is obtained from different varieties of brown seaweed.

alginate—used as a thickening agent in cosmetic preparations. Alginate may be used as microcapsules and is obtained from marine extracts.

alginic acid—*see* algin.

alkyl benzoate, C_{12-15} (C_{12-15} alcohol benzoate)—an emulsifier used in sunscreens, it also acts as a solubilizer for oxybenzone, and provides a good skin feel. This is a mixture of synthetic alcohols.

alkyl ethyl hexanoate, C_{12-13} (C_{12-13} alkyl ethyl hexanoate)—an emollient, it can help soften and smooth the skin.

allantoin—a botanical extract said to be healing, calming, and soothing, it can also help protect the skin from harmful external factors (e.g., wind burn). It is considered an excellent temporary anti-irritant and is believed to stimulate new tissue growth, helping heal damaged skin. Allantoin is appropriate for sensitive, irritated, and acne skins. Derived from the comfrey root, it is considered non-allergenic.

allantoin acetyl methionine—a chemical compound used primarily for its anti-seborrhoeic and healing properties. It also soothes irritated skin and can promote the healing of acne lesions. In hair care it would be found in anti-dandruff shampoos, as well as conditioners and sprays (as an anti-static). In skin care cosmetics, allantoin acetyl methionine may be found in products for acne and/or seborrhoeic conditions.

allyl methacrylates crosspolymer—a polymer delivery system. According to the manufacturer, it is sufficiently versatile to deliver a wide range of reactive ingredients, such as retinol. It can also successfully deliver volatile ingredients, such as fragrances, and easily soluble ones, such as the sunscreen chemical avobenzone.

almond flour—used primarily in soaps for a thicker consistency and a scrubbing action.

almond meal—used in cosmetic scrubs as an exfoliant. It does not have any other direct effect on the skin. It comes in different sieve sizes: #1, very fine, through #10, very large. Almond meal is made from the almond shell.

almond oil, bitter (*Prunus amygdalus amara*)—serves as an emollient and a carrier, providing an elegant skin feel and promoting spreadability in creams, lotions, and bath oils. Obtained from the bitter almond, it supposedly stays fresh longer than oil obtained from sweet almonds. It is the volatile essential oil distilled from almonds, and is also used in fragrances and flavors. When used in high concentrations, it is known to cause strong allergic reactions, including headaches.

almond oil, sweet (*Prunus amygdalus dulcis*)—serves as an emollient and a carrier, providing an elegant skin feel and promoting spreadability in creams, lotions, and bath oils. Sweet almond oil's main constituent is olein with a small proportion of linoleic acid glyceride. It is obtained from sweet almonds that have undergone a cleaning and crushing process, leaving them in powder form. The powder is then cold-pressed and left to "rest" for one to two weeks. After the resting period, the almond oil is filtered and often bleached. Sweet almond oil is the triglyceride oil (vegetable oil) derived from almonds, and is very similar in composition to olive oil.

almond powder—*see* almond flour.

almond protein—has moisture-binding properties. It is derived from almond meal.

almondermin—the basic trade name for two different complex compounds both containing sweet almond nut extract, marshmallow (*althaea officinalis*) extract, linseed oil, and xanthan gum. According to manufacturers, almondermin has moisturizing, smoothing, and soothing properties and leaves skin with a velvety feel. It is also said to improve skin brightness and transparency, giving the skin a more refreshed look. Among almondermin's active constituents are galatruonic and glucuronic acids, rhamnose, galactose, xylose, and glycose, as well as a series of peptides. It is considered suitable for all skin types, and can be found in hydrators, sun and post-sun products, as well as anti-aging preparations and some hair care items.

aloe extract—a popular botanical recognized for centuries as having beneficial medicinal properties including antibiotic, anti-inflammatory, and wound healing. These benefits apply to skin care as well. Aloe vera is frequently used in cosmetics for its moisturizing, soothing, and calming properties. It is excellent for dry and sensitive skin, as well as for the treatment of sunburns and other minor burns, insect bites, and skin irritations. Aloe extract is obtained from aloe vera leaves and is also referred to as aloe vera gel. *See also* aloe vera.

aloe juice—also referred to as aloe vera gel. Technically, the term *aloe juice* applies to a diluted version of aloe vera gel. *See also* aloe vera.

aloe vera—an emollient and film-forming gum resin with hydrating, softening, healing, anti-microbial, and anti-inflammatory properties. It is most widely recognized for its moisturizing capacity. Aloe vera supplies moisture directly to the skin tissue. Other properties include moisture regulation and an apparent ability to absorb UV light. It has a slightly relaxing effect on the skin, making it valuable for sensitive, sunburned, and sun-exposed skins. Aloe vera was popular in traditional medicine to heal burns. It is often used in gels to refresh and calm irritated skin, hence its popularity in sun preparations for cooling and soothing. In addition, it is found to be effective in emulsions formulated for regulating dry skin. There is some indication that aloe vera has a synergistic effect when used in conjunction with other anti-inflammatory substances. Concentrations over 50 percent have been shown to increase the blood supply to the area of application. Although aloe vera's important constituents are minerals, polysaccharides, amino acids, and carbohydrates, it is about 99.5 percent water. Its benefit in a skin care product depends on the appropriate concentration, as different concentrations result in different benefits and end products. An almost odorless and nearly colorless extract, it is derived from the sap of the aloe leaf. It is used in cosmetics in a gel form (also referred to as an extract) or in a diluted version referred to as aloe vera juice.

aloe vera gel—the mucilage obtained from aloe vera leaves. *See also* aloe vera.

alpha bisabolol—*see* bisabolol.

alpha hydroxy acid (AHA)—the family name for a group of naturally occurring acids often referred to as "fruit acids." AHAs are used in cosmetics as moisturizers, emollients, and exfoliants. They are also employed to treat such conditions as photodamage and hyperpigmentation, and at the medical level, eczema, and ichthyosis. Their activity and associated benefits are dependent on the type of AHA used, the concentration employed, and the pH of the formula. The benefits attributed to AHAs include a reduction of fine lines and superficial wrinkles, a lightening of surface pigmentation, and softer, suppler skin with improved hydration. These noted benefits are a result of AHA activity to normalize the stratum corneum by reducing its thickness through exfoliation, and the creation of a more compact structure; increased skin hydration because of the natural moisturizing properties; an ability to activate hyaluronic acid, which in turn will retain a greater amount of moisture in the skin; and an increase in dermal thickness because of increased hydration and a normalization of skin functions. There are six key AHAs found in various plants and fruits: glycolic acid found in sugar cane juice; lactic acid from sour milk and tomato juice; malic acid found in apples; tartaric acid from grapes and wine; and citric acid found in lemons, pineapples, oranges, and other fruits. Pyruvic acid is also an AHA. AHAs used in cosmetic formulations are synthetically derived. The exfoliating and hyperkeratinization-reducing properties of some AHAs make them prime ingredients for acne-oriented products, for reducing actinic keratosis, and for improving the appearance of aging skin. Also, their emollient and hydration properties help dry and aged skin. Of all the AHAs, glycolic and lactic acid, and their salts, are the most popular for use in skin care. They are considered the most effective, with this efficacy validated through a large number of scientific studies. Between the two, glycolic acid is regarded as somewhat more effective for the normalization of skin functions. Controversy has surrounded the long-term use and effect of AHAs, primarily glycolic and lactic acids. This resulted in a 1998 statement issued by two leading cosmetic industry organizations and governing bodies, the Cosmetic Ingredient Review (CIR) and Personal Care Products Council formerly called the Cosmetic Toiletries and Fragrance Association (CTFA). They assert that glycolic and lactic acids, as well as their respective glycolate and lactate derivatives, can be safely incorporated into retail cosmetic products at concentrations less than or equal to 10 percent with the product's final pH not to be below 3.5. They also note that in their directions for use, manufacturers should include a statement about the daily use for sun protection.

Key AHAs: Comparison of relative molecular size

Glycolic Acid	Lactic Acid	Malic Acid	Tartaric Acid	Citric Acid
CH_2OH	CH_3	$COOH$	$COOH$	$COOH$
CH_2OH	$CHOH$	CH_2	$CHOH$	CH_2
	$COOH$	$CHOH$	$CHOH$	$HOC-COOH$
		$COOH$	$COOH$	CH_2
				$COOH$

Comparison of relative molecular sizes of key AHAs.

Copyright © 2015 Milady, a part of Cengage Learning®. All Rights Reserved.

alpha hydroxy acetic acid—*see* glycolic acid.

alpha hydroxy caproic acid—when added to sunscreen preparations, can prevent the skin peeling that results from excessive sun exposure.

alpha hydroxy ethanoic acid—*see* glycolic acid.

alpha-isomethyl ionone—used to mask odor in a formulation.

alpha linolenic acid—also known as omega-3. *See also* linolenic acid.

alpha lipoic acid (ALA)—also known as thioctic acid. It is a powerful and versatile anti-oxidant that acts by neutralizing free radicals. It also appears to demonstrate an anti-oxidant activity similar to that of vitamin C having the capacity to help revitalize other anti-oxidants (including vitamins C and E) as well as coenzyme Q10, thereby prolonging their activity. Some evidence exists that it may be able to activate cell signaling. Used medically for diabetes, in skin care it is found in anti-oxidant and anti-aging cosmetics.

alpha tocopherol—the most commonly employed form of vitamin E. *See* vitamin E.

alpha tocopheryl ferulate—a depigmenting agent that may be particularly effective in lightening hyperpigmentation resulting from UV exposure. It is said to inhibit melanin formation by suppressing tyrosinase activity. Alpha tocopheryl ferulate is obtained by reacting an alpha tocopherol ester with ferulic acid. Ferulic acid, like alpha tocopherol, is an anti-oxidant. It is also a UV absorber. *See also* tocopherol.

alteromonas ferment extract—a skin conditioner suitable for dry or damaged skin, and also considered anti-inflammatory. It is obtained through the fermentation of *Alteromonas macleodii* a marine bacterium.

althea extract (*Althaea officinalis*) (**marshmallow extract; marshmallow root extract**)—a botanical that is said to have emollient, soothing, and healing capabilities when incorporated into skin care formulations. It is considered particularly beneficial in aftershave preparations and in products that treat sunburns and dry skin. This is a natural hydroglycolic plant extract from the althea root.

alum—*see* potassium alum.

alumina—also known as aluminum oxide. Depending on the formulator's needs it can be used as an abrasive, or for its absorbent, anti-caking, bulking, opacifying, or viscosity-controlling properties.

aluminum PCA—has astringent and antiseptic properties.

aluminum acetate solution (Burow's solution)—has astringent and antiseptic properties, and is used in astringent lotions and protective creams. This is a mixture of alkali metal acetate, acetic acid, and dibasic aluminum acetate with boric acid as a formulation stabilizer. Some cosmetic companies try to avoid using this ingredient because of its metal content and the benefits of metal-based products on the skin are questioned by some manufacturers. Prolonged and continuous use can produce skin rashes and severe skin sloughing.

A

aluminum hydroxide—an inorganic compound used to make a product less transparent. It is also used by formulators as a humectant, and to soften, smooth, and protect the skin. In addition it helps control product viscosity. Often found in facial masks and make-up preparations.

aluminum magnesium hydroxy stearate—an additive and formulation stabilizer generally used in water-in-oil emulsions. It helps improve the suspension of insoluble particles or pigments in formulations, and is particularly useful when manufacturers desire a colorless gel.

aluminum starch octenyl succinate—an SPF enhancer, particularly when used in combination with titanium dioxide. It is hydrophobic (lacking affinity for water) and can be used to reduce the feeling of greasiness in a product.

aluminum stearate—a saline form of stearic acid used as a thickener and emulsifier, and to regulate the stability and suspension of a cosmetic formulation.

aluminum sulfate—a common aluminum salt used in astringents. It is very similar to aluminum.

amino acid—used in cosmetic formulations to enhance water retention and skin moisture. Because of their reduced size, amino acids can penetrate deeper into the stratum corneum's cell layers than proteins, such as collagen, which have a higher molecular weight. The ingredient's "feel" on the skin will depend on the amino acid composition of the protein used. In the past, the most commonly used amino acids were derived from animal collagen. Today, because of consumer demand, vegetable substitutes are more popular, and ongoing investigations are seeking alternative sources. Although amino acids are fundamental skin components, the skin does not utilize topically applied amino acids to produce new skin, as the role of amino acids in skin formation is an extremely complex process.

γ-amino-β-hydroxy butric acid (gamma amino beta hydroxy butric acid)—studies indicate that when used in conjunction with vitamin E, it has an anti-aging effect. It appears to impact microcirculation, which in turn accelerates skin metabolism and generally improves skin condition.

ρ-amino benzoic acid (PABA)—a sunscreen chemical. *See* PABA.

aminobutyric acid—an amino acid with water-binding properties and possible anti-inflammatory capacities.

aminoethyl propanol—an alcohol with anti-bacterial and topical antiseptic properties generally used as a pH adjuster in cosmetics.

aminomethyl propanol—an alcohol used as a pH adjuster in cosmetics. It also acts as an emulsifier and may be used as a gelling agent. It is primarily used in hair preparations.

aminoserine—*see* serine.

ammonium acryloyl dimethyl taurate/VP copolymer—a thickener.

ammonium alpha hydroxy ethanoate—*see* ammonium glycolate.

ammonium bituminosulfonate—also known as ichthyol; ichthammol; sodium shale oil sulfonate. *See* sodium shale oil sulfonate.

ammonium caseinate—a binder and emulsifier incorporated into cosmetics as a polymer. It is a water-soluble protein powder, derived from milk. *See also* polymer.

ammonium chloride—used as a thickener and as an additive in non-alcoholic toners. According to cosmetic formulators, the ammonium component provides the tingling or stinging sensation that some people associate with toners or aftershaves, and which, in regular toners, is usually provided by the alcohol content. Ammonium chloride's use is the result of preference in formulation feel.

ammonium cocoyl isethionate—a mild surfactant, with a high-foaming capacity, it can create a lubricating lather and impart a soft skin feel. It is derived from natural coconut oil.

ammonium glycolate—a cleanser used in shampoos and liquid soaps. Ammonium glycolate is also a neutralized version of glycolic acid commonly incorporated in glycolic acid-based cosmetics to reduce the irritation typically associated with the use of free glycolic acid. Ammonium glycolate has moisturizing properties as well. *See also* glycolic acid.

ammonium glycyrrhizinate—a conditioner, it is also used as a flavoring agent, particularly for lipsticks.

ammonium hydroxide—used in cosmetic preparations as an alkali to neutralize excessive acidity in a formulation.

ammonium lactate—when topically applied, it is found to thicken the viable epidermis while reducing the thickness of the stratum corneum layer. It is a neutralized version of lactic acid. *See also* lactic acid.

ammonium laureth sulfate—a surfactant with foaming capabilities. It can also serve as an emulsifying agent and is frequently found in skin cleansers. As a member of the ether sulfate group, it is considered less irritating than its lauryl counterpart, ammonium lauryl sulfate.

ammonium lauryl sulfate—a surfactant with emulsifying capabilities. Given its detergent properties, at mild acidic pH levels it can be used as an anionic surfactant cleanser. It is considered one of the most irritating surfactants, causing dryness and skin redness. Today, it is either combined with anti-irritant ingredients to reduce sensitivity or replaced with a less irritating but similar surfactant, such as ammonium laureth sulfate.

ammonium polyacryldimethyltauramide—a thickener and stabilizer. It is particularly effective at the high pH required by water-soluble sunscreen formulations.

ammonium polyacryloyldimethyltaurate—a polymer used to stabilize emulsions and control formulation viscosity.

amniotic fluid—some consider this simply an animal protein serving as a surface film-forming agent with moisturizing properties. Others claim it is nourishing, has anti-toxic properties, acts as an epithelial stimulant, and can diffuse through the skin. Research indicates that amniotic fluid seems to have a positive effect on wound healing and cellular regeneration. Advocates of its use point out that animal sacrifice is not required to obtain the substance because the amniotic fluid (the fluid surrounding the cow embryo in utero) can be extracted from live animals in their third to sixth month of gestation, supposedly without harm to the animal or fetus.

amodimethicone copolyol—a silicone product with skin-softening and conditioning properties.

amphoteric 2—an extremely mild surfactant commonly used in baby shampoos. It can also serve as an excellent emulsifier.

amydimethyl PABA—*see* pentyl dimethyl PABA.

amyl cinnamal—used as a fragrance. Although it is naturally occurring in some plants, it is most often synthetically derived when used in cosmetic products.

anemone extract (*Anemone sp.*)—a botanical ingredient with soothing and anti-inflammatory properties, as well as an ability to heal superficial wounds. These attributes would make it appropriate for sensitive, delicate, and acne skin. There are about 70 species of anemones. Most frequently used are wood anemone (*Anemone nemorosa*) and the pasque flower (*Anemone pulstilla*). Some varieties of anemone are known to cause swelling and blistering. The extract is obtained from the whole herb.

A

angelica (*Angelica sp.*)—in both extract and essential oil form, this botanical is described as tonic, detoxifying, and purifying for the blood and lymph systems. It is also considered soothing. Angelica's principal constituents are volatile oil (about 1 percent), valeric acid, angelic acid, sugar, a bitter principle, and a resin called angelicin that is stimulating to the skin. The essential oil of the root contains terebangelene and other terpenes. The oils of the seeds contain methyl-ethylacetic acid and hydroxy myristic acid. Angelica extracts are made from the seeds, and more often, the roots.

anhydrous lanolin—an emollient and emulsifying agent. Its level of comedogenicity depends on how it has been processed for cosmetic use. *See also* lanolin.

anise extract (*Pimpinella anisum*)—used as a fragrance. No therapeutic value has been ascribed to the external application of this botanical. Anise's composition is 80 to 90 percent anethole and methyl claricol. The extract is obtained by steam distillation of the anise seeds. The extract may cause allergic reactions and produce hives, scaling, and blisters when applied directly to the skin.

ρ-anisic acid—also known as 4-methoxybenzoic acid. A phenolic acid, generally used as a fragrance, it also has preservative (anti-microbial) capacities. In addition, clinical studies indicate it may be able to inhibit tyrosinase. It is naturally occurring in anise seed.

annatto extract (*Bixaorellana*)—used in creams and sun products as a colorant and a highlighter. The orange color it provides is obtained from the plant's dried fruit, specifically the pulp.

apple extract (*Pyrusmalus*)—claimed to have soothing and anti-inflammatory properties and to be beneficial for dry skin. In addition to the enzyme amylase, fresh apples and apple juice contain malic acid (up to 90–95 percent of the fruit's total acid content) and tartaric acid, both of which can provide a degree of natural exfoliating activity. As vitamin and enzymatic actions are easily destroyed, the value of the enzymatic action and vitamin content of the fruit in cosmetic preparations is entirely dependent on the product's formulation.

apricot oil—*see* apricot kernel oil.

A

apricot kernel oil—an emollient with a non-greasy feel. It provides good slip and lubricity to a product. Primarily used as a carrier, apricot kernel oil is rapidly absorbed by the skin, and once absorbed, acts as a good occlusive and moisturizing agent. It is popular for use in cosmetics given its skin-softening action. This oil has a high vitamin E content that some claim can aid the skin in retaining elasticity, clarity, and suppleness. Apricot kernel oil is a triglyceride in the same category as avocado oil, olive oil, and sesame oil, and consists of approximately 75 percent oleic acid, 20 percent linoleic acid, and unsaturated fatty acids esterfied with glycerin. Apricot kernel oil is considered by some chemists to be a natural replacement for mineral oil. It is extracted from the apricot kernel by expression and is far less expensive than almond oil, which it very closely resembles and therefore can substitute.

apricot powder—a natural peeling material incorporated into soaps and scrubs.

apricot seeds—the seeds are ground and then incorporated into soaps and scrubs as a natural peeling material.

apricot stone (ground)—*see* apricot powder.

arachidonic acid—an ingredient with skin-smoothing, emollient, and healing properties. Arachidonic acid is an omega-6 essential fatty acid naturally occurring in the skin and considered critical for appropriate skin metabolism. It is a constituent of vitamin F.

arachidyl alcohol—an emollient and a thickener. It is often incorporated into cosmetics to prevent moisture loss and improve skin smoothness.

arachidyl glucoside—an emulsifier that may also be used to enhance the quality of a cosmetic cream or lotion in terms of its smoothness, creaminess, and thickness.

arachidyl propionate—aids in the rapid spreadability of a cosmetic preparation. It has a non-oily feel and a high sheen. It is a non-comedogenic, semisolid ester that liquefies at body temperature. Some consider it a possible replacement for lanolin.

arachis oil (peanut oil)—a carrier oil used in cosmetic products designed for sensitive and delicate skin. *See also* peanut oil.

arbutin—used primarily for its anti-oxidant and bleaching properties. Arbutin is the active constituent of bearberry, and found in other plant sources, including wheat. It acts as a tyrosinase inhibitor by converting to hydroquinone, and thus can prevent melanin formation.

areca nut extract (*Areca catechu*) (**betel nut**)—described as astringent, anti-bacterial, and aromatic. It may also have potential tissue regeneration capabilities. Key constituents include tannin, gallic acid, and a number of alkaloids. In skin care, it is said to tighten pores, help control oiliness, and increase capillary strength. It is claimed to be 25 percent more astringent than witch hazel. Areca nut extract is more often employed in products for oily skin and skin toners.

argan oil—emollient and skin conditioning. It also protects and moisturizes the skin. Its constituents include tocopherol, phenolic acid, carotenes, and essential fatty acids. It is obtained from the nut of the argan tree.

Argania spinosa **kernel oil**—emollient and skin conditioning. It is the fixed oil expressed from the kernels of the argan tree. *See also* argan oil.

arginine—also known as l-arginine. This is an amino acid with antistatic, masking, hair- and skin-conditioning properties. *See also* amino acid.

arginine/lysine polypeptide—a polypeptide used for improving the look and feel of dry skin, it is obtained by combining the amino acids l-arginine with l-lysine.

arginine PCA—in a cosmetic preparation, it appears to have the ability to increase the skin's oxygen consumption and to improve moisturization.

Arlacel (165)—a very good, acid-stable emulsifier. It keeps the oil and water molecules together to maintain a product's integrity and has no effect on the skin. Arlacel is a trade name for a glyceryl stearate and PEG 100 stearate mixture, sometimes also listed as a combination of glyceryl monostearate and POE stearate.

armoise oil—a mixture of natural essential oils said to have antimicrobial properties and the ability to act as a cosmetic preservative. For this mixture to be effective in a cosmetic preparation, a 2 percent concentration is required. Mixtures such as this in leave-on products may cause skin sensitivity if not carefully formulated.

arnica extract (*Arnica montana*)—a botanical credited with a wide variety of properties, including antiseptic, astringent, anti-microbial, anti-inflammatory, anti-coagulant, circulation-stimulating, healing, and stimulating. Some claim it promotes the removal of wastes from the skin, aids in the promotion of new tissue growth, and is anti-allergenic. Traditionally used for acouperose condition, arnica extract is also considered excellent for an acne condition. It is effective in gels and creams designed to treat damaged, reddened, or tired skin. Important constituents include arnicin, a volatile oil, tannin, phulin, sesquiterpenes, flavonoids, and coumarins. The flowers of this perennial herb are said to contain more arnicin than the rhizome and are the preferred segment of the plant used. Repeated applications may produce severe inflammation and great care must be exercised in its use as some people are particularly sensitive to the plant.

arnica oil—credited with healing properties. *See also* arnica extract.

artichoke extract (*Cynara scolymus*)—sources claim that artichoke extract helps heal skin irritations, is anti-inflammatory and beautifying. Studies indicate that artichoke extract leaves dry skin more vital, smoother, and firmer with an improvement at the dermal level. In cases of oily skin, it seems to help regulate oiliness, clear the skin, and make pores appear smaller. It is also believed to help even out skin tone and improve blemished complexions. Important constituents include tannin, pectin, and glucoside compounds.

ascophyllum algae—a type of algae. *See also* algae extract.

ascophyllum nodosum extract—an algae extract used to help enhance the look and feel of dry or damaged skin. *See also* algae extract.

ascorbic acid (**vitamin C**)—ascorbic acid and its derivatives, such as ascorbyllinoleate, are said to have skin-lightening and anti-oxidant properties. Its stability is a main concern when incorporating it into cosmetic formulations. *See also* vitamin C.

l-ascorbic acid ethylene oxide—a compound with skin-lightening properties. Tests indicate that it inhibits melanin formation.

ascorbic acid phosphate magnesium salt—*see* magnesium ascorbyl phosphate.

ascorbyl glucoside—according to the manufacturer, it functions as a time-release version of vitamin C (ascorbic acid), and therefore is more stable than traditional ascorbic acid. It is considered to have skin-lightening and anti-hyperpigmentation properties, thanks to an ability to suppress melanin production. Its skin-brightening capacities are attributed to an apparent ability to reduce pre-existing melanin levels (as in the case of freckles or age spots). Ascorbyl glucoside could also help promote collagen synthesis and help reduce skin inflammation. It is found in anti-aging, anti-wrinkle, and sun care products. *See also* vitamin C.

ascorbyl linoleate—an ascorbic acid derivative. It can serve as a skin-lightening agent or inhibit skin darkening by preventing melanin formation.

ascorbyl palmitate—used as a preservative and an anti-oxidant in cosmetic creams and lotions to prevent rancidity. Ascorbyl palmitate facilitates the incorporation of ingredients such as vitamins A, C, and D into cosmetic formulations. It has no known toxicity.

ascorbyl polypeptide—an ingredient that allows for better incorporation of vitamin C into cosmetic preparations.

ascorbyl tetraisopalmitate—an emollient, with anti-oxidant and skin-conditioning properties. It is derived from l-ascorbic acid (vitamin C).

asebiol—said to regulate excessive oil gland activity, aid in emulsifying excess sebum, possess skin-softening properties, and promote surface skin peeling. This is a mixture based on hydrolized yeast extract containing lipopeptides and phospholipids to which sulfuric amino acids, water-soluble vitamin B, urea, methionin, and cysterin have been added.

ash bark extract (*Fraxinus excelsior*)—astringent and skin conditioner. The bark contains both esculin and fraxin, which are known to reduce capillarian permeability, giving the extract vasculo-protective properties, and making in it potentially beneficial for fragile or couperose skin. In addition, these two glucosides appear to have anti-oxidant activity that helps prevent the degradation of hemoglobin. Such properties would make ash bark extract also appropriate for use in eye creams designed to reduce the appearance of dark circles under the eyes.

l-aspartic acid—an amino acid used as a skin-conditioning agent. *See also* aspartic acid.

aspartic acid—an amino acid used to enhance skin smoothness. It is usually present in products for dry skin. Aspartic acid is a nonessential amino acid naturally occurring in animals, plants, sugarcane, sugar beets, and molasses. A synthetic version is more commonly used for commercial applications.

astaxanthin—an anti-oxidant. Molecularly, astaxanthin is similar to beta-carotene, but in clinical studies it appears to demonstrate stronger anti-oxidant properties, including an ability to inhibit lipid peroxidation and an anti-inflammatory capacity. It is used in cosmetics for its anti-oxidant properties, and for possible UV protection abilities. Astaxanthin is a naturally occurring pigment, part of the carotenoid group, and found in many foods. It is what provides salmon and certain crustaceans (e.g., shrimp, crab, lobster) with their reddish tint. Astaxanthin can also be synthetically produced.

astrocaryum butter—emollient and skin conditioner. It has film-forming capacities to help the skin retain moisture.

atelocollagen—a skin conditioner and moisturizing emollient, it is a protein obtained when telopeptides are enzymatically removed from collagen. Its physical properties are almost identical to those of natural, unsolubilized collagen.

Australian tea tree oil (*Melaleuca alternifolia*)—*see* tea tree oil.

avens extract (*Geum urganum*)—a botanical credited with antiseptic and skin-clearing properties. For therapeutic properties, the extract is obtained from the roots of the herb.

avobenzone (**BMDM,** butyl methoxydibenzoylmethane)—a sunscreen chemical that offers broad-range protection against UVA rays. It is associated with some photoinstability, which can be overcome in the overall sunscreen formulation. It is approved for use up to 3 percent in the United States and 5 percent in the European Union. Avobenzone is noted to rarely be photosensitizing. *See also* butyl methoxydibenzoylmethane.

avocado oil—can function as an emollient and as a carrier oil in a cosmetic preparation, helping transport active substances into the skin. It is bactericidal and soothing, particularly to sensitive skin. There is some research indicating that avocado oil may mobilize and increase the collagen of connective tissue. This would keep the skin moist and smooth, and help in the treatment of minor skin conditions. Avocado oil has also demonstrated sun screening characteristics and has been given the highest ranking by the *Encyclopedia of Chemical Technology* for sunscreen effectiveness when compared to other naturally derived oils such as peanut, olive, and coconut. In cosmetic formulations, it is also employed to help stabilize oil-in-water emulsions and can be effectively used in cleansing creams, moisturizers, lipsticks, makeup bases, bath oils, sunscreen, and suntan preparations. Avocado oil enjoys the highest penetration rate among similar oils (corn, soybean, olive, and almond). It consists mostly of oleic, linoleic, and linolenic acids. Other constituents include palmitic and palmitoleic acids, lecithin, phytosterol, carotinoids, and a high concentration of vitamins A, D, and E. This oil is obtained from the ripe avocado fruit and is generally expressed from the seed.

avocado oil (*unsaponifiable*)—has excellent penetration and sunscreening properties. *See also* avocado oil.

azulene—renowned as an anti-inflammatory, calming, and soothing agent. Excellent for sensitive skin, azulene is a German chamomile derivative with a characteristic deep blue color. Careful, it stains! *See also* chamomile.

A

B

babassu oil—also known as babaçu oil. A superior emollient, babassu oil is recommended for use in sunscreen products. It can also benefit combination skin as it is appropriate for dry skin areas and does not exacerbate the oiliness of an already oily T-zone.

bacaba pulp oil—emollient and moisturizing. This botanical has a high oleic acid content, as well as omega-6 (linoleic acid).

baking soda—*see* sodium bicarbonate.

balm—*see* balm mint extract.

balm of Gilead (*Commiphora meccanensis, Commiphora opobalsamum*)—helps in treatment of eczema and dry skin.

balm mint extract (*Melissa officinalis*) (**balm; melissa**)—folklore ascribes the following properties to balm: "revivifying a man completely, effective for treating nervous disorders, strengthen the brain, relieves languishing nature."[1] Modern research, on the other hand, is a bit more specific, attributing balm mint with calming, soothing, healing, antispasmodic, tightening, anti-bactericidal, and circulation stimulating properties. It can be beneficially incorporated into acne treatment formulations and post-sun preparations, as well as products for blemished or sensitive skins. Balm mint's effectiveness is because of its constituents, which include citral, citronella, linalol, geraliol, and aldehydes. Its strong aroma makes it a popular fragrance component. It is derived from the plant's leaves or leaf juice.

balm mint oil (**lemon balm; melissa oil**)—the general properties attributed to this oil include sedative, antispasmodic, and antiseptic. It is indicated for acne skin and for individuals with dermatitis and eczema. Constituents include caffeic acid, rosemarinic acid, salicylic acid, luteolin, asparagine, glucose, maltose, and amino acids such as proline, asparogine, glutamic acid, valine, serine, alanine, and methionine. The recommended use level for this oil is 1 to 10 percent of a formulation's total composition. Balm mint oil has a very low yield and thus is very expensive. Because of this, it is widely adulterated, usually with citronella and lemongrass. The oil is obtained from the leaves

---

Grieve, M. (1971), *A Modern Herbal*, Dover Publications, Inc., New York.

and tops of *Melissa officinalis*. There are some indications that balm mint oil may cause skin irritation.

balsam Peru (*Myroxylon pereirae*)—a botanical attributed with strong medicinal actions. It is considered anti-bacterial, anti-fungal, and anti-parasitic, and is preferred by some to sulfur ointments. It is recommended for cases of scabies and skin problems such as acne and eczema. Balsam Peru can also be employed in a cosmetic to mask odor, lending a vanilla and cinnamon-like scent to a preparation. Its main constituents are a colorless, aromatic, oily liquid called cinnamein; a dark resin known as peruviol; a small quantity of vanillin; and cinnamic acid. It is extracted from the trunk of a large and beautiful tree, akin to mahogany. Every part of the tree, including the leaves, abounds in a resinous juice. It may cause skin irritation.

B

balsam tolu oil (*Myrospermum toluiferum*)—valuable to perfumers as a fixative. Its botanical actions are mostly indicated for internal use and its value in external applications is not clear. It is described as a stimulant. This oil is constituted of about 80 percent amorphous resin, with cinnamic acid and a little vanillin, benzyl benzoate, and benzyl cinnamate. It is sometimes used instead of balsam Peru. It is obtained by making V-shaped cuts in the tree.

bamboo extract (*Bambusa arundinacea*)—used in cosmetics for its moisture-binding properties. Bamboo extract's function in a product can depend on the extract's source. For example, the extract obtained from bamboo leaves or stems can improve the skin's overall condition in terms of look, feel or texture, while the sap extract is emollient.

banana fruit extract (*Musa sp.*)—banana fruit is considered astringent and thus provides a tightening sensation to the skin. The fruit extract is classified as skin conditioning, improving the appearance of dry skin. Among banana's constituents are iron, potassium, tryptophan, vitamins B_6, and B_{12}.

banana oil—a carrier oil. The banana family is of more interest for its nutritional value rather than for its botanical properties. The use of plantain juice as an antidote for snake bites has been reported in parts of Southeast Asia since 1916. *See also* banana fruit extract.

baoab (*Adansonia digitata*)—highly emollient and soothing. It is said to enhance skin elasticity and have an immediate skin-firming effect. The seed oil or an extract obtained from the pulp, seed, or leaf are often used in cosmetic formulations. The baoab tree is most commonly found in Africa and India.

barberry extract (*Berberis vulgaris*)—its herbal properties have been reported as anti-inflammatory, antiseptic, and beneficial for application to cutaneous eruptions. The common barberry is a bushy shrub cultivated for its fruit, but the stem bark and root bark are used for cosmetic applications. Barberry bark's main constituent is berberine, a bitter alkaloid. Other constituents include oxyacanthine, bergamine, other alkaloidal matter, a little tannin, wax, resin, fat, albumin, gum, and starch.

bardane extract (**burdock**)—*see* burdock root extract.

barium sulfate—an emulsion stabilizer for sunscreen formulations. Outside of sunscreen preparations, this inorganic salt is most commonly used in non-cosmetic soaps.

barley extract (*Hordeum vulgare*)—an emollient that is also beneficial for restoring the condition of dry skin.

barley oil—a carrier oil with soothing properties.

basil oil (*Ocimum basilicum*)—its properties are noted to include stimulating, tonic, purifying, and anti-microbial. Basil oil's constituents include methyl chavicol, eucalyptol, linalool, and estragol. It is often used as a carrier oil and for fragrance, and may have some application in acne preparations.

bay leaf oil (*Pimenta acris*)—it is most often used for fragrance purposes. Oil obtained from the plant's leaves is used as an odor-masking agent. Fifty to sixty-five percent of the oil obtained from the fruit is composed of phenols including eugenol, myrcene, chavicol, methyleugenol, methyl chavicol, citral, and l-phellandrene.

bayberry (*Myrica cerifera*)—its properties are described as astringent, anti-bacterial, and stimulant. Bayberry's application is primarily to treat acne and damaged skin. The parts of the plant used are the dried bark of the root and the wax. Volatile oil, starch, lignin, gum, albumen, tannic and gallic acids, acrid and astringent resins, a red coloring substance, and an acid resembling saponin are all constituents that have been found in the stem bark and the root. The wax consists of the glycerides of stearic, palmitic, and myristic acids, and a small quantity of oleaic acid. Bayberry is another name for the wild cinnamon found in the West Indies and South America that yields oil of bayberry.

bean oil (*Phaseolus vulgaris*)—a carrier. It is also found to be soothing and relieves itching. Bean oil is said to be good for skin with an acne condition.

bearberry extract (*Arctostaphylos uva-urusi*)—the leaves have a powerful astringency and probably also an antiseptic and anti-inflammatory effect. Some sources cite skin-lightening properties as well given its arbutin content. The main constituent of bearberry leaves is a crystallisable glucoside called arbutin. Other constituents include methyl-arbutin, ericolin, ursone, gallic acid, ellagic acid, and probably also myricetin. The bearberry plant is a small shrub, and the dried leaves are the only part of the plant used in cosmetics.

bee balm oil (*Monarda didyma*)—antiseptic and a bacterial growth inhibitor, in traditional medicine bee balm oil was used to treat skin infections and small wounds. It is also a tonic, leaving the skin feeling refreshed. Considered beneficial for oily and acne skin, and for seborrheic skin conditions, it can also be used as a fragrance, as its scent is similar to that of bergamot. Thymol (a phenol) is one of its primary constituents.

beech tree extract (*Fagus sylvatica*)—herbologists claim that when used in proper form, beech tree extract increases protein synthesis and the enzymatic activity of keratinocytes. Beech tar is attributed with stimulating and antiseptic properties, making it valuable for application in various skin diseases. The oil is a carrier, and used in the same fashion as other fixed oils. Well-ripened beech nuts, called "mast," yield 17 to 20 percent of a non-drying oil similar to hazel and cottonseed oils.

beer yeast (natural)—*see* yeast.

bee pollen wax—*see* beeswax.

beeswax—one of the oldest raw ingredients used in cosmetic preparations. It is traditionally used as an emulsifier for water-in-oil emulsions and is now also used to regulate a formulation's consistency. Beeswax is used as part of the wax composition of solid and paste products such as creams, lipsticks, and pomades. When on the skin's surface, it can form a network rather than a film, as is the case with petroleum. Though there is no scientific proof for it, beeswax is credited with anti-inflammatory, anti-allergic, anti-oxidant, anti-bactericidal, germicidal, skin-softening, and elasticity enhancing properties. As an anti-oxidant, beeswax has some free-radical scavenging ability. Depending on its source, beeswax can be considered a non-comedogenic ingredient. It rarely causes sensitivity, and allergic reactions to beeswax are low.

beeswax (**white**)—regular beeswax that has been bleached. Unbleached beeswax is yellow. *See also* beeswax.

beeswax (**liquid paraffin**)—*see* beeswax.

beet powder (*Beta vulgaris*)—used mostly for color when obtained from the root. It can also act as an anti-oxidant and a binder for other ingredients. If the powder is obtained from the plant's leaves, it does not have colorant properties and is most likely to be used for its binding abilities.

behenic acid—a long-chain fatty acid used in product formulations to form a viscous emulsion. It is considered a non-comedogenic raw material.

behenoxy dimethicone—an emollient, pigment dispersant, lubricant, and moisture barrier silicone. It is used in small quantities to give a smooth slip on the skin.

behenyl alcohol—a binder and an emulsion stabilizer. It is also used to increase a formulation's viscosity. This is a mixture of fatty alcohols.

behenylerucate—an occlusive skin-conditioning agent. It is considered non-comedogenic.

behenoyl stearic acid—an emulsifier.

behenyl alcohol—may be used for any number of purposes in a cosmetic formulation, including as an emollient, a binder, an emulsion stabilizer, or to increase a product's viscosity. It may be derived either synthetically or from plants.

behenyl triglyceride—a skin-conditioning agent. It is considered a non-comedogenic raw material.

bentonite (bentonite clay)—used to regulate the viscosity and suspension properties of a cosmetic formulation. It also acts as an overall formula stabilizer. Bentonite's water-absorption capabilities allow it to form a gelatinous mass. Considered a non-comedogenic raw material, bentonite is a colloidal aluminum silicate clay.

bentonite clay—*see* bentonite.

benzalkonium chloride—a preservative with anti-microbial and deodorant properties. It can also be used as a surfactant. With continuous use, it may cause occasional allergic reactions.

benzethonium chloride—a preservative that works against algae, bacteria, and fungi. In skin care preparations, it is safe for use at concentrations of 0.5 percent.

benzoic acid—a preservative primarily for use against molds and yeasts. Its performance is classified only as fair against bacteria. Benzoic acid is used in concentrations of 0.05 to 0.1 percent. Although it has a low sensitizing rate, it may cause an allergic reaction in persons sensitive to similar chemicals.

benzoin—a fragrant essential oil with bactericidal, anti-irritation, and anti-itching properties. It is considered a good ingredient for reducing skin redness and is a preservative of fats. Although its primary constituent is benzoic acid, it also contains canillin and an oily aromatic liquid. This balsamic resin is extracted by cutting deeply into the trunks of trees that grow primarily in Indonesia and Thailand.

benzophenone-2—a UV-absorber that helps protect against product degradation because of UV-light exposure. It can also mask odor associated with a formulation's composition.

benzophenone-3 (oxybenzone)—an oil-soluble UV absorber and filter with absorption rates within the UVA and UVB peak ranges. It has an approved usage level of up to 6 percent in the United States and 10 percent in the European Union. Benzophenone-3 enhances SPF and is popular among sunscreen formulators given a concern over potential safety problems associated with more traditional sunscreen chemicals. However, some reports associate it with causing photocontact allergy. It is considered a non-comedogenic raw material.

benzophenone-4 (sulisobenzone)—a commonly used, FDA-approved sunscreen chemical with UVA-absorbing properties and an approved usage level of 5 to 10 percent. It protects a formulation from the effects of UV-light exposure.

benzophenone-8 (dioxybenzone)—an FDA-approved sunscreen chemical with UVA-absorption capabilities. It also can protect product degradation arising from UV-light exposure. It has an approved usage level of 3 percent in the United States.

benzotriazolyl dodecyl p-cresol—a UV-light absorber. It helps protect a product from deterioration because of UV-light exposure.

benzoyl peroxide—an antibacterial ingredient commonly used in acne treatments. It functions by forcing an oxidant (peroxide in this case) into the philosebaceous orifice where it releases oxygen, thereby diminishing the *P. acnes* population. This reduces the level of free fatty acids and skin infection. Benzoyl peroxide may cause skin irritation in people with sensitive skin.

benzyl alcohol—a preservative against bacteria, used in concentrations of 1 to 3 percent. It can cause skin irritation.

benzyl benzoate—an anti-microbial. It can also act as a solvent, helping dissolve other substances in the product, and as a perfuming ingredient. It is the ester of benzyl alcohol and benzoic acid.

benzyl laurate—an emollient ester that is easily emulsified and leaves the skin feeling silky. It is non-toxic, non-irritating, non-viscous, and non-oily. It also reduces the oiliness of mineral oil and solubilizes sunscreen actives.

B

benzyl nicotinate—can increase skin oxygenation—thanks to vaso-dilatation properties—and help stimulate the healing process of wounded skin. It is an ester form of niacin (vitamin B), benzyl alcohol, and nicotinic acid.

benzyl PCA—a synthetically manufactured humectant. It helps the skin hold and retain water.

benzyl salicylate—a fragrance found naturally occurring in carnations and in certain members of the primrose family. Although it can be derived for cosmetic use from natural essential oils, such as jasmine oil, neroli, and ylang-ylang, it can also be synthetically manufactured.

3-benzylidene camphor—a sunscreen chemical with UVB-filtering and absorption capacities with an approved usage level of up to 2 percent in the European Union.

benzylidene camphor sulfonic acid—a UV filter and UV absorber with an approved usage level of up to 6 percent in the European Union.

bergamot oil (*Citrus bergamia*)—used as a perfuming ingredient in cosmetic products, it is also considered an antiseptic, calming, healing, and wound-healing. In addition, studies indicate benefit for treating fungal infections of the skin. Sun exposure after applying pure bergamot oil, or a compound with a high bergamot oil concentration to the skin, may cause hyperpigmentation and a skin rash. When used in perfumes, the photosensitizing properties of bergamot are responsible for the hyperpigmentation seen behind the ear and on the neck area near the ear. Manufacturers indicate that bergamot oil can be useful for treating acne, and oily and severely dry skins. The oil extracted from the rind of citrus fruits is referred to as bergamot orange. Its constituents include α-pinene, limonene, α-bergaptene, β-bisabolene, linlool, nerol, geraniol, and α-terpineol.

beta-carotene—a known anti-oxidant. It has demonstrated photo protection properties particularly when taken internally. It is also used as a yellow-orange color additive. Beta-carotene is a caratinoid and a precursor to vitamin A. It is beneficial for dry and flaking skin. Naturally occurring in fruits and vegetables that contain orange-yellow pigment, such as apricots, carrots, mangoes, and oranges, beta-carotene can also be synthetically manufactured.

beta-glucan—said to stimulate collagen formation. Incorporated into anti-aging cosmetics in order to reduce the appearance of fine lines and wrinkles. *See also* glucans; polyglucan.

18 beta-glycerrhentinic acid (glycyrrhetic acid)—a triterpenic acid credited with anti-inflammatory, decongestant, and redness-reducing properties. It can also act as an epithelial regenerator. It is used effectively in milks, creams, and gels for the treatment of sensitive skins. It is obtained from the hydrolysis of glycyrrhizic acid. *See also* glycyrrhizic acid.

beta hydroxy acid (BHA)—refines skin texture by reducing stratum corneum thickness through surface exfoliation. BHAs are excellent for use in acne products because of their ability to exfoliate excessive dead cell accumulation around the orifice of the sebaceous follicle. Salicylic acid is the most commonly used beta hydroxy acid. *See also* salicylic acid.

betaine—a surfactant, humectant, and excellent skin conditioner. It is also used to build product viscosity and as a foam booster. It is found mostly in skin cleansers, shampoos, and bath products.

beta-lipo hydroxy acid—also known as LHA. A salicylic acid derivative that can help acne skin, particularly to prevent relapses when acne has been successfully treated. It is a keratolytic that helps prevent the formation of microcomedones. Beta-lipo hydroxy acid also appears to improve the skin's tolerance to tretinoin when used in conjunction with the retinoid.

betony extract (*Stachys officialis*)—traditionally used in dermatological disorders as a soothing and anti-itching treatment. It is recommended for problem prone skin.

BHA (butylated hydroxy anisole)—a preservative with anti-oxidant capabilities, not to be confused with beta hydroxy acids (BHAs).

BHA—*see* beta hydroxy acid.

BHT—also known as butylated hydroxy toluene. It is an anti-oxidant that also has preservative and masking capabilities.

bilberry fruit extract (*Vaccinium myrtillus*)—also known as European blueberry; huckleberry. It is astringent, anti-inflammatory, anti-oxidant, has a slight muscle-relaxing capacity, and in clinical studies it has shown an ability to protect collagen against degradation. Much of this action is attributed to its anthocyanin content. Anthocyanin (also known as an anthocyanoside) is a blue, red, or violet flavonoid (also found in currants, grapes, beets, and eggplant). Anthocyanin-containing plant extracts demonstrate powerful anti-oxidant activity, an ability to promote collagen biosynthesis and prevent collagen degradation. They also appear to reinforce capillaries, reducing capillarian permeability and fragility. The anti-inflammatory properties come from an apparent ability to prevent the production of inflammatory chemicals such as histamines. In

B

addition to anthocyanins, the plant's constituents include sugars, a variety of vitamins, tannins, pectins, quercetin, catechins, and acids. One formulatory challenge is the fact that as the fruit ripens, the anthocyanin seems to increase while the activity of the leaf constituents seems to fall.

blueberry juice (*Vaccinium sp.*)—depending on the species of blueberry from which the juice is obtained, this ingredient's activity can include astringent and skin conditioning (*Vaccinium angustifolium*), and humectant (*Vaccinium virgatum*). Blueberries contain polyphenols and anthocyanin, vitamins A, B, C, E, and K as well as minerals such as magnesium, potassium, and zinc.

Biophytex—a manufacturer's name for a combination of plant extracts, including butchers broom, horse chestnut, and Indian water nave. It is reported to have calming, desensitizing, and minor healing properties.

biosaccharide gum-1—skin conditioner and humectant. This is a derivative of sorbitol. *See also* sorbitol.

biotin (**biotine; vitamin B$_7$/vitamin H**)—anti-seborrhoeic, some cosmetic manufacturers claim biotin has healing properties and as such, is a good ingredient for treating acne skin. Biotin is also part of the B complex group of vitamins (specifically vitamin B$_7$). A deficiency of this vitamin has been associated with greasy scalp and baldness. Its deficiency in humans is considered extremely rare, and the value of external applications through the use of cosmetic products is questionable.

birch (*Betula sp.*)—birch and birch derivatives have been described as astringent, antiseptic, cleansing, softening, and circulation stimulating, and they are believed to have curative properties in cases of skin diseases. In folklore, birch has been used for its healing effects on rashes and in cases of hair loss. Birch's important constituents include glanonoids, hyperoside, tannin, saponins, and quercetin. Even though some manufacturers list this ingredient as simply "birch," a proper description should be more specific, such as birch bark extract, birch leaf extract, or birch sap. Actual clinical data is scant in substantiating its therapeutic effects, as well as those of its derivatives. *See also* birch bark extract.

birch bark extract—described as having anti-irritant and antiseptic properties, and effective in acne treatment. It is used to make sunburn products, soothing lotions, and aftershaves. The oil is astringent and is mainly used for its curative effects, especially in cases of acne and eczema. In folkloric medicine, birch bark extract was considered good for bathing skin eruptions. Destructive distillation of the bark's white epidermis yields an empyreumatic oil known as oil of birch tar, *Oleum rusci*, or dagget. This is a thick, bituminous, brownish-black liquid with a pungent, balsamic odor. It contains a high percentage of methylsalicilate, creosol, and guaiacol and is almost identical to wintergreen oil.

birch leaf extract—believed to have antiseptic and astringent properties and to help heal skin irritations. It is used in traditional medicine for skin rashes. The leaves, which have a peculiar, aromatic, yet agreeable odor and a bitter taste, secrete a resinous substance with acid properties. They contain flavonoids, tannins, and essential oils.

birch sap—claimed to help retain moisture in the skin.

bisabolol—a botanical used for its anti-inflammatory and soothing properties. It is derived from chamomile and/or yarrow.

bis-digylceryl polyacryladipate-2—a synthetic substitute for lanolin, it is a skin softener.

bishydroxyethyl bicetyl malonamide—a skin conditioner.

bismuth oxychloride—an inorganic color additive. It is used mostly in makeup manufacturing and rarely in skin care formulations. It may also be used for pearlization in cosmetics.

bismuth oxychloride and mica and silica—a combination of minerals that diffuse and scatter light. It may be used in makeup and cosmetic preparations, such as eye creams, to provide a "blurring" effect, thereby reducing the visibility of wrinkles, skin imperfections, and dark circles around the eyes.

bitter almond extract—an emollient and a carrier, it may cause irritation and negative skin reactions. *See also* almond oil, bitter.

bitter orange extract (*Citrus aurantium*)—a botanical credited with soothing properties. It is obtained from the peel of bitter oranges and it has a more delicate fragrance than sweet orange. *See also* orange extract.

black catechu—*see* acacia.

black cohosh extract (*Cimicifuga racemosa*) (**black snakeroot, rattleroot, squaw root, bugbane**)—said to have astringent, calming, skin-protecting, anti-microbial, humectant, emollient, anti-inflammatory, and anti-spasmodic properties. Cosmetic ingredient suppliers indicate it for use in anti-aging preparations. Black cohosh's primary constituent is a resin known as cimicifugin or macrotin; it also contains recemostin. Therapeutic properties come from the use of its root, and this is the part of the plant most often used.

black currant extract (*Ribes nigrum*)—it can be used in cosmetic products for astringent and skin-smoothing activities, as well as for its perfuming and emollient properties. Some report it to be anti-inflammatory. Although the whole plant may be used, including the fruit, leaves, bark, and roots, the properties of the extract can depend on the part of the plant from which the extract is derived.

black currant seed oil—may be an effective ingredient for enhancing the skin's ability to develop normal barrier functions and the protective effect of the corneum layer. Black currant seed oil contains fatty, linoleic, and linolenic acids. When applied to dry skin, it may increase the skin's own content of these previously lacking components.

black pepper oil—its cosmetic application is unclear, though it may be used on skin inflammations and superficial wounds. This oil is obtained from a small-grain black pepper shrub found primarily in the hilly parts of Jamaica.

black tang—*see* seaweed extract.

black tea extract—*see* tea extract.

black walnut extract—an antiseptic, non-comedogenic raw material. *See also* walnut.

black willow bark extract (*Salix nigra*)—used as an exfoliating ingredient, given its salicylic acid content. *See also* willow extract.

blackberry extract (*Rubus villosus*)—regarded as excellent for its astringent and tonic properties because of the high tannin content of the root bark and the leaves. The leaf extract can be used beneficially for acne conditions.

blackthorn (*Prunus spinosa*)—the ability to identify its activity in a cosmetic formation depends on the part of the plant and form used. For example, the flower extract has emollient, moisturizing, and general skin-conditioning properties. The flower water is considered a tonic. If the fruit's juice is used, the activity can be tonic, as well as astringent and skin conditioning. Finally, the wood bark extract is where blackthorn's anti-oxidant (free-radical scavenging) properties lie, and is astringent, like other parts of the plant. Blackthorn is also considered to be healing and soothing for the skin. Its constituents include flavonoids, sugar, tannin, organic acids, vitamin C, pectin, and trace elements.

bladderwrack—*see* fucus algae; seaweed extract.

blessed thistle extract (**holy thistle**)—tonic and stimulating properties have been attributed to this herb. It is an effective extract for problem-prone skin, such as skin with papules and pustules. In antiquity, this plant was believed to aid in the healing of skin sores and to reduce itching. Blessed thistle contains a volatile oil and a bitter, crystalline neutral body called cnicin, said to be analogous to salicin in its properties. It is one of many varieties of thistle.

bloodroot—*see* tetterwort extract.

blue centaury extract—*see* cornflower extract.

BMDM—*see* avobenzone; butyl methoxy dibenzoyl methane.

Boerhavia diffusa **root extract (hogweed, horse purslane, red spiderling, tar vine)**—anti-inflammatory, soothing, anti-fungal, and skin protecting. It is claimed to be suitable for irritated and sensitive skin. Some manufacturers cite the ingredient to be particularly appropriate for after-shave products.

bois de rose oil—a fragrance with a light camphor scent. This essential oil is obtained by means of steam distillation of the chipped wood from the tropical rosewood tree. *Bois de rose* oil has no known toxicity.

boldine—attributed with strong anti-oxidant properties. It has also demonstrated an ability to protect against UVB rays. Boldine is a constituent of the boldo plant (*Peumus boldus* Mol.) native to Chile, and is found in the plant's leaves and bark.

borage extract (*Borago officinalis*) (**borago**)—its topical application is described as anti-inflammatory. It is beneficial for sensitive skin and allergic reactions. Borage contains potassium and calcium, combined with mineral acids. This is a hardy annual plant of which the leaves—and to a lesser degree, the flowers—are used.

borage seed oil (**borage oil**)—an effective anti-irritant, it has demonstrated hydrating properties and an ability to improve cases of pruritis and xerosis. It is a rich source of gamma-linolenic acid. *See also* borage extract.

boric acid—an effective preservative against yeast. It is used in concentrations of 0.01 to 1.0 percent and has fair to good antiseptic properties. It may also be used as a buffer and denaturant. Boric acid is prepared from sulfuric acid and natural borax. It can cause skin rashes and irritation if used in high concentrations. The use of boric acid in cosmetic preparations is no longer very popular.

borneol—utilized in perfumery for its peppery odor. Borneol is a naturally occurring substance found in coriander, ginger oil, oil of lime, rosemary, strawberries, thyme, citronella, and nutmeg. Its toxicity is similar to that of camphor. *See also* camphor.

boron nitride—a synthetically manufactured white, talc-like powder that can reflect light, giving a product a sparkle effect. It is primarily used in color cosmetics to provide subtle shimmer; however, it can also be found in skin care formulations for enhancing product smoothness and slip.

boxwood (*Buxus sempervirens*)—skin conditioner. It also has absorbent properties. Boxwood's constituents include saponins, chlorophyll, tannin, and wax. The sap can cause itching or irritation.

bran extract—used in peels and scrubs for its mild abrasive qualities.

Brazil nut oil (*Bertholletia excelsa*)—used in skin care products as an emollient and skin conditioner to help keep the skin soft, smooth, and supple. Brazil nut oil is composed of linoleic acid, oleic acid, palmitic acid, and stearic acid. Studies indicate it also contains high levels of beta-tocopherol providing it with antioxidant properties.

Brazilian babassu nut oil—*see* babassu oil.

brewer's yeast—*see* yeast.

brewing grain extracts—said to be anti-inflammatory with some anti-irritant properties. Brewing grain extracts are reported to be anti-fungal, to inhibit certain types of erythema, and relieve skin itching. The grains include barley and wheat.

British gum—*see* dextrin.

2-bromo-2 nitro-1,3 propane diol—also known as bronopol. This preservative is effective against a broad range of microorganisms but performs best against fungi and yeast. Used in concentrations of 0.01 to 0.1 percent, it is non-toxic, non-irritating, and non-sensitizing to humans. It is safe as a cosmetic ingredient up to and including 0.1 percent concentrations (except under circumstances where its reaction with amines and amides can result in the formation of nitrosamines or nitrosamides). It has a slightly higher-than-moderate sensitizing potential in leave-on cosmetic preparations. It is unstable at high temperatures and inactive in formulations containing sulfur.

bronopol—*see* 2-bromo-2 nitro-1,3 propane diol.

brown seaweed—*see* seaweed.

buckthorn—*see* cascara sagrada extract.

bupleurum falcatum root extract—credited with anti-inflammatory properties based on its saikosaponin content, and some ingredient suppliers indicate an anti-cellulite application as well.

burdock—*see* burdock root extract.

burdock root extract (*Arctium lappa*)—credited with anti-bacterial and anti-fungal properties and an apparent ability to help regulate/normalize oil production. Traditionally used in the treatment of mild acne conditions. When applied externally as a compress, burdock leaves are considered highly effective for relieving bruises and inflammation. Burdock's constituents include inulin, mucilage, sugar, a crystalline glucoside called lappin, fixed and volatile oils, and some tannic acid. Extracts from the fruit (commonly though mistakenly referred to as the seeds) are also considered beneficial for treating chronic skin diseases. The dried root and root extract are the official therapeutic segments of burdock.

buriti pulp oil (*Mauritia flexuosa*)—emollient, anti-oxidant and free-radical scavenging. Rich in carotenoids (including beta-carotene) and essential fatty acids (particularly oleic and palmitic acids), it is often used to help regenerate the skin's hydrolipid barrier. Beneficial for use on burned or sunburned skin, it is also said to be nourishing, moisturizing, and able to improve skin elasticity. It is incorporated into products for aging, dry and very dry skin, eczema, sun care preparations, and lip and hair care products.

Burow's solution—*see* aluminum acetate solution.

butchers broom extract (*Ruscus aculeatus*)—studies indicate vaso-constrictive properties but there are no clear benefits identified for its application in skin care. Some sources cite it as having slimming, anti-cellulite and diuretic effects, potentially because of an indication for edema, as well as anti-itching properties. Its constituents include flavonoids that help strengthen blood vessels and capillaries, as well as saponins, sterols, and coumarins. Butchers broom is a low, shrubby evergreen plant of which the herb and the root are used.

butyl alcohol—an emulsion stabilizer and occlusive skin-conditioning agent. It is the mono-octadecyl ether of glycerin.

butyl methoxydibenzoylmethane (**BMDM, avobenzone**)—when incorporated as an active ingredient, butyl methoxydibenzoylmethane is listed as avobenzone, a sunscreening agent with broad-range UVA protection. However, when listed among other ingredients, either with the full nomenclature or the abbreviation BMDM, it is most likely being used as a UV absorber, helping maintain a product's stability in face of UV exposure. For example, when placed in clear glass or plastic containers, the color of some emulsions will fade because of UV penetration through the container's clear material. By adding BMDM, a formulator can help reduce or eliminate the possibility of a product's fading or succumbing to other associated UV instability. *See also* avobenzone.

butyl oleate—an ester of butyl alcohol and oleic acid with lubricant, moisturizer, and emollient properties.

butyl paraben—a preservative against fungi and yeast, with little sensitizing effect. It is generally used in combination with other preservatives to increase the preservative activity spectrum. Butyl paraben is effective only in the acid pH range. *See also* parabens.

butyl phenyl methylpropional—a fragrance.

butyl stearate—a stearic acid used in very small quantities in cosmetic preparations as an emulsifier for creams and lotions. It has been shown to cause allergic reactions.

butylated hydroxyanisole—*see* BHA.

butylated hydroxytoluene—*see* BHT.

butyl diadipate—an emollient and pH-adjusting agent with good penetrating properties.

butylene glycol—a solvent with good antimicrobial action. It enhances the preservative activity of parabens. Butylene glycol also serves as a humectant and viscosity controller, and to mask odor.

1,3 butylene glycol—a solvent and viscosity-decreasing agent commonly used in cosmetic and toiletry preparations.

butylphenyl methlypropional—a synthetic fragrance ingredient that gives a strong floral scent, but is also considered potentially allergenic.

C

cactus extract—an emulsifier for creams and lotions that, as an active substance, is described as good for sunburns and other minor burns, insect bites, skin irritations, swelling, and inflammation. It has been used in traditional medicine for edema. Its sticky, gelatinous quality makes it valuable for face masks, particularly the clear, peel-off types. The main constituents of cactus include cactin, flavonoids, amino acids, and polysaccharides.

caffeine—has a lipolytic effect on fatty cells, able to break down lipids and release fatty acids. Given this ability and its draining properties, caffeine is used for skin firming and tightening. It is often incorporated into body product formulations targeting cellulite and slimming, as well as in eye creams that claim to reduce puffiness. Among its constituents are tannin and the alkaloid methylxanthine. Caffeine is a bitter-tasting, odorless white powder that occurs naturally in coffee, cola, guana paste, kola nuts, and tea. It is obtained as a by-product of decaffeinated coffee.

cajeput oil (*Melaleuca leucadendron*)—healing, antiseptic, stimulating, and mildly counterirritant. It is used for acne and other skin problems, such as psoriasis and eczema. The principal constituent of this oil is cineol, at an average level of 45 to 55 percent. Also present is solid terpineol as well as valeric, butyric, and benzoic aldehydes. It is similar in odor to camphor and eucalyptus. Cajeput oil is extracted from the leaves and twigs of the cajeput tree.

calamine—has mildly astringent and cooling qualities, and is particularly useful for sunburned or irritated skin. Calamine is a mineral solution composed primarily of zinc oxide with the addition of approximately 0.5 percent ferric oxide.

calamint (*Calamintha officinalis*) (**calamintha**)—considered to reduce bruising. Calamint contains a camphoraceous, volatile, stimulating oil that is common with other mints. It is obtained from a bushy plant closely related to the thyme family and ground ivy.

calamintha—*see* calamint.

calcium alginate—used as a visual accent in cosmetics. This is an alginate gel impregnated with an oily core material that can be pigmented or neutral in color. It can also be used to mask odor and adjust product viscosity.

calcium chloride—an astringent. It also helps improve the reaction among certain ingredients used in cosmetic formulations. This inorganic salt is no longer commonly used in skin care products and is being replaced with potassium chloride.

calcium hydroxide—an inorganic base used to adjust the pH of a product, it can also serve as a topical astringent and alkali in solutions or lotions. It can burn the skin and eyes.

calcium pantetheine sulfonate—a skin-conditioning ingredient with apparent anti-inflammatory properties. Clinical studies indicate an ability to inhibit tyrosinase activity and melanin synthesis. It is most commonly used in moisturizers, anti-aging, and SPF products, though it can also be found in cosmetics for skin whitening or lightening.

calcium pantothenate—used as an emollient and to enrich creams and lotions in hair care preparations. This is the calcium salt of pantothenic acid found in liver, rice, bran, and molasses. It is also found in large amounts in royal jelly.

calcium thioglycolate—used almost exclusively in depilatory creams and hair products. This is a calcium salt of thio-glycolic acid. It may cause skin irritation.

calendula extract (*Calendula officinalis*) (**marigold**)—an emollient said to have healing, wound-healing, soothing, antiseptic, anti-itching, and anti-inflammatory properties. It can be effectively used in cases of oily and/or delicate skin as well as for acne. The extract is obtained from the calendula blossom. *See also* marigold extract.

calendula hydrolysates—a calendula derivative. *See also* calendula extract.

Calophyllum inophyllum **seed oil**—an anti-oxidant with UV-absorption capacities. It can also be used as an anti-microbial and a skin conditioner. Its properties are said to include the improvement of cell regeneration. It is often incorporated into anti-aging and regenerating creams, sun and post-sun creams. This occurs in the same family as *Calophyllum tacamahaca*. *See also* tamanu oil.

Calophyllum tacamahaca **seed oil**—*see* tamanu oil.

camelina sativa seed oil—emollient and skin conditioning, it is used in anti-aging cosmetic products for its reported ability to improve skin elasticity and suppleness. Among its constituents are alpha-linolenic acid, linoleic acid, and tocopherol.

camellia kissi seed oil—an occlusive emollient also used to soften and smooth dry skin. Manufacturers of this ingredient credit it with cell regeneration properties and an ability to restore skin elasticity, making it appropriate for calming, and wound healing. It is attributed with some anti-oxidant capacity based on its vitamin content (vitamins A, B, C, and E). Most often found in moisturizers, night creams, and skin cleansers.

camellia oil—used as a non-greasy emollient for skin care products. Camellia oil plays an important role in anti-oxidation as a result of its high content of oleic acid. It is derived from the seeds of *Thea sasanqua nois* variety.

camellia seed oil—an easily absorbed carrier oil, that does not leave a greasy feeling on the skin. It contains fatty and essential fatty acids, including oleic acid. Camellia seed oil also contains vitamin E, providing it with some anti-oxidant properties. Ingredient manufacturers cite it as beneficial for dry, aging, and sunburned skin. It is used in both skin and hair care preparations.

camellia seed powder—an ingredient used for its abrasive action.

camellia sinensis leaf extract—*see* green tea extract.

camphor (*Cinnamomum camphora*)—credited with anesthetic, anti-inflammatory, antiseptic, astringent, cooling, and refreshing properties, and thought to be slightly stimulating to blood circulation and function. Once absorbed by the subcutaneous tissue, it combines in the body with glucoronic acid and is released through the urine. Camphor is effective for oily and acne skin treatment, and has a scent similar to eucalyptus. In high concentrations, it can be an irritant and numb the peripheral sensory nerves. Natural camphor is derived from an evergreen tree indigenous to Asia, although now its synthetic substitute is often used.

camphor benzalkonium methosulfate—a UV filter and UV absorber. It also has anti-microbial properties.

camphor oil—*see* camphor.

candelilla wax (*Euphorbia cerifera*)—binds oils and waxes, and gives body to a formulation. It is also used as a film former. It is obtained from candelilla plants and is similar to carnauba wax.

candlenut—*see* kukui nut oil.

canola oil—has good emolliency and lubricity. Canola oil is a rapeseed oil extract considered to be a natural replacement for mineral oil.

capryl isostearate—an emollient.

caprylic/capric triglyceride (**Tricaprylin**)—an emollient with good spreading properties. It promotes penetration and does not leave visible traces of oiliness on the skin. It is effectively used in creams, lotions, and oil formulations.

C

caprylol collagen amino acids—a liquid with an anti-acne effect. *See also* amino acid; collagen.

capryloyl collagenic acid—a lipoamino acid found to have similar anti-bacterial properties as benzoyl peroxide when tested against *S. aureus, S. epidermidis,* and *P. acnes* bacteria. Test results show it to be most effective in treating mild cases of acne vulgaris, though it demonstrates some positive results against moderate and severe acne cases as well. Although it reduces inflammatory lesions, it does not affect comedones and cysts. When treatment is suspended, there is a mild relapse of the acne lesions.

capryloyl salicylic acid—a skin conditioner. This is an ester of salicylic and caprylic acids.

caprylyl/capryl glucoside—a surfactant used in cleansing preparations, primarily shampoos.

caprylyl glycol—an emollient with moisturizing properties that may also be used as a cosmetic stabilizer. When found in combination with phenoxyethanol these two ingredients work together as an anti-microbial.

caprylyl methicone—used for its occlusive properties. It can help retain water on the surface of the skin.

caramel—used as a coloring agent. It provides products with a slight touch of brown. Some sources also state that it acts as a soothing agent in skin care preparations. Caramel is a concentrated solution obtained from heating sugar or glucose solutions.

caraway oil (*Carum carvi*)—a carrier oil credited with the ability to alleviate bruises, and believed to have tissue-regenerating properties. It is said to be beneficial for acne and oily skin. Caraway is a member of the group of aromatic, umbelliferous plants, such as anise, cumin, dill, and fennel, characterized by carminative properties. Carvene (also found in dill and cumin oils), an oxygenated oil, and carvol are the principal constituents of caraway oil. Caraway oil is obtained from the distillation of the seeds, and may cause allergic reactions and skin irritation.

carbocysteine—an amino acid. It can be used to help control sebum production. *See also* amino acid.

carbomer 934, 940, 941, 980, 981—high molecular-weight, cross-linked polymers. They are used as thickening and suspending agents, and as emulsion stabilizers in cosmetic formulations. They are often used with triethanolamine, sodium hydroxide, or other alkaline compounds to crosslink the polymer. White, slightly acidic powders, carbomers react with fat particles to form thick, stable, oil-in-water emulsions. *See also* carbomer entry in Chapter 4 of Part 1.

Carbopol—a trade name for carbomer. *See also* carbomer.

carboxyethyl-γ-aminobutyric acid—described as an amino acid-based ingredient promoting cellular growth.

carboxymethyl cellulose (cellulose gum)—a thickener. Used in cosmetic formulations when a reactant is not required or desired. Often used in bath preparations, beauty masks, hand creams, and shampoos. It is considered a non-comedogenic raw material.

carboxymethyl chitin—moisturizing. It is derived from the exoskeleton of shrimp and crab. *See also* chitin.

carboxypolymethylene—a binder, film-former and emulsion stabilizer. It can also help increase product viscosity. *See also* carbomer.

carboxyvinyl polymer—provides viscosity, and is suitable for thickening and stabilizing emulsions or dispersions in cosmetics. Its incorporation into cosmetic formulations results in very clear gel preparations. It is a synthetic resin.

cardamom oil (*Elettaria cardamomum*)—credited with antiseptic, stimulating, and deodorant properties. This is a large perennial herb that yields cardamom seeds containing volatile oil, fixed oil, potassium salt, a coloring principle, starch, nitrogenous mucilage, ligneous fiber, an acrid resin, and ash. The volatile oil contains terpenes, terpineol, and cineol.

carmine—a crimson pigment. This is the aluminum lake of the coloring agent cochineal, a natural pigment derived from the dried female insect *Coccus cacti*. Carmine may cause allergic reactions.

carnauba wax—used to firm and texturize cosmetic preparations, and give them a less fluid consistency. Carnauba wax also forms a protective layer on the skin's surface. It has the highest melting point among natural plant waxes and does not usually cause allergic reactions. This wax is obtained from leaves and leaf buds of the Brazilian wax palm.

carnitine—a skin-conditioning agent, surfactant, and formulation viscosity-increasing substance. Carnitine is used primarily in hand and body preparations.

carnitine hydroxycitrate—an amino acid said to help break down fat stored in the cells more effectively than caffeine, making it beneficial for use in slimming and body-contouring products.

carnosine—an anti-oxidant that works to prevent cellular damage because of free radical activity. Studies indicate an ability to boost the immunological functions. Carnosine is a naturally occurring amino acid. In cosmetics, it has anti-aging and skin-conditioning applications.

C

carob extract (*Jacaranda procera, Caroba balsam, Ceratonia Siliqua*)—its botanical property is reported as anti-infectious. In the small leaves—carob extract's source—caroborelinic acid, carobic acid, steocarobic acid, carobon, and carobin have been found.

carotene—used to provide a red-orange color in cosmetic formulations. It is the primary yellow coloring component of butter, carrots, and egg yolk. Carotene is found in plants as well as in many animal tissues. *See also* beta-carotene.

carotene oil—a red-orange colored oil containing carotene, used for coloring. A carrot extract.

carrageenan—*see* carrageen extract.

carrageen extract (*Chondrus crispus*) (**Irish moss**)—a very common thickener that, in its sodium salt form, has jellifying properties. It can help maintain the skin feeling soft and in good condition. Carrageen is a polysaccharide of red algae origin with a seaweed-like odor and is considered non-toxic. *See also* seaweed extract.

carreghane extract (**red algae**)—*see* seaweed extract.

carrot extract (*Daucus carota*)—there are some indications that, when obtained from carrot leaves, the extract may have cleansing and healing properties because of its strong antiseptic qualities. The root contains no less than 89 percent water. The juice also contains beta-carotene, sugar, a little starch, extractine gluten, albumen, volatile oil, vegetable jelly or pectin, saline matter, malic acid, and carotin. Carrot's botanical properties depend on its volatile oil. *See also* beta-carotene.

carrot oil—used since the sixteenth century for skin diseases for its attributed cleansing, purifying, and draining properties. This carotene-rich emollient has been indicated for acne skin conditions, dermatitis, skin irritation, skin rashes, and wrinkles. It is derived from the carrot root.

carrot oleoresin—has good conditioning properties. This ingredient is found more often in hair care products.

carrot root extract—*see* carrot extract.

carrot seed oil—contains beta-carotene and vitamin A, providing anti-oxidant properties. It is also beneficial for treating dry, damaged skin. *See also* carrot oil, beta-carotene.

cascara sagrada extract (*Rhamnus purshiana*) (**buckthorn; sacred bark**)—used to add a skin-soothing factor in lotions and creams. It can also be incorporated into a skin care product to protect the skin from harsh external conditions, as well as to improve the skin's overall condition. It may also be used as a perfuming component. The extract is prepared from this shrub's bark, which includes glucosides among its constituents.

casein amino acids—hydrolyzed milk protein. It is used as an emulsifier in many cosmetics. It also binds water for moisturization. *See also* amino acids; milk protein.

castor isostearate succinate—used by cosmetic formulators to replace lanolin. It is classified as a natural ingredient.

castor oil—a highly emollient carrier oil that penetrates the skin easily, leaving it soft and supple. It also serves to bind the different ingredients of a cosmetic formulation together. Castor oil is high in glycerin esters of ricinoleic acid (an unsaturated fatty acid). It is rarely, if ever, associated with irritation of the skin or allergic reactions. It is obtained through cold-pressing from seeds or beans of the *Ricinus communis* (castor oil) plant. Impure castor oil may cause irritation, as the seeds contain a toxic substance that is eliminated during processing. Its unpleasant odor makes it difficult to use in cosmetics.

caviar—*see* roe extract.

cedar—*see* cedarwood oil.

cedarwood oil (*Thuja occidentalis*) (**cedar; thuja**)—credited with antiseptic, sedative, and astringent properties. It is used as a fixative in fragrances because it blends well with other oils. This clear oil is also valuable for use on skin eruptions and to relieve itching. It is good for acne and oily skin, and could be helpful in cases of dermatitis, eczema, and psoriasis. Two types of cedarwood oil exist: Atlas cedarwood oil from Morocco (*Cedrus atlantica*) and one derived from the *Juniperus virginiana* (or red cedar) that is a juniper of the United States (its oil, however, is very similar to true cedarwood). The oil may cause skin irritation when used in high concentrations. Cedarwood oil is obtained from recently dried, leafy, young twigs.

celandine (*Chelidonium majus*)—also known as tetterwort, this plant is a member of the poppy family. Attributed with anti-spasmodic properties, and can help reduce inflammation. It can, however, also cause irritation. Celandine contains numerous alkaloids, including chelidonine, sanguinarin, alpha- and beta-homo chelidonine, berberine, and cheleryhrine, some of which may help improve blood flow. Among its other constituents are resin and protease enzymes. It may also serve as a "natural" colorant. It may be incorporated into eye care products to improve the appearance of tired eyes.

cellular protein—*see* protein.

cellulose—a thickener and an emulsifier. It is obtained from plants.

cellulose (**microcrystalline**)—used as an emulsifier in cosmetic creams. It is the chief constituent of plant fiber.

cellulose fiber—used as a thickener, suspending agent, and binder.

cellulose gum—a thickener, binder, and emulsifier equivalent to cellulose fiber. It is resistant to bacterial decomposition and provides a product with uniform viscosity. It can prevent skin moisture loss by forming a film on the skin's surface, and also help mask odor in a cosmetic product. Constituents are any of several fibrous substances consisting of the chief part of a plant's cell walls (often extracted from wood pulp or cotton). *See also* carboxymethyl cellulose.

cera alba—*see* beeswax (white); beeswax.

ceramides—a family of naturally occurring lipids that act primarily in the skin's uppermost layer, forming a protective barrier and reducing natural transepidermal water loss. Ceramides repair the stratum corneum layer in cases of dry skin, improve skin hydration, and increase the feeling of softness. They are beneficial for stressed, sensitive, scaly, rough, dry, aged, and sun-damaged skin. Ceramides play an essential role in the structure of superficial epidermal layers and form an integral part of the intercellular membrane network. They help generate and sustain the skin's barrier function. This is extremely important: if the stratum corneum's hydration is maintained, then it functions more normally in terms of flexibility and desquamation, its integrity is upheld, and the skin is less susceptible to irritation. Ceramide production decreases with age, accentuating any tendency to dry skin. When incorporated into a skin care preparation, the topical application of ceramides could benefit the stratum corneum if the ceramides manage to fill the intercellular spaces and if they are hydrolyzed by the correct extracellular enzymes on the skin. Such application also can stimulate ceramide production in the skin, thereby increasing the skin's natural lipid content and reinforcing the skin's protective barrier, measured through transepidermal water loss. Topically applied ceramides have been shown to capture and bind water, necessary for the skin to remain supple, smooth, and hydrated. Natural ceramides are obtained from animals and plants. While ceramides can be synthetically manufactured, it is hard to obtain an identical equivalent to those found in nature, making them expensive raw materials.

cereal lipoplastidins—coconut oil that has been mixed with a number of cereal grain extracts such as rice, bran, and/or oat.

cereal germ oil—a carrier oil.

cereal seed oil—a carrier oil.

ceresin—regulates the viscosity, suspension properties, and overall stability of a skin care preparation. It is used in protective creams as a beeswax and paraffin substitute. This white-to-yellow waxy mixture of hydrocarbons is obtained by the purification of ozokerite. Ceresin may cause allergic reactions.

ceresin wax (ceresin)—a thickener and a binder with non-comedogenic properties. *See also* ceresin.

ceteareth, ceteareth 4, 12, 19, 20, 30—all are used for their emollient, emulsifying, anti-foaming, and/or lubricant properties in cosmetic formulations. Ceteareth is obtained from a combination of cetyl alcohol and stearyl alcohol. Ceteareth-4 is the polyethylene glycol ether of cetearyl alcohol, and ceteareths-20 and -30 are also good solubilizing agents.

cetearyl alcohol (cetostearyl alcohol)—an emulsifying and stabilizing wax produced from the reduction of plant oils and natural waxes. Also used as an emollient and to give high viscosity to a finished product. Cetearyl alcohol is a mixture of fatty alcohols consisting primarily of cetyl and stearyl alcohols.

cetearyl glucoside—an emulsifier and surfactant.

cetearyl isononandate—an emollient with a high hydrophobic effect.

cetearyl octanoate—an emollient. This ingredient can be either a palm kernel or coconut derivative, and has a high degree of water repellency. It is used in non-comedogenic moisturizers. In nature, it occurs on the feathers of water birds.

cetearyl olivate—an olive-oil derived emulsifier. It is said to also reduce transepidermal water loss. It is often used in conjunction with sorbitan olivate.

cetearyl palmitate—an emollient. When incorporated into a skin care product, it leaves the skin with a velvety feel. This ingredient has replaced spermaceti wax.

ceteth—used as a surface active agent in cosmetics. It is a compound of derivatives of cetyl, lauryl, stearyl, and oleyl alcohols mixed with ethylene oxide.

ceteth 20—an emulsifier for oil-in-water creams and lotions.

cetostearyl alcohol—*see* cetearyl alcohol.

cetrimonium bromide—also known as cetyl trimethyl ammonium bromide. This is a quaternary ammonium salt that can prevent the proliferation of bacteria, fungi, and yeast in cosmetic preparation, while also act as an emulsifying agent.

cetrimonium chloride—also known as cetyl trimethyl ammonium chloride. Can be incorporated into a cosmetic preparation for any number of formulatory needs including as an anti-static, an emulsifier, and a surfactant. It can also be used as a preservative and anti-microbial against the proliferation of bacteria, fungi, and yeast.

cetyl alcohol—a versatile ingredient that can serve as an emollient, emulsifier, thickener, binder, foam booster, or emulsion stabilizer, depending on the formulation and need. It is derived from coconut or palm oil as well as being synthetically manufactured. It is considered by some sources to be a non-comedogenic material.

cetyl alcohol 40—a preservative and carrier similar to cetyl alcohol.

cetyl dimethicone—a silicone-based emollient and occlusive skin-conditioning agent.

cetyl dimethicone copolyol—an emulsifier and emollient used in cosmetic preparations to form water-in-oil emulsions that have viscosity but also rub out easily. These types of preparations are used in sunscreen formulations where good spreadability and waterproofing are valued characteristics. Used in moisturizers, these emulsions provide a good moisture barrier and reduce the speed of transepidermal water loss.

cetyl esters—used in formulations to give body to emulsions. They are also formulation stabilizers and thickeners. Cetyl esters are produced by combining various fatty esters with cetyl palmitate. They are generally indistinguishable from natural spermaceti wax in terms of composition and properties, and are its synthetic version.

cetyl ethylhexanoate—an emollient that helps make the skin feel softer, smoother, and more supple. It can be naturally derived or synthetically manufactured.

cetyl hydroxyethyl cellulose—similar to hydroxyethyl cellulose, but might yield slightly different thickness and absorption properties within a formulation. *See also* hydroxyethyl cellulose.

cetyl palmitate (synthetic spermaceti)—its chemical structure is the same as whale spermaceti. It may be used to thicken, produce viscose emulsions, give stability, and add texture to emulsions. It is similar to cetearyl palmitate.

cetyl PEG/PPG-10/1 dimethicone—used to improve the appearance of dry skin, it is also an emulsifier and surfactant.

cetyl phosphate—a mild emulsifier with a low irritancy potential.

cetyl ricinoleate—an emollient and emulsion stabilizer considered to be a non-comedogenic ester.

cetyl trimethylammonium bromide (cetrimonium bromide)—*see* cetrimonium bromide.

cetyl trimethylammonium chloride (cetrimonium chloride)—*see* cetrimonium chloride.

chamomile extract (*Anthemis nobilis; Matricaria chamomilla*)— has clinically proven anti-inflammatory and repairer properties.

It is also considered bactericidal, anti-itching, soothing, antiseptic, purifying, refreshing, and hypoallergenic with the ability to neutralize skin irritants. There are various forms of chamomile, including Roman chamomile (*Anthemis nobilis*) and German chamomile (*Matricaria chamomilla*). German chamomile tends to be more potent than Roman because of its higher azulene content. Active constituents include azulene, bisabolol, and phytosterol. The chamomile plant is aromatic, and its flower heads are used to obtain aqueous-alcoholic extracts and the blue chamomile oil. Chamomile is considered a non-comedogenic raw material and can be particularly useful in aftershaves and eye treatment preparations, as well as in products for dry skin.

chamomile oil—considered a capillary wall constrictor, an anti-allergenic agent, and antiseptic, cooling, analgesic, emollient, and healing. It is considered useful for treating burns and skin inflammations as well as dermatitis, and beneficial for acne, dry, or supersensitive skins. The active principles are a pale blue volatile oil (which can turn yellow with time), a little anthemic acid, tannic acid, and a glucoside. The volatile oil, obtained through distillation, is lost in the preparation of the extract. The whole plant is odoriferous and of value, but the flower heads are primarily credited with therapeutic benefits. Because the chief botanical virtue of the plant lies in the central disk of the yellow florets and in the cultivated double form of the white florets, the botanical properties of the single, wild chamomile are considered to be the most powerful.

chamomile flower oil—*see* chamomile oil.

chaparral extract (*Larrea divaricata*)—attributed with anti-inflammatory, anti-oxidant, and anti-microbial properties, it can also be used for fragrance. This desert shrub, native to the southwestern United States, produces a sticky resin on its stems and leaves that provide natural UV protection for the plant. It is uncertain whether this translates to a skin benefit. Some sources, however, cite UV-protection capacities. It is used in products that treat acne, eczema, psoriasis, and contact dermatitis. Chaparral's primary constituent is nordihydroguaiaretic acid (NDGA), an anti-oxidant.

chaulmoogra oil (*Taraktogenos kurzii*)—a soothing and anti-inflammatory oil. It is considered by some to be healing, with good application in acne cases. It contains chaulmoogric acid and palmitic acid. Its fatty oil constituent has been found to yield glycerol, a very small quantity of phytosterol, and a mixture of fatty acids. Chaulmoogra oil can be irritating and can have an unpleasant odor. It is obtained from the seeds of *Taraktogenos kurzii*.

Chenopodium quinoa **flower/leaf extract**—a skin conditioning botanical obtained from the flowers and leaves of the quinoa plant. Nutritionally, quinoa is rich in protein, vitamins E and B, calcium, amino acids, and iron. It also contains phytosterols and flavonoids. Studies indicate that quinoa has water-retention capacities, and can act as a gelling agent, emulsifier, and foaming agent. Quinoa oil is noted for an omega-6 content as well.

chestnut extract (*Castanea sativa*)—because of its high tannin content, the extract from the bark is claimed to have an astringent effect when applied topically.

China clay—*see* kaolin.

Chinese angelica root—*see* angelica.

chios gum mastic clay—a trade name for mastic gum. *See* mastic gum.

chitin (chitine)—a moisture retainer and film-forming agent. This is a naturally occurring polysaccharide found in the shells of crustaceans, such as shrimp and crab, as well as in some fungi and algae. *See also* chitosan.

chitine—*see* chitin.

chitosan—a film-forming polysaccharide that can aid the skin's moisture content and moisture-retention capacity by preventing transepidermal water loss. In addition, it appears to help bind other ingredients (for example, to increase liposome stability), thereby increasing the availability of active ingredients to the skin. Anti-bacterial properties are also associated with chitosan, as well as an ability to enhance the microbiological stability of a preparation. Some studies show that it can help improve the water-resistance properties of sun protection creams and lotions, and the longevity of a fragrance's scent (the perfume adheres more strongly to the skin and evaporates more slowly, over a longer period). It acts as a skin conditioner, improving skin softness and suppleness. It may be found in moisturizers, sunscreens, and acne preparations, in addition to hair care products. It is the decarboxylated form of chitin and can hold water without creating a feeling of tackiness in a cosmetic preparation. According to some chitosan suppliers, the use of shrimp shells is one of the most important sources. They consist of 30–35 percent protein, 30–35 percent minerals, and 15–20 percent chitin, with some traces of lipids, dyes, and soluble proteins. *See also* chitin.

chitosan ascorbate—a synthetically produced ingredient that combines the film-forming and binding properties of chitosan with the anti-oxidant properties of ascorbic acid. It is manufactured by combining chitosan with ascorbic acid and sodium. *See also* chitosan and ascorbic acid.

chlorella vulgaris extract—an algae extract that helps protect and improve the condition of the skin. It is thought to have strong anti-oxidant properties. It may be used in skin care preparations to enhance skin smoothness and prevent collagen and elastin degradation. Certain studies also indicate an ability to increase skin firmness. Among its constituents are carotenoids, amino acids (including lysine, proline, glycine, and alanine), and vitamin B_{12}. It would likely be most beneficial in anti-aging and skin-protecting formulations. Manufacturers of this ingredient list it as appropriate for use in products designed to protect, restructure, firm, tone, and invigorate the skin, as well as in anti-wrinkle and anti-stretch mark preparations. It is extracted from the *chlorella vulgaris* algae. *See also* algae extract.

chlorhexidine—used as a topical antiseptic in liquid cosmetics. It is strongly alkaline and may cause irritation.

chlorhexidine digluconate—a preservative generally used in concentrations of 0.01 to 0.1 percent to protect against bacteria. It is unstable at high temperatures. Chlorhexidine digluconate is more widely used in Europe than in the United States. *See also* chlorhexidine.

chlorhexidine dihydrochloride—a preservative, it functions primarily as an anti-microbial, helping control the proliferation of bacteria, fungi, or yeast in a product.

5 chloro-2 methyl-4 isothiazolin 3 one and 2-methyl 4 5-hydroxy-2styryl-4-pyrones—a skin-lightening agent because of its ability to inhibit melanin formation. It is stable and non-irritating to the skin.

chlorophenesin—a preservative with fungistatic and bactericidal properties.

chlorophyll—used as a natural coloring agent. It is credited with skin-soothing and healing properties thanks to its phytol content, and has a mild deodorizing effect. Chlorophyll is the green coloring matter found in all living plants and seen in plant leaves.

chlorophyllin copper complex—a color additive obtained from chlorophyll. *See also* chlorophyll.

chloroxyethanol—a preservative with low sensitizing potential.

chloresteric esters—a cholesterol derivative. *See also* cholesterol.

cholesterol—a moisturizer and emollient that acts as a powerful emulsifier in water-in-oil systems. Cholesterol is a fat-like substance found in plant and animal cells. It is also present in the secretion of the sebaceous glands and, therefore, is a component of the fat on the skin's surface. It is considered a non-comedogenic raw material. It may sometimes be obtained from sheep's wool wax.

choleth 24—an emulsifying agent, considered a non-comedogenic raw material. It is often employed for its moisturizing action. It is a polyethylene glycol ether of cholesterol.

chondroitin sulfate—reported to increase water-binding properties when used with hydrolyzed protein and to enhance the moisturizing effects of creams and lotions. In the skin, chondroitin sulfate is a glycosaminoglycan component.

Chondrus crispus extract (brown seaweed)—*see* seaweed extract.

chromium compounds—these are oxides used primarily for green eye shadows and greenish mascaras. Chromium compounds may cause allergic reactions when applied to the skin.

chromium hydroxide green—a color additive used primarily in makeup preparations. *See also* chromium compounds.

chromium oxide green—a color additive used primarily in makeup preparations. *See also* chromium compounds.

cimicifuga racemosa root extract—*see* black cohosh extract.

cinchena—*see* cinchona extract.

cinchona extract (*Cinchona ledgeriana*) (**cinchena; quinquina**)—a major source of quinine. Cinchona extract has long been known for its tonic, antiseptic, and astringent properties. It also has been commonly used as a remedy for malaria and fever in tropical areas. It is obtained from the bark of various Latin American plant species belonging to the *Linnaean* genus. If used in large quantities, cinchona will cause headache and nausea in those allergic to it.

cinnamic acid—has sunscreen capabilities. Some manufacturers use it to replace PABA because of its lower allergic and phototoxic reaction incidence. Cinnamic acid is found in cinnamon leaves and cocoa leaves, and is an essential oil of certain mushrooms. It may cause allergic skin rashes.

cinnamon oil (*Cinnamomum zeylanicum*)—said to have a stimulating effect on the skin. It can also be used for fragrance. Widely recognized for its tonic and antiseptic properties, cinnamon oil is very important in traditional pharmacopoeia. Cinnamon oil is used in a wide variety of skin care and make-up preparations. It is obtained from distillation of the plant's leaves. It can cause irritation if used in high doses.

cinnamon bark oil—has similar properties to those of cinnamon oil, but this distillation of the plant's bark is considered of much higher quality than extractions from the plant's leaves. Use in high doses or in high concentrations could produce skin irritations. *See also* cinnamon oil.

cinnamon leaf oil—*see* cinnamon oil.

cinnamyl alcohol—naturally occurring in cinnamon bark, it can also be synthetically manufactured. It is used in cosmetics as a fragrance or flavoring agent.

cinoxate (2-hydroxy-p-methoxycinnamate)—an FDA-approved sunscreen chemical with an approved usage level of 1 to 3 percent. Studies indicate it causes photosensitivity.

cinquefoil extract (*Potentilla anserina*) (**five leaf grass; silverweed**)—an astringent ingredient with anti-inflammatory and healing properties. It can be valuable for problem skin. Cinquefoil is a creeping plant with large yellow flowers. The extract is obtained from the herb and root of the plant.

citral—a naturally occurring aroma compound used to provide a lemon-type fragrance. Citral is a constituent of lemon oil, lemongrass oil, lime oil, ginger oil, verbena oil, and other plant-derived essential oils.

citric acid—has astringent and anti-oxidant properties. It can also be used as a product stabilizer, pH adjuster, and preservative with a low sensitizing potential. It is not usually irritating to normal skin, but it can cause burning and redness when applied to chapped, cracked, or otherwise inflamed skin. It is derived from citrus fruits.

citric oils—refers to one or a combination of oils from citrus fruits such as orange oil, lemon oil, grapefruit oil, and the like.

citronella—used primarily as a fragrance (perfuming and masking), it also has tonic properties. It is derived from the essential oil of the *Cymbopogon nardus* plant, and its constituents include geraniol (approximately 60 percent), citronellal, camphene, limonene, linalool, and borneol.

citronella java oil—antiseptic and widely used in soaps and deodorizers. It may also have insect repellent properties. This herb distillation may cause a skin rash when used in cosmetics.

citronellol—a constituent of plant essential oils. Found abundantly in eucalyptus oil. It is used for masking odor or providing a fragrance component to a cosmetic product.

Citrus aurantium amara—also known as bitter orange. *See* bitter orange.

clary sage oil (*Salvia sclarea*)—could be beneficial in products designed for use around the eyes because of its soothing and anti-inflammatory properties. It is used to refresh the skin and can also mask odors. In addition, its fragrance may have aroma therapeutic value, such as promoting cell regeneration for normal, dry, and sensitive skin types.

clay—as a general ingredient category, it may include bentonite, beetum, and China clay. Most frequently used for its ability to absorb oil or water, it is also employed as a bulking, stabilizing, and viscosity-controlling agent. Clay can help clarify liquids, act as an emollient, and serve as a poultice. It is found as a color component in face powders, face masks, body powders, and makeup foundations. It does not cause skin allergies.

clay-earth—*see* clay.

clay sediments—*see* clay.

cleavers extract (*Galium aparine*)—said to be useful in treating eczema. Cleavers extract is recommended for normal to dry skins.

clematis—the extract from the plant's roots and stems has anti-inflammatory action. However, the leaves and flowers, when crushed, irritate the eyes and produce inflammation when applied directly to the skin. Clematis is a perennial plant.

climbing ivy extract—*see* ivy.

clove oil (*Eugenia caryophyllus, Caryophyllus aromaticus, Syzygium aromaticum*)—considered a powerful antiseptic and wound-healing agent with a strong germicidal effect. Clove oil is also indicated as a topical, local anesthetic. Depending on the part of the small evergreen tree from which the oil is derived (buds, flowers, leaves, or stems) it may also be tonic, astringent, improve skin texture and feel, and help mask odor. Eugenol is a key constituent of clove oil and is associated with many of its therapeutic benefits. This oil may cause strong skin irritation when used in high concentrations, although in diluted forms, it is generally harmless.

clove bud oil—has similar properties to clove oil, though it is most often used for its odor-masking properties. Distillates from dried buds are considered of higher quality than those obtained from the stems and leaves. Clove oil derived from the plant's leaves is sometimes used to adulterate the oil obtained from the bud.

clover extract (*Trifolium sp.*)—the fluid extract is used as an antispasmodic. A short-lived perennial plant, clover produces abundant blossoms that are used in herbal oils and extracts. Extract obtained from cloverleaf and clover root is considered antioxidant and able to improve the skin's general condition.

clover blossom extract—credited with astringent properties and an ability to mask odor. *See also* clover.

club moss extract (*Lycopodium clavatum*)—the spores of club moss have traditionally been used as an external dusting powder for various skin diseases and wounded surfaces. The tops of the plants are cut as the spikes approach maturity, and the powder is shaken out and separated with a sieve.

cocamide DEA—a thickener and viscosity builder for cosmetic surfactant systems. It is added to lauryl sulfate-based liquid cleansers to help stabilize the lather and improve foam formation.

cocamidopropylamine oxide—a cleansing agent that also acts as a surfactant, conditioner, viscosity builder, and foam booster. It is derived from coconut oil.

cocamidopropyl PG-dimonium chloride phosphate—an antimicrobial and anti-fungal that is very mild to the skin. *See also* coconut oil.

cocamidopropyl betaine—a surfactant derived from a coconut oil salt. It is particularly effective in shampoos, foam baths, shower foams, and other preparations where high, creamy foam and good skin tolerance are desired. *See also* coconut oil.

C

cocoa butter—softens and lubricates the skin. This yellowish vegetable fat is solid at room temperature but liquefies at temperatures between 90°–100°F (32.2°–37.8°C). Thus, it is frequently used in lip balms and massage creams because of its favorable melting point (i.e., close to body temperature). Cocoa butter is considered comedogenic and may cause allergic reactions.

coco-caprylate/caprate—a light and cosmetically elegant emollient obtained from vegetable sources.

cocoampho carboxyglycinate—used as a cleansing agent, skin softener, and lubricant, and commonly incorporated into soaps and creams. It is a solid fat from cocoa plant seeds.

cocoglucoside—a very mild cleansing agent, naturally derived from coconut oil and fruit sugar.

cocoglyceride—used for its emollient, emulsifying, and skin-conditioning properties. *See also* hydrogenated cocoglyceride.

coconut alcohol—a multi-function ingredient that may be incorporated into a cosmetic as an emollient, emulsifier, stabilizer, or surfactant, or to help control a product's viscosity. Its actual function in a product will depend on the specific formulation.

coconut oil—used as a cream base, it is a raw material for soaps, ointments, massage creams, and in sunscreen formulations. Soft white or slightly yellow in color and semisolid in consistency, coconut oil is a grouping of primarily short-chain fatty acids bonded with glycerine and expressed from coconut kernels. It is stable when exposed to air. Coconut oil may be irritating to the skin and cause skin rashes. It is also considered comedogenic.

cocoyl sarcosine—used as a cleansing agent. It can also serve as a surfactant.

codium tomentosum extract—hydrating and can help protect the skin against harmful external factors. It is cited as being beneficial for incorporation into a wide variety of cosmetics including moisturizers and skin-hydrating serums, body creams, anti-aging creams, and lip balms. *Codium tomentosum* is a green seaweed, and the extract contains polysaccharides. *See also* seaweed.

coenzyme Q10—*see* ubiquinone.

***Coffea arabica* fruit extract**—also known as CoffeeBerry˙ extract. It is a powerful, natural anti-oxidant with anti-aging and skin-lightening properties. The extract is obtained from the whole fruit, rather than from the seed or bean, as in the case of coffee seed oil.

coffee seed oil (*Coffea arabica*)—extracted from green coffee beans, it is rich in essential fatty acids including linoleic acid. It can also be used as a masking agent for odor. Depending on how the ingredient is used, coffee seed oil may also be beneficial for draining and slimming. The oil is obtained from the coffee seed/bean. *See also* caffeine.

***Coleus barbatus* extract** (**coleus**)—also known as *Coleus forskohlii.* A member of the mint family, it appears to have cleansing and soothing properties. In traditional medicine it was used to relieve scorpion bites, centipede stings, and more commonly, skin rashes. Among its natural constituents is forskolin. It grows wild in Nepal, India, and Thailand.

collagen—very popular in skin care formulations for its strong hydration potential and its ability to bind and retain many times its weight in water. This water-binding and retention ability makes collagen effective for use in skin moisturizers as a skin-protecting agent. It will not leave a feeling of tackiness or dryness on the skin, especially when used in hydrolyzed or soluble forms. As a film former, collagen aids in reducing natural moisture loss, thereby helping hydrate the skin. In skin care preparations, it enhances the humectancy of a topical product, contributes sheen, builds viscosity, and leaves the skin smooth and soft. It is not water soluble, and has been very popular in cosmetic formulations for more than 30 years. Collagen is rich in proline and hydroxyproline, and is considered a "commercially pure" protein. Originally

C

derived from animal connective tissue, which is similar to the collagen produced by the body in the skin and bones, today for cosmetic use it is either synthetically derived or bioengineered. Also considered an anti-irritant, collagen does not cause allergic reactions when used on the skin. It is very stable, bland in odor, and light in color. This is one of the most effective and economical proteins available to cosmetic formulators.

collagen amino acids—a mixture of amino acids resulting from the complete hydrolysis of collagen. It has a higher moisture-binding capacity than collagen alone, thereby improving the moisturizing efficacy of skin creams and lotions. Its moisture-binding capacity is because of the very large number of hydrophilic groups per unit weight. *See also* collagen.

collagen amino-polysiloxane hydrolyzate—*see* collagen.

collagen fiber—anti-irritant and hydrating. When used in particular sponge versions, it can serve as a delivery system for active ingredients. Its lack of solubility in water and other commonly used cosmetic ingredients has restricted its range of application.

collagen hydrolysates (hydrolyzed animal protein; hydrolyzed collagen)—collagen that has been processed to achieve a lower molecular weight than regular collagen. This can facilitate the use of collagen in cosmetic formulations and improve its properties. This is one of the most common forms of collagen used in cosmetic formulations. *See also* collagen.

collagen (soluble)—demonstrates enhanced moisture uptake and, therefore, is more effective than collagen. This is a clear liquid form of collagen preferred for use in cosmetics because, when incorporated into a formulation, it does not separate as regular collagen can. When incorporated into detergents, soluble collagen significantly reduces the amount of amino acids extracted from the skin when washing with the detergents and water. Soluble collagen is perhaps the most widely used and recognized high molecular-weight protein in skin care formulations. *See also* collagen.

colloidal oatmeal—an anti-itching skin protectant with soothing properties. Its lipid content gives it enhanced lubricity and emolliency. Colloidal oatmeal has consistently been recommended for use on infants, adults, and the aged in bath, lotion, and poultice preparations designed for topical application on damaged skin. The addition of colloidal oatmeal into bath water diminishes inflammation and irritation that frequently occur in eczema cases when bathing with soap alone. It is used in cleansing creams, soaps, and bath products. *See also* oat.

colloidal silver—used as a preservative. *See also* silver.

colloidal sulfur—*see* sulfur.

colostrum—a naturally occurring substance, colostrum is a fluid secreted by the mammary glands just after giving birth. When combined with elastin, it leaves a colloidal film that mimics natural elastin.

coltsfoot extract (*Tussilago farfara*)—has astringent, emollient, conditioning, and moisturizing properties. Studies indicate a possible skin-lightening effect. Coltsfoot extract contains a high concentration of mucilage, making it useful for soothing delicate and/or easily inflamed skin. The leaves are the primary plant part used, but the flower stems are also utilized. Cystine is among its noted constituents.

comfrey extract (*Symphytum officinale*)—is credited with healing, astringent, and emollient properties. It is used in cases of swelling and bruising, cuts, papules, and pustules. Comfrey extract was traditionally used topically for soothing and anti-itching treatment, as well as for eczema and sunburns. The whole plant is considered excellent for soothing pain in any tender, inflamed, or suppurating part. Comfrey root's chief constituent is mucilage. It also contains 0.6 to 0.8 percent of allantoin and a bit of tannin. Some say that certain alkaloids found in comfrey are toxic. The roots and leaves are generally collected from wild plants.

coneflower extract (*Echinacea angustifolia*)—*see* echinacea.

copper—copper-based ingredients are often used as coloring agents in cosmetics. Copper itself is nontoxic, but soluble copper salts, notably copper sulfite, are skin irritants. In the body, copper combines with certain proteins to produce a variety of enzymes, which in turn serve as catalysts for different functions. For example, copper plays a role in the keratinization process. In normal skin, this catalytic action is completed in 8 to 12 hours, however more than three days may be required in cases of copper deficiency. Through such enzymatic activity, copper is involved in melanin production, as decreased pigmentation has been observed in cases of copper deficiency. Such enzyme-based action also links copper to maintaining and repairing the skin's connective tissues (collagen and elastin), as well as to wound healing.

copper aspartate—has occlusive and skin-conditioning properties, and may be able to protect the skin from damaging external agents. It is the copper salt of aspartic acid. *See also* copper.

copper chlorophyll—used to provide color to a cosmetic product. It is a synthetic ingredient.

copper gluconate—cited as having skin-conditioning and skin-protecting functions. *See also* copper.

copra oil—*see* coconut oil.

Corallina officinalis—in powder form it is can be used to control product viscosity and as a binder. *Corallina officinalis* extract can help improve the overall skin condition. This is a variety of red algae. *See also* algae extract and seaweed.

cordyceps sinensis extract—emollient, humectant, and skin conditioning. Clinical studies indicate potential anti-oxidant and anti-aging effects. The extract is obtained from the *cordyceps sinensis* fungus.

coriander oil (*Coriandrum sativum*)—used in the appropriate mixture and dosage, it can work with other natural oils and extracts as a preservative. It also serves as a deodorant. Coriander oil is produced from the distillation of the fruit (the so-called seeds), which contains about 1 percent of volatile oil, the active constituent. The fruit also contains malic acid. Coriander oil can cause allergic reactions.

corn cob meal—used in face and bath powders. It is made from the ear of Indian corn.

corn germ oil—a skin softener derived from the germ of the seed of the corn plant.

corn meal—used as a thickening agent. It is a coarse corn flour prepared by milling the corn kernel. *See also* corn starch.

corn oil—used as a carrier oil, it has average emollient properties. Although not particularly prone to cause allergies, it is also not widely used in cosmetic formulations. It is considered somewhat comedogenic. Corn oil is obtained from the wet milling of corn.

corn seed extract—found in creams, lotions, and revitalizing ampules. *See also* corn seed fraction.

corn seed fraction—credited with increasing skin metabolism. It is rich in amino acids, sugar, vitamin B, and phytates. It can be used in creams, lotions, and post-sun preparations.

corn starch—used as a thickener in cosmetics and in face powders. Corn starch absorbs water and is soothing to the skin. It can cause allergic reactions such as inflamed eyes, stuffy nose, and perennial hay fever. A natural material obtained from corn kernels.

cornflower extract (*Centaurea cyanus*)—used in folklore as a tonic and stimulant with action similar to that of blessed thistle. A type of water distilled from cornflower petals was formerly thought of as a remedy for weak eyes. Cornflower extract has been used in Europe since ancient times to treat bites. It is considered beneficial for normal skin and skin care products designed for use around the eyes. Healing properties, particularly in cases

C

of bruises, are attributed to cornflower extract obtained from the plant leaves. Important constituents include gentiopricrin, erythrocentaurine, nicotinic acid compounds, essential oil, and oleanolic acid.

cornflower water—*see* cornflower extract.

Corylus avellana **seed oil**—*see* hazelnut oil.

cotton seed oil (hydrogenated)—a carrier. This oil is used in the manufacture of soaps, creams, and baby creams. Although it is known to cause allergies and be mildly irritating, it is widely used in cosmetics. It is considered somewhat comedogenic. Expressed from various species of cotton.

cotton thistle extract (*Onopordum acanthium*)—may aid in protecting the skin against damage because of environmental aggression. Some studies indicate an ability to help repair the epidermis, stimulate skin repair, stabilize and regulate skin hydration, and enhance the skin's natural barrier function. It can be found in a variety of cosmetic products including moisturizers and anti-aging preparations. Product manufacturers also indicate use for treating sunburned skin and skin that has undergone dermatological treatments such as peels and dermabrasion.

coumarin—considered a blood thinner, it can also increase blood flow. Some sources cite anti-oxidant capacities, as well. It is a specific plant constituent and is what creates the fragrance of freshly mowed hay. Coumarin is found in such plants as cherries, lavender, licorice, and sweet clover.

crambe abyssinica seed oil—a non-greasy emollient, it improves skin feel and moisturization. It is a member of the mustard family.

cranberry seed oil (*Vaccinium macrocarpon*)—plays a role in skin moisturization by helping protect the skin's lipid barrier. It is also nourishing, and said to help promote the absorption of fatty acids by the skin. Its constituents include vitamins A and E, omegas-3, -6, and -9, and phospholipids and phytosterols. Its application includes use in cosmetic creams or lotions for dry, dehydrated, and aging skin.

crane's bill extract (*Geranium maculatum*)—credited with astringent and tonic properties. Constituents include gallic and tannic acids. The leaves and roots are the parts used.

cream—emollient and skin conditioning. Cream contains lecithin, sterols, and oils, plus 18 to 40 percent butterfat. It is the yellowish part of cow's milk.

cresin—*see* ozokerite.

cryolidone—a PCA derivative. Cryolidone increases resistance to heat following UV radiation. As it provides a cooling effect on the skin, it is suggested as an ingredient for post-sun and aftershave products.

cucumber extract (*Cucumis sativus*)—credited with moisture-binding, moisture-regulating, soothing, tightening, anti-itching, refreshing, softening, healing, and anti-inflammatory properties. This extract can be used in aftershave preparations, eye treatment products, and treatments for oily skin. It is also effective in emulsions as a tightening agent for tired, stressed skin, and in sun preparations as a refresher. It contains amino acids and organic acids that are claimed to strengthen the skin's acid mantle. Other important constituents include minerals and mucins. The fruit is the part of the plant used.

Cucumis melo—the Latin name for melon, including honeydew, cantaloupe, and sugar melon. The fruit, root, or seed extracts—as well as the juice and water of melon—are all known to maintain the skin in good condition. Melon water is also humectant, while melon juice is considered to have soothing properties. Among the constituents of melon are vitamins A and C, pectin, flavonoids, volatile oils, and fructose (a sugar). Cantaloupe is specifically noted for having astringent properties.

cupuaçu seed butter (*Theobroma grandiflorum*)—also known as cupuassu seed butter. Emollient and moisturizing, it also improves skin softness. Cupuaçu butter contains phytosterols, and appears able to regulate the balance and activity of stratum corneum lipids. It is also reported to have a high water-absorption capacity, making it particularly beneficial for dry skin. The butter is extracted from the seeds of the Cupuaçu tree, native to Brazil.

curcumin—*see* turmeric.

cyclohexasiloxane—a silicone-based emollient.

cyclomethicone—provides a silky, smooth feel to skin care products, and is considered a non-comedogenic emollient. This is a form of silicone that can deliver active ingredients and also serve as a vehicle for delivering fragrance.

cyclopentasiloxane—incorporated into a formulation for its emollient and solvent activity.

cyclotetrasiloxane—a silicone-based emollient. *See also* cyclomethicone.

cymbopogon nardus—*see* citronella.

O-cymen 5-OL—a bactericide used in hand and body preparations. It is a phenol derivative.

C

cypress extract (*Cupressus sp.*)—an extract derived from the leaves and twigs of the cypress tree. *See also* cypress oil.

cypress oil—said to have antiseptic, astringent, healing, soothing, and anti-spasmodic properties. Cypress oil is also claimed to be useful in treating acne and in inhibiting oil gland secretion. It can also be used as a fragrance. This oil, which can range from clear to yellow to brown, is generally obtained from a distillation of cypress cones.

cysteic acid—an amino acid that is used in skin care cosmetics as a skin conditioner.

cysteine—an essential amino acid obtained by fermentation. Cysteine is a component of the skin's natural moisturizing factor and can help normalize oil gland secretion because of its sulfur content. It is also said to promote wound healing. In addition, studies indicate that cysteine helps increase levels of glutathione (an anti-oxidant) in the body. It is considered beneficial in treating oily skin.

C

D

D&C colors—refer to color entry in Chapter 4 of Part 1.

D-alpha-tocopherol—*see* vitamin E.

daisy extract (*Bellis perennis*)—said to be tonic, astringent, and skin conditioning. Daisy was a component in a popular fourteenth-century wound ointment. This application continued through the centuries, using daisy alone or in combination with oxeye daisy. The flowers and leaves are found to have a certain amount of oil and ammoniacal salts.

damiana leaves extract (*Turnera aphrodisiaca*)—the cosmetic properties of this spicy, aromatic extract are not clear, but they could be tonic, astringent, and potentially anti-spasmodic. The leaves, which are the part used, produce a greenish volatile oil that smells like chamomile, and damianin, an amorphous bitter principle, resins, and tannin. Among damiana's constituents are flavonoids, phenolic glucosides, and phytosterols.

dandelion extract (*Taraxacum officinale*)—has tonic properties, refreshes the skin, and corrects pH balance. It apparently also aids in increasing the respiratory capacity of skin tissue. Dandelion extract is said to be beneficial for dry skin and can also be found in acne preparations. The plant root, rather than the flower, is used in cosmetic preparations as the juice of the root is the more powerful part of the plant. The main constituents of dandelion root are taraxacin, a crystalline, bitter substance; and taraxacerin, an acrid resin. Other constituents include inulin, gluten gum, potash, citric acid, sterols, and vitamins B and C. Dandelion is used in many patented medicines.

DEA (diethanolamine)—an organic alkali used in formulations to neutralize organic acids and thus adjust pH. It is usually listed on ingredient labels preceding the compound that it is neutralizing. Oleth-3 phosphate, for example, is a powerful emulsifier, but it is very acidic when it is made, so manufacturers use DEA to neutralize it and improve the nature of a formulation.

DEA cetyl phosphate—an emulsifying agent that gives a rich, velvety feel to a product. It can be used as a primary or secondary emulsifier, depending on the concentration. This is the diethanolamine salt of cetyl phosphate.

DEA dihydroxypalmityl phosphate—an emulsifier.

DEA oleth-3 phosphate—an emulsifier. This is the diethanolamine salt of a complex mixture of phosphoric acid esters and oleth-3.

DEA oleth-10 phosphate—an emulsifying agent used primarily in moisturizing preparations. This is the diethanolamine salt of a complex mixture of phosphoric acid esters and oleth-10.

DEA ρ-methoxycinnamate (octocrylene)—a chemical UV absorber that exhibits excellent UV absorption and has an approved usage level of 8 to 10 percent. Because of its water solubility, it is not generally used in waterproof formulations. Octocrylene is the INCI and over-the-counter drug name for this sunscreen chemical.

decarboxycarnosine HCL—a skin conditioning and anti-static agent. It can be found in such cosmetic preparations as eye lotions, moisturizers, and night creams.

decene/butene copolymer—used to control product viscosity.

decyl alcohol—can be used for any number of functions, including as an emollient, a foam-booster, a surfactant and a viscosity controller, as well to mask odor and as a fixative in perfumes. Decyl alcohol occurs naturally in sweet orange and ambrette seed. It is also derived commercially from liquid paraffin.

decylglucoside—a mild, foaming cleansing agent.

decyloleate—an emollient with good penetrating properties that helps improve product spreadability and provides a formulation with good feel on the skin. It is a component of the sebum of human skin. For use in cosmetics, it is obtained from olive oil or produced synthetically. It is also produced synthetically and from olive oil.

decylpolyglucose—a non-ionic surfactant with good foaming properties. It is extremely mild to the eyes and skin. It can be obtained from naturally derived raw materials from renewable sources, though this depends on the supplier.

dehydroacetic acid—a preservative with low sensitizing potential. This is a weak acid used as a fungi- and bacteria-destroying agent in cosmetics. The presence of organic matter decreases its effectiveness. It is not irritating or allergy causing when applied on the skin.

deoxyribonucleic acid—*see* DNA.

dermasomes—liposomal preparations containing cosmetic ingredients (usually actives) entrapped within lipid spheres. Dermasomes provide increased penetration and absorption, improved product efficiency at lower usage levels, and targeted and time-released delivery.

devil's claw (*Harpagophytum procumbens*)—said to have anti-bacterial, anti-inflammatory, and moisture-binding capabilities. The plant's root contains mucilage.

dextran—a polysaccharide with water-binding properties. It is also used to control product viscosity. Some studies indicate a capacity to enhance the anti-aging activity of formulations containing weak acids, as well as to reduce possible skin irritation arising from such acids.

dextran sulfate—clinical studies indicate a possible capacity to reduce edema. It is cited as a binder and skin conditioner.

dextrin (**British gum; starch gum**)—absorbs moisture. It is also used as a binder to control product viscosity and reduce the density of a cosmetic. This powder is produced from corn starch and modified by means of a bacterial process. It may cause an allergic reaction.

dextrose—*see* glucose.

d-glucono-1,5-lactone—the chemical name for gluconolactone. *See* gluconolactone.

DHA—*see* dihydroxyacetone.

DHPH—*see* dipalmitoyl hydroxyproline.

diatomaceous earth—in purified form, it is used for powders and as an abrasive agent in peeling formulations. If improperly formulated, it may be too abrasive as a peeling agent. Diatomaceous earth is a fine-grain, almost white powder consisting mostly of amorphous silicic that is obtained by crushing the silicic acid structures of mono-cellular sea algae.

diazolidinyl urea—an antiseptic and deodorizer. It is also a broad-spectrum preservative against bacteria and fungi. Generally, it is used in concentrations of 0.03 to 0.3 percent. It has been found that diazolidinyl urea is a stronger sensitizer than imidazolidinyl urea for people sensitive or allergic to formaldehyde.

dibehenyl fumarate—a wax with thickening and film-forming properties that is used as a coemulsifier.

di-C$_{12-15}$ alkyl fumarate—an emollient.

dicaprylyl ether—a skin-conditioning agent.

dicaprylyl maleate—a derivative of malic acid, with emollient and skin-conditioning properties. It can also be used as a solvent in cosmetic preparations. It is synthetically manufactured.

dicetyldilinoleate—a non-irritating emollient that provides slip, emollience, and a smooth, satiny feel to a cosmetic preparation. It leaves the skin feeling soft, supple, and without greasiness.

D

It is claimed that dicetyldilinoleate helps normalize the epidermal lipid structure and promotes the formation of soft, flexible, and healthy looking skin. It may also act as a vehicle for the delivery of active topical substances. This ingredient can be effectively incorporated into creams, lotions, skin oils, and makeup bases that contain sunscreens. Dicetyldilinoleate can be used as a replacement for partially hydrogenated animal and vegetable tallows, cocoa butter, and isopropyl lanolate. It is based on omega-6 linoleic acid, a naturally occurring vegetable derivative.

dicetyldimonium chloride—an ammonium salt that can be used in a cosmetic formulation for its anti-static, emulsifying, surfactant and hair-conditioning properties.

dicetyl phosphate—used in cosmetic preparations as an emulsifier and surfactant.

dichlorobenzyl alcohol—a preservative and antimicrobial, particularly effective in protecting against yeasts and molds.

diethanolamine—*see* DEA.

diethanolamine p-methoxycinnamate—*see* DEA p-methoxycinnamate.

diethylamino hydroxybenzoyl hexyl benzoate—a UV filter that helps protect against UVA and demonstrates good photostability.

diethyllauramide—*see* lauramide DEA.

diethylene glycol monoethylene ether—*see* ethoxydiglycol.

diethylhexyl butamido triazone—a sunscreen chemical that acts as a UV filter and absorber.

digalloyl trioleate—an FDA-approved sunscreen chemical with an approved usage level of 2 to 5 percent. A chemical UVB absorber, digalloyl trioleate, is no longer available as it apparently exhibits a poor UV absorption profile.

diglycerin—can increase the water content in the top layers of the skin. Formulators may select this ingredient for its humectant properties, and also when needing a skin-conditioning agent or a solvent. It is synthetically manufactured.

dihydroxyacetone (DHA)—a self-tanning agent used in cosmetics designed to provide a tanned appearance without the need for sun exposure. It is also a UV protector and a color additive. As a self-tanning agent, it reacts with amino acids found on the skin's epidermal layer. Its effects last only a few days as the color it provides fades with the natural shedding of the stained cells. Reportedly, it works best on slightly acidic skin. DHA, when combined with lawsone, becomes an FDA Category I (approved) UV protectant. In 1973, the FDA declared that DHA is safe and suitable for use in cosmetics or drugs that are applied to color the skin, and has exempted it from color additive certification.

2-dihydroxyethyl-2-hydroxy-6,10,14-trimethylpentadecane—facilitates the penetration of vitamin E into the skin. It has also demonstrated free-radical scavenging abilities and can function as a blocker of UV rays.

diisoarachidyl dilinoleate—a liquid wax emollient that provides good product spreadability. It may replace mineral oil in skin care preparations.

diisoarachidyl dodecanedioate—an emollient. This liquid wax provides a feel similar to heavy mineral oil but without the associated greasiness and oiliness. It may, therefore, be used as a partial or total replacement for mineral oil in formulations where improved tactile properties are sought. Diisoarachidyl dodecanedioate leaves a protective, though not completely occlusive, film on the skin. Its qualities suggest use in special cleansing preparations; rich, soft creams; and sunscreens. It is considered a potentially excellent vehicle for the delivery of active topical substances. It is non-irritating in skin and eye tests.

diisocetyl dodecanedioate—an emollient that enhances skin feel and texture. It also may be incorporated into a cosmetic preparation as an emulsifier or surfactant.

diisopropyl adipate—a low-viscosity emollient. It increases a preparation's spreadability.

diisopropyl dimerate—a chemical modifier that lowers the irritation potential of ingredients incorporated into a formulation.

diisopropyl sebacate—can be used in cosmetic formulations for its emollient properties. It is also used as a solvent, particularly for fragrances.

diisostearyl dimer dilinoleate—an occlusive skin-conditioning agent primarily used in makeup and hand and body preparations.

diisostearyl malate—a film former and a secondary emollient used mostly in makeup or other formulations involving suspensions.

dimethicone—a form of silicone used to give products lubricity, slip, and good feel. It can also serve as a formulation defoamer and help reduce the feeling of greasiness that some creams leave on the skin immediately upon application. In addition, dimethicone is reported to protect the skin against moisture loss when used in larger quantities. It improves product flow and spreadability. In combination with other ingredients, dimethicone becomes a good waterproofing material for sunscreen emulsions, and helps reduce the greasiness often seen in high-SPF preparations.

dimethicone copolyol—provides soft feel and helps reduce irritation caused by soap. It is used to improve the skin feel of some sunscreen preparations. It is a modified form of dimethicone. *See also* dimethicone.

dimethicone copolyol isostearate—acts as a skin softener and gives a formulation high lubricity. *See also* dimethicone.

dimethicone copolyol phosphate—an emulsifier.

dimethicone copolyol polyacrylate—a water-resistant emulsifier with film-forming properties.

dimethicone/PEG-10/15 crosspolymer—incorporated into a cosmetic product for its film-forming capacities. It can also help reduce a formulation's transparency. Formulators may select this ingredient as an emulsion stabilizer or to increase emulsion viscosity.

dimethicone crosspolymer—used to increase a formulation's viscosity, or to stabilize an emulsion. It can also help disperse solid ingredients in a liquid.

dimethicone/vinyl dimethicone crosspolymer—a thickener that can absorb skin oils, leaving a dry, silky feel.

dimethiconol esters—fatty wax that liquefies when rubbed on the skin. *See also* dimethicone.

dimethiconol hydroxystearate—an oil-phase compound with non-occlusive hydrophobic film formation on skin. *See also* dimethicone.

D

dimethiconol stearate—a non-occlusive hydrophobic waterproofing base used in sunscreens and other skin care applications. *See also* dimethicone.

dimethyl MEA (DMAE)—also known as dimethylaminoethanol. Studies indicate skin-firming properties, and an ability to reduce the appearance of fine lines and wrinkles as well as dark circles under the eyes. It is considered anti-aging, and anti-inflammatory, and has exhibited free-radical scavenging activity.

dimethyl isosorbide—a carrier, solvent, and viscosity controller. Its particular skin-penetrating ability opens the possibility of enhancing active substance efficacy in optical products. Its physical characteristics and solubility properties are superior to those of propylene glycol, glycerin, or ethyl alcohol.

dimethyl oxazolidine—improves the activity of a formulation's preservative. It is non-toxic at approved cosmetic-use levels.

dimethyl siloxane—*see* dimethicone.

dimethyl aminoethanol—*see* dimethyl MEA.

dimethylisosorbide—*see* dimethyl isosorbide.

dimethylsilanol hyaluronate—has very strong skin-hydrating activity. It appears to provide regenerating, restructuring, and repairing action for tissue supplement and, therefore, is said to improve skin elasticity and firmness. It is incorporated into anti-aging products and those for skin maintenance such as night, sun, and protective creams.

di-n-octyl carbonate—functions as a solvent and can be used to facilitate solubility and spreadability of such sunscreen components as benzophenone-3 and methylbenzylidene camphor. It is also used as a dispersing agent.

dioctyladipate—an emollient. It allows transepidermal respiration through occlusive-type films. It has a very low irritancy level.

dioctyl malate—a light film former and emollient used in skin care formulations.

dioctyl maleate—a film former and emollient derived from maleic acid.

dioctylcyclohexane—an emollient used as a squalene substitute.

dioctyl sodium sulfosuccinate—a mild surfactant used as a cleansing agent.

dioxybenzone—*see* benzophenone-8.

dipalmitoyl hydroxyproline (DPHP)—an anti-aging ingredient with moisturizing properties, it is said to enhance skin firmness, protect elastin fibers, and act as a carrier of hydroxyproline through the skin. It is a vegetal derivative. *See also* hydroxyproline.

D

dipeptide-2—primarily used as a skin conditioner to improve the look and feel of dry skin. It is also thought to help improve lymphatic drainage. It is considered to be a natural moisturizing factor, able to promote skin healing and maintain epidermal integrity. Given these characteristics, it is used in anti-aging products as well as in eye creams said to help reduce puffiness and the appearance of dark circles. This is a peptide based on the amino-acids valine and tryptophan.

dipotassium phosphate—used as a buffering agent to control the degree of acidity in solutions.

di-PPG myristyl ether adipate—an emollient that can also provide better delivery of active ingredients to the skin. Its film-forming capabilities help it enhance the skin's ability to retain active ingredients. In addition, it can disperse physical sunscreens such as titanium dioxide and zinc oxide. It also provides excellent skin-softening action.

diphenylsiloxy phenyltrimethicone—reduces a product's tendency to foam. It can also be used to improve the overall condition of skin and hair.

dipotassium glycyrrhizinate—a liquorice derivative that helps reduce skin redness and inflammation, thanks to its anti-irritant, calming, and soothing properties. It can be incorporated successfully into sensitive skin products, while also appearing to help improve oily skin.

dipropylene glycol—may be incorporated into a cosmetic for a variety of purposes including to mask odors or to perfume a product. In addition, it can help decrease product viscosity and serves as a solvent for essential oils and fragrance oils.

dipropylene glycol monomethyl ether—*see* PPG 2 methyl ether acetate.

disodiumcocoyl glutamate—a cleansing agent, it will most often be found in skin cleansing products, soaps, and shampoos.

disodium EDTA—a preservative used in concentrations of 0.1 to 0.5 percent.

disodium laureth sulfosuccinate—a very mild surfactant, appropriate for baby and child care products. It reduces the irritation properties of high-foaming surfactants when used in the same product formulation.

disodium lauriminodipropionate—a surfactant with cleansing and foaming properties.

disodium lauroamphodiacetate—an anti-static agent and foam-boosting. Formulators may incorporate it into a product for its cleansing and hair conditioning action. In addition, disodium lauroamphodiacetate can help control product viscosity and serve as a surfactant that enhances the water solubility of other surfactants in a product.

disodium lauryl sulfosuccinate—similar in activity to disodium lauroamphodiacetate, it helps boost foam, and acts as a surfactant while helping enhance the water solubility of other surfactants in a product. In addition, it is a cleansing agent, with degreasing and skin-conditioning properties. It is reported to be mild, with low irritation potential, and would most often be found in cleansing products for skin or hair.

disodium mono-oleamido MIPA sulfosuccinanate—*see* dioctyl sodium, sulfosuccinate.

disodium phosphate—a hydroscopic inorganic salt, it absorbs moisture that is then released to the skin. In dry climatic conditions, however, it may draw moisture from the skin and release it to the air, aggravating dryness. Without water, disodium phosphate may cause slight irritation. It can also be used in a cosmetic as a fragrance, and to adjust pH or keep pH stable. Finally, it can be selected to reduce corrosion of metallic materials used for product packaging.

DL-alpha-tocopherol—*see* vitamin E.

DMDM hydantoin—a popular preservative with moderate sensitizing potential, it is used to control against mold, mildew, and bacterial spoilage. This preservative is similar to imidazolidinyl urea, as both act by releasing formaldehyde into the formulation. Cosmetic expert panels have determined that DMDM hydantoin has an excellent safety record for use in both leave-on and wash-off cosmetic preparations. Maximum-use concentrations are set at 0.2 percent in the U.S. and 0.6 percent in the European Union. DMDM stands for dimethylimidazolidine, though in a listing the acronym is rarely spelled out.

DNA (freeze-dried) (pure biological) (pure vegetal) (deoxyribonucleic acid)—a surface film-forming protein with moisturizing action. DNA's large macromolecules do not enable it to penetrate the skin. In addition, its affinity with the stratum corneum layer keeps it anchored to the skin's surface, where it serves to protect and retain skin moisture. Although the use of DNA was particularly popular in the 1980s, its incorporation into cosmetic products since then has practically disappeared. It is usually used in a potassium salt form obtained from fish sperm.

drometrizole trisiloxane—a UV absorber/UV filter, it provides UVB- and some UVA-spectrum protection.

echinacea (*Echinacea angustifolia*)—also known as coneflower. Echinacea is well known for its ability to boost the body's immune system. It is described as having antiseptic and anti-bacterial properties rendering it helpful in treating skin lesions and in shortening skin healing time. It also has anti-itching, soothing, and moisturizing properties when used in skin care products. It is commonly used in acne preparations. The main constituents of both the oil and the resin, derived from the wood or bark of the plant are inulin, inuloid, sucrose, betaine, phytosterols, and fatty acids such as oleic, cerotic, lizolic, and palmitic.

ECM—*see* extra cellular matrix.

EDTA—helps boost a formulation's preservative system and is also a chelating agent.

egg lecithin—emollient and particularly recommended for sensitive skin. *See also* egg protein; egg yolk extract.

egg oil—recommended for sensitive skins. It is extracted from the egg yolk using vegetable oil. *See also* egg protein; egg yolk extract.

egg protein—creates a film, thereby acting as a moisture-retention agent allowing the skin to build up a supply of water. This moisturizing process tightens and softens the skin only temporarily as the skin cannot utilize the protein contained in an egg. Egg protein is primarily used in facial masks. It may cause skin rashes and other reactions in those with an allergy to eggs.

egg extract—a protein. Egg white provides emollient, humectant, and skin-conditioning properties. Egg yolk has emulsifying capabilities and may be used in products for sensitive skin. It contains lecithin sterols and vitamin A. Egg extract provides a temporary tightening effect on the skin. *See also* egg protein.

egg powder—used in many cosmetics to produce a temporary tightening effect on the skin. It is found in a variety of products including face masks, creams, and bath preparations. *See also* egg extract.

Egyptian rose extract—*see* rose extract.

eicosapentaenoic acid—also known as EPA. With emollient and skin-conditioning properties, this omega-3 fatty acid helps repair and maintain the skin barrier functions. It is said to improve the structure and function of the skin cell membrane. In addition, it may also have anti-irritant and anti-inflammatory properties.

elastin—a surface protective agent used in cosmetics to alleviate the effects of dry skin, enhance skin flexibility, improve skin feel, increase and improve the tension of the skin, and influence the formation of tropocollagen fibers when used in combination with soluble collagen. Preparations containing elastin and peptides derived from it are reported to promote wound healing. Reportedly, in such systems, elastin can absorb lipids from the skin, and when applied to scars, increase the structural glycoproteins and elastin available in the scar tissue. Elastin is an elastic structural protein found in the dermis together with collagen, and is difficult to obtain in pure form. Collagen and elastin are similar, although elastin has a different amino acid composition and is found in lower concentrations. Its molecular size is also much smaller than collagen's, and as a result, there is a tendency to believe that it penetrates the surface epidermal layers, thereby improving overall skin appearance, softness, and suppleness. Elastin is often used in moisturizing products and those products for aging or mature skin.

elastin (hydrolyzed)—a modified form of elastin that has better solubility, and thus is more convenient for use in cosmetic formulations than regular elastin. *See also* elastin.

elastin hydrolysates—moisturizing and able to promote water retention in the skin. *See also* elastin (hydrolyzed).

elastin polypeptides—an elastin derivative that can be used as an active ingredient carried by liposomes.

elder extract (*Sambucus sp.*)—also known as elderberry. It is a botanical that is credited with astringent, antiseptic, and emollient properties. It is useful to treat problem or inflamed skin. Ointments made of elder leaves have been domestic remedies for bruises, swelling, and wounds. Elder leaves are also an ingredient in many cooling ointments. The bark, leaves, flowers, and berries have all been used botanically, though use of the bark is now considered obsolete. Manufacturers report that presently the flower is the preferred segment of the plant.

elder flower extract—mildly astringent and a gentle stimulant. It is principally used as a vehicle for eye and skin lotions. It is reported to be particularly beneficial in treatment of dry skin. In the nineteenth century, elder flower water was commonly used to clear the complexion of freckles and sunburn and to keep the skin in good condition. The most important constituent of elder

E

flower is a trace of semisolid volatile oil, present in a very low percentage, which possesses the scent of the flower in a high degree. *See also* elder extract.

elecampane (*Inula helenium*) (**horseheal; scabwort**)—its herbal properties for topical use are described as astringent and antiseptic. In the past, it was used for treating skin problems in people and animals. Its common name, scabwort, comes from the belief that it cured sheep affected with the scab. It gets its other name, horseheal, from its reputed virtues in curing skin diseases suffered by horses. Elecampane's therapeutic value is attributed to its abundant content of inulin, a polysaccharide found in plants. It can also be used to mask odor. The extract used for therapeutic purposes is preferably obtained from the root of a two- to three-year-old plant. When the plant is older, the root becomes too woody for extraction.

elm bark (*Ulmus sp.*)—credited with astringent, healing, and soothing properties that can benefit surface skin problems.

elm extract—described as a problem skin extract given its healing and reputed cicatrizant properties. Extracts from elm leaves have been recommended by herbologists to wash wounds, bruises, and sore eyes.

emulsifying wax—an emulsifier and thickening agent used to thicken a formulation. Unlike some waxes (for example, beeswax), this is not a true wax. It is a chemical mixture of emulsifiers and fatty alcohols that permits the formulation of stable creams.

emulsifying wax NF—this is the same as emulsifying wax and is considered a non-comedogenic raw material. NF is the abbreviation for a reference called National Formulary. It denotes quality compliance with the pharmaceutical monogram.

English daisy extract—said to reduce swelling. *See also* daisy extract.

English oak extract—*see* oak bark extract.

ensulizole—one of the chemical names for phenylbenzimidazole sulfonic acid. Used as a sunscreen ingredient and also to protect a product from deterioration caused by UV light. *See also* phenylbenzimidazole sulfonic acid.

enzymes—*see* enzyme entry in Chapter 4.

epidermal lipid extract—an example of a vague ingredient description found on some product labels. Literally, this would be an oil or fat extracted from the epidermis. It is not specific enough to allow one to determine if it refers to lipids that blend with those in the human skin or if lipids extracted from animal epidermis are being used.

Epilobium angustifolium **extract**—a botanical with potential anti-microbial and anti-irritant properties. This is a member of the evening primrose family and is commonly known as willowherb or fireweed.

ergocalciferol—also known as vitamin D2. *See also* vitamin D.

erythrityl triethylhexanoate—can be incorporated into a skin care formula for a variety of purposes, including as an emollient and a solvent. It can also maintain the skin in good condition.

erythrulose—used in self-tanning formulations to promote a tanned color. This is a natural ketosugar, commonly found in raspberries, and is said to give best results when used in combination with DHA. It works through a chemical reaction with amino acids found in the skin's keratin. It is considered non-toxic and is found in self-tanning creams and lotions as well as bronzers.

escin—a saponin occurring in the seed of the horse chestnut tree. *See also* horse chestnut extract.

esculin—used as a skin protectant in ointments and creams. This is a glucoside compound originally obtained from the leaves and bark of the horse chestnut tree. *See also* horse chestnut extract.

esculoside—utilized in formulations for the treatment of cellulite. Esculoside is apparently beneficial for impaired microcirculation.

ethanol—*see* ethyl alcohol.

ethanol acetamide—*see* acetamide MEA.

ethoxydiglycol—a solvent for essential oils, fragrance materials, and terpene oils. It is used often in nail enamels but can also be incorporated into skin care products as a humectant. Ethoxydiglycol is non-irritating, non-penetrating, and non-comedogenic when applied to the skin.

ethoxydiglycol behenate—used to enhance a product's final consistency and creaminess.

ethoxydiglycol oleate—an emollient.

ethoxyethanol—*see* ethylene glycol monomethyl ether.

ethoxylated plant sterols—*see* plant sterols.

ethyl alcohol—also known as ethanol, and commonly known as rubbing alcohol. Ethyl alcohol is ordinary alcohol and is used medicinally as a topical antiseptic, astringent, and anti-bacterial. At concentrations above 15 percent, it is also a broad-spectrum preservative against bacteria and fungi, and can boost the efficacy of other preservatives in a formulation. Cosmetic companies tend to use alcohol SD-40 in high-grade cosmetic manufacturing as they consider ethanol too strong and too drying for application

E

on the skin. Obtained from grain distillation, it can also be synthetically manufactured. *See also* alcohol.

ethyl 4-(bis[hydroxypropyl]) aminobenzoate—an FDA-approved sunscreen chemical with an approved usage level of 1 to 5 percent.

ethyl arachidonate—an emollient with healing and smoothing properties that is also reported as appropriate for use in indoor tanning preparations. It is the ester of ethyl alcohol and arachidonic acid. A modified form of ethyl arachidonate can reduce the possibility of irritation that can result from using straight ethyl arachidonate.

ethyl cellulose—a binder, film former, and thickener. It is used in suntan gels, creams, and lotions. This is the ethyl ether of cellulose.

ethyldihydroxypropyl ρ-aminobenzoate—*see* ethyl dihydroxypropyl PABA.

ethyl ether—a solvent that may cause skin irritation. Although considered a non-comedogenic raw material, it is rarely used in cosmetics.

ethyl linoleate (vitamin F)—an emollient and an essential fatty acid. *See also* vitamin F.

ethyl linolenate—an emollient reportedly used in indoor tanning preparations. It is not very popular as it may pose rancidity problems. It may also be used as an ingredient to enhance the fragrance of a product.

ethyl macadamiate—an emollient fatty acid derived from the ester of ethyl alcohol and macadamia nut oil. Its primary constituents are ethyl oleate and ethyl palmitoleate. It can be used as an alternative to silicone-based ingredients such as dimethicone.

ethyl palmate—a moisturizer and emollient derived from palm oil. Ingredient manufacturers note that it is easily absorbed by the skin, leaving it with a smooth and silky feel.

ethyl paraben—a preservative with minimal sensitizing potential. *See also* parabens.

ethylene acrylate copolymer—a film former, binder, and viscosity-increasing agent. It is a synthetic polymer. *See also* acrylates.

ethylene glycol monomethyl ether (ethoxyethanol)—considered a non-comedogenic raw material. It is used as a solvent in nail products and as a stabilizer in cosmetic emulsions. It is able to penetrate the skin and may cause skin irritation.

ethylene glycol monostearate (glycol stearate)—a non-comedogenic raw material that provides a pearly look and consistency to clear preparations. *See also* glycol stearate.

ethylenediamine tetraacetic acid—*see* EDTA.

2-ethylhexyl 2-cyano-3, 3-diphenylacrylate—also known as octocrylene. It is a UV absorber. *See also* octocrylene.

ethylhexyl dimethyl PABA—formerly referred to as octyl dimethyl PABA. It is an FDA-approved sunscreen chemical with an approved usage level of 1.4 to 8 percent in both the United States and the European Union. In the 1970s, it was the most popular sunscreen chemical because it is one of the best UVB absorbers. Its use, however, has been replaced by octyl methoxycinnamate as a result of the PABA-free trend in sunscreen products. A PABA derivative, it can cause skin irritation and photocontact allergy.

ethylhexyl glycerin—a skin conditioner and preservative derived from glycerin.

2-ethylhexyl 2-hydroxybenzoate—*see* octyl salicylate.

2-ethylhexyl isostearate—a chemical reactant used in cosmetic formulations to reduce the amount of anti-oxidants needed for that particular formulation. It is also used as an emollient for high-quality skin care preparations. This is an isosteric acid derivative.

2-ethylhexyl methoxycinnamate—*see* octyl methoxycinnamate.

ethylhexyl methoxycinnamate—also known as octinoxate and octylmethoxycinnamate. It is an FDA-approved sunscreen chemical with an approved usage level of 2 to 7.5 percent in the United States and up to 10 percent in the European Union. Currently, this is the most popular sunscreen chemical, worldwide, for sun products. It has an excellent UV absorption capability, a good safety profile, broad solubility in oils, insolubility in water, and rarely causes photoallergy. These attributes all add up to make it an almost perfect sunscreen chemical. Considered a non-comedogenic raw material, it is derived from balsam of Peru, cocoa leaves, cinnamon leaves, and storax. This is the INCI name for what has been listed in the past as octylmethoxycinnamate. For a time, both nomenclatures were in use, with ethyl hexyl methoxycinnamate becoming the standard.

ethylhexyl ρ-methoxycinnamate—provides excellent UVB protection with some limited UVA absorption, as well. *See also* octylmethoxycinnamate.

2-ethylhexyl ρ-methoxycinnamate—*see* octylmethoxycinnamate.

ethylhexyl-ρ—*see* octylpalmitate.

ethylhexyl palmitate—*see* octylpalmitate.

2-ethylhexyl salicylate—also known as ethylhexyl salicylate and octyl salicylate. It is a UVB absorber. *See also* ethylhexyl salicylate.

ethylhexyl salicylate—an FDA-approved UVB sunscreen chemical, it absorbs within the entire UVB range. It has an approved usage level of 3 to 5 percent in both the United States and the European

E

Union, and is a good solubilizer for benzophenone-3. In suntan lotions, it is used as a preservative and anti-microbial. This is a salt of salicylic acid occurring in wintergreen leaves and in other plants. It is also synthetically manufactured. It is considered a non-comedogenic raw material. This is the INCI name for octyl salicylate.

ethylhexyl triazone—the INCI name foroctyltriazone. It is a UV filter and absorber. Clinical studies show high photostability and very high UVB-absorption capacity, particularly when compared to other popular UV filters. Studies also indicate that even low concentrations of ethylhexyltriazone in a sun care preparation can contribute significantly to the final product's SPF. It appears to perform particularly well in synergy with zinc oxide.

eucalyptol—considered an antiseptic. This is a monoterpene compound that provides the fragrance associated with the essential oil of eucalyptus. Eucalyptol is also used to fragrance cosmetic preparations. *See also* cajeput oil; eucalyptus oil.

eucalyptus extract (*Eucalyptus globulus*)—possibly a mild astringent with antiseptic properties. It may also act as an insect repellent. *See also* eucalyptus oil.

eucalyptus oil—described as having antiseptic, disinfectant, antifungal, and blood-circulation activating properties. It is also used as a fragrance. Native to Australia, it was regarded as a general cure-all by the Aborigines and later by the European settlers. It has a long tradition of use in medicine, and is considered one of the most powerful and versatile herbal remedies. It is said that eucalyptus oil's anti-septic properties and disinfectant action increase as the oil ages. The most important constituent of the oil is eucalyptol. The essential oil is obtained from eucalyptus leaves. Eucalyptus oil may cause allergic reactions.

eugenol—a botanical fraction. It is anti-bacterial, anti-inflammatory, and pain relieving. It can also be used as a local, topical anesthetic and antiseptic. In a cosmetic formulation, it can mask odor or provide fragrance. Eugenol is a yellow, oily liquid and is generally associated with clove oil. However, it is also found in nutmeg, cinnamon, and bay leaf.

euglena gracilis extract—a freshwater-algae extract that is attributed with skin-toning and firming abilities. Ingredient suppliers indicate that it can help boost cellular metabolism during skin repair phases, and thus recommend it for use in night creams and lotions.

Euterpe oleracea—*see* açai pulp oil.

Euterpe oleracea **pulp oil**—*see* açai pulp oil.

Euterpe oleracea **pulp powder**—*see* açai pulp powder.

evening primrose oil (*Oenothera biennis*)—its therapeutic botanical properties are described as astringent and helpful for skin irritations. Incorporated into certain preparations at a 10 percent concentration, it appears to improve cases of pruritis and xerosis. Evening primrose oil improves the skin's hydration and its ability to develop normal barrier functions. Evening primrose oil contains a high amount of gamma linoleic acid, which is one of the essential fatty acids vital for maintaining the normal functioning of the epithelial barrier membrane.

evergreen clematis (*Clematis vitalba*)—anti-inflammatory and astringent. Its constituents include mucilage, chlorophyll, and vitamins. Stems and leaves are the parts used.

everlasting oil (*Helichrysym italicum*)—said to be anti-inflammatory, astringent and fungicidal. It reportedly decreases UVB-induced erythema on sunburned skin. If applied prior to sun exposure, everlasting oil may help prevent sunburn. The photoprotective activities of this oil are largely because of the action of its flavonoids content. *See also Helichrysum italicum.*

extra cellular matrix (ECM)—described as a mixture of bioactive substances including collagen, glycosaminoglycans, heparan sulfate, dermatan sulfate, chondroitin sulfate, and the glycoproteins laminin and fibronectin. It has the ability to stimulate the cells to actually help repair the skin. In general, it is believed to improve cellular function. It is used primarily in products for wrinkled or mature skin.

eyebright extract (*Euphrasia officinalis*)—an herb credited with astringent, anti-inflammatory, and tonic properties. As indicated by its name, it has traditionally been used in eye care preparations to decrease and counteract eye area inflammation and potential irritations. Some manufacturers claim that when combined with horsetail and lady's mantle, it works to counter skin wrinkling around the eye area. Important constituents of eyebright extract include tannin, mineral salts, and iridic glycosides. The extract is prepared from the plant after it has been cut just above the root.

E

fango—*see* mud.

fango mud—a redundancy; *fango* means mud in Italian. *See* mud.

farnesol—described as a substance of high biological potential, capable of acting in the skin as a true bioactivator. A biological precursor and fatty alcohol, farnesol is one component of vitamin K. It is said to help smooth wrinkles, normalize sebum secretion, and increase the skin's elasticity, tissue tension, and moisture-binding capability. It is able to penetrate the epidermis. In humans, farnesol is found in the skin and is involved in sterol biosynthesis. It is also used for its deodorant, odor-masking, and skin-soothing properties. In clinical studies, farnesol has demonstrated anti-microbial activity, though it is unclear if this remains the case once incorporated into a cosmetic formulation. It is widely present in vegetables and found in many essential oils (for example, acacia, lilac, lily of the valley, rose, orange blossom, oak moss, and sandalwood).

farnesyl acetate—a tonic, also used for perfuming. A variety of beneficial effects on the skin's metabolic process have been noted with the use of compounds consisting of a mixture of farnesyl acetate, farnesol, and panthenyl triacetate. Studies indicate that a combination of farnesyl acetate and panthenyl triacetate can help reduce sebum production in oily skin.

FD&C colors—refer to color entry in Chapter 4.

fennel extract (*Foeniculum vulgare*)—described as a cleanser and detoxifier indicated for oily skin types. The principal constituents of fennel oil are anethol and fenchone, plus d-pinene, phellandrine, anisic acid, and anisic aldehyde. Anethol, also a main constituent of anise oil, may produce hives, scaling, and blisters when applied directly to the skin. The therapeutic properties of fennel oil are most probably because of fenchone, and so only the varieties of fennel that contain a good proportion of fenchone are suitable for therapeutic use. Fennel oil is obtained from a distillation of the seeds.

fenugreek extract (*Trigonellafoenum-graecum*)—considered an emollient, anti-inflammatory, and healing ingredient. It can also be used to mask odor or add fragrance to a product. It was traditionally used in treatments for irritated skin. The seeds of this annual herb have been used through the ages and were held in high regard among the Egyptians, Greeks, and Romans for medicinal and culinary purposes.

fern (*Dryopteris sp.*) (**shield fern**)—healing, cleansing, and skin conditioning. Its chief constituents include tannin, filicic acid, and filamaron. Fern oil and the powdery fern extract are obtained from the plant's rhizome.

ferric ferrocyanide—an inorganic blue pigment with no known toxicity. Used as a colorant, it is commonly known as Prussian blue.

ferulic acid—a plant-derived anti-oxidant and free-radical scavenger, it protects the skin against UVB-induced redness. When incorporated into formulas with ascorbic acid and tocopherol, ferulic acid can improve their stability and double the photoprotection capacities offered by the formulation. In clinical studies, ferulic acid exhibits good permeation capacities through the stratum corneum, which can be attributed to its lipophilic properties.

feverfew extract (*Chrysanthemum parthenium*)—used for its esters and borneol as a counterirritant. It is claimed to relieve the pain and swelling caused by insect bites. Feverfew is a perennial, herbaceous plant.

fibronectin—a cosmetic ingredient described as a surface protective agent with a moisturizing and protective effect. Produced by many types of cells, fibronectin is a glycoprotein and an important component of the skin's basal layer. Research suggests fibronectin plays a significant role in maintaining a healthy basal layer. Fibronectin's function in the skin is to strengthen the attachments among collagen and elastin fibers, fibroblasts, and other cells in the dermis with connective tissues. Its presence may also be important to cell growth. There is some evidence that fibronectin may act as a cell regenerator by reversing abnormal cell formation and growth. It constitutes 1 to 3 percent of the total cellular protein of fibroblasts.

fibronectin (hydrolyzed)—a humectant and moisturizing agent for skin creams and lotions. *See also* fibronectin.

ficain enzyme—also known as ficin enzyme. Its enzymatic activity can make it an effective exfoliant, and it is also said to have anti-oxidant benefits. Derived from fig sap, it belongs to the same enzymatic group as papain, derived from papaya.

field poppy extract—therapeutic properties are described as pain and spasm soothing.

figwort extract (*Scrophularia nodosa*)—traditionally used in cases of superficial burns, including sunburn, cutaneous eruptions, swelling, and inflammations. There are a number of varieties

F

of figwort, including common, yellow, balm-leaved, water, and knotted, all appearing to have similar properties. The extract is obtained from the plant's leaves.

fir needle extract—attributed with astringent properties. Suppliers indicate it is appropriate for incorporation into creams and lotions.

fir needle oil—can be used to add fragrance, and also for antiseptic and stimulating properties. Suppliers indicate that when incorporated into massage oils it can help pep up poor circulation and soothe muscle pain. Constituents of this oil include careen, limonene, terpinolene, borneol, and piperitone. It is obtained from the steam distillation of fur tree needles.

firmogen—provides an astringent, strengthening, and lightening effect. Its use in cosmetic formulations results in smoother skin feel. Firmogen is a biological substance, blending polysaccharides with hydrolyzed enzymatic proteins.

fish collagenic protein—a transparent, uncolored gel used in moisturizers.

fish glycerides—a fish oil used primarily in soaps.

five leaf grass—*see* cinquefoil extract.

flavonoids—a general category of plant derived anti-oxidants. *See also* bioflavonoids and full entry in Chapter 4.

flavonastaes—an enzyme. *See also* enzyme.

flowers extract—probably used as a fragrance. Such a listing is an all-encompassing statement that does not allow one to identify the type of flowers used and, therefore, prohibits determining any therapeutic value.

folic acid—generally used as an emollient. *In vitro* and *in vivo* skin studies now indicate its capacity to aid in DNA synthesis and repair, promote cellular turnover, reduce wrinkles, and promote skin firmness. There is some indication that folic acid may also protect DNA from UV-induced damage. Folic acid is a member of the vitamin B complex and is naturally occurring in leafy greens.

fragrance—refer to fragrance entry in Chapter 4.

frankincense (*Boswellia thurifera*)—described as anti-inflammatory and a mild antiseptic that brings relief to dry and sensitive skins and helps heal all types of wounds. Its astringent properties are said to help balance oily or overactive skin. This is one of the oldest essential oils in use, and dates back to ancient Egypt.

fructan—moisturizing and anti-inflammatory, it is also used to help improve skin barrier function. It is a fructose derivative. *See also* fructose.

F

fructose—a naturally occurring sugar in fruits and honey. It has moisture-binding and skin-softening properties.

fruit oil extract—a blend used in perfumery.

fucus—*see* fucus algae.

fucus algae (*Fucus vesiculosus*) (**bladderwrack, fucus seaweed**)—a succulent giant kelp attributed with some anti-oxidant, preservative, and fragrance value. Anecdotal evidence indicates it has skin toning and anti-cellulite properties as well as an ability to improve elasticity. Its essential oil exhibits anti-microbial activity, as it contains compounds similar to traditional preservatives. Clinical studies are indicating that fucus extract be beneficial for use in anti-aging cosmetic formulations. Fucus algae is cited as being rich in vitamin B. *See also* seaweed extract.

fucus seaweed—*see* fucus algae.

fullerenes—also known as fullerines; buckyball. Fullerenes are soluble carbon molecules that are studied and incorporated into cosmetics for their anti-oxidant and free-radical scavenging properties. Some manufacturers cite significantly greater anti-oxidant potential than vitamins C and E and an ability to retain their anti-free radical activity under a variety of external conditions such as heat, strong ultraviolet radiation. They are most commonly used to minimize potential reactions through an interaction with the immune system. Fullerenes are generally incorporated into anti-aging and skin rejuvenation formations. The most common form of fullerenes is C60; other forms include C70, C76, and C84. They are the result of nanotechnology and its application in skin care.

fullerines—*see* fullerenes.

fumaria officinalis **flower/leaf/stem extract**—an extract derived from the mixture of flowers, leaves, and stems of the *fumaria officinalis* plant (commonly known as fumitory). It is attributed with skin-conditioning properties. *See also* fumitory herb extract.

fumaric acid—used to add fragrance to products and to decrease product pH. It can also help keep the pH stable. It is generally used in cleansers. Fumaric acid is naturally occurring in plants, such as lichen and Iceland moss, and in animals. For example, the skin produces fumaric acid when exposed to light. It can also be synthetically manufactured.

fumitory herb extract (*Fumaria officinalis*)—credited with curative properties because of its purifying powers. Historically, it was attributed with bleaching and skin-clearing properties as well. The leaves yield a juice credited with medicinal properties because of its fumaric and malic acid content. This small annual plant is considered a common weed.

F

G

galactoarabinan (GA)—a multi-functional ingredient with humectant and exfoliating properties. In aqueous solutions, GA can deposit a clear film, creating or helping to create an occlusive environment, preventing transepidermal water loss and enhancing the functionality of a formulation's active ingredients. In humid conditions GA acts as a moisture binder, and in dry conditions, it is able to retain moisture, further inhibiting moisture loss from the skin. Additionally, GA can improve particle dispersion and the uniformity of emulsion droplets resulting in a more stable emulsion and potentially more efficacious formulation, particularly in the case of sunscreens. *In vitro* and *in vivo* studies indicate possible benefit to the immune system given an ability to enhance Langerhans cell proliferation and cytokine production. GA has been shown to boost AHA exfoliation activity without increasing skin irritation, and it also exhibits its own exfoliant properties independent of AHA presence in a formulation, thereby helping reduce the appearance of fine lines and wrinkles. GA is a polysaccharide found in all plants and is the dominant sugar of the western larch tree.

galactomannan—a polysaccharide. *See also* senna.

galbanum (*Ferula galbaniflua*)—depending on the form used (gum, gum extract, or resin oil), galbanum is used as a perfuming agent. It can also exhibit anti-microbial and tonic properties.

gallic acid—a potential bleaching agent and anti-oxidant, it is also astringent and potentially anti-microbial and anti-fungal. Scientists are finding that gallic acid may serve as a skin-lightening agent by inhibiting the action of the tyrosinase and peroxidase enzymes. Some studies indicate that it is more effective than hydroquinone when combined with the proper ingredients. It is also incorporated into anti-aging formulations for its ability to prevent mucopolysaccharide deterioration. It is a constituent of witch hazel and oak bark, among many other plants; however, it is generally obtained from nutgalls for commercial purposes.

gamma aminobutyric acid (**GABA**)—an amino acid claimed to help improve skin elasticity. *See also* aminobutric acid.

gamma linoleic acid—*see* linoleic acid.

G

174

Gardenia florida **fruit extract**—has skin-conditioning, refreshing, and coloring properties.

garlic extract (*Allium sativum*)—antiseptic and bactericide. It is sometimes externally applied in ointments and lotions to reduce hard swellings and to treat problem skin (acne, for example). The active properties of garlic depend on a pungent, volatile, essential oil that is obtained by distillation with water. This oil is an allyl sulfide found in the onion family, and it is rich in sulfur but contains no oxygen. The common garlic is included in the same group of plants as the onion.

garlic oil—considered a healing oil with bacteriostatic and bactericidal action. It is incorporated into skin care formulations for skin healing and to aid in clearing problems such as eczema and acne. *See also* garlic extract.

garlic sage—*see* germander extract.

gelatin—used as a natural sealant against moisture loss and as a formulation thickener. The films produced by gelatin are tacky when moist and hard, and brittle when dry. It is obtained by the partial hydrolysis of mature collagen derived from the skin, connective tissue, and bones of animals. It does not have the water-binding ability of soluble collagen.

gellan gum—used as a gelling agent, thickener, and stabilizer in cosmetic preparations.

genistein—an isoflavone commonly found in soy. It has demonstrated UV-protection properties through anti-oxidant activity. Studies indicate genistein can promote collagen synthesis, making it applicable in anti-aging cosmetics. *See also* isoflavones.

gentian extract (*Gentiana sp.*)—credited with cooling, antiseptic, and anti-inflammatory properties. Studies indicate that the gentian root also has skin-lightening capacities, thanks to an ability to inhibit melanocyte tyrosinase production. All known gentian species are remarkable for their intensely bitter properties but are considered valuable tonic medicines. The root is the principal part used for medicinal and cosmetic purposes. Dried gentian root contains gentian, gentiamarin, and bitter glucosides together with gentianic acid (gentisin) and gentiopicrin.

geraniol—perfuming and with tonic properties. It is a primary constituent in many essential oils, including citronella, lavender, lemongrass, orange flower, and ylang-ylang.

geranium burbon oil—*see* geranium oil.

geranium oil (*Pelargonium sp.*)— refreshing, anti-irritant, mildly tonic, and astringent. Although good for all skin types, it is particularly beneficial for oily and acne skins, and to those with inflammatory tendencies. The cell-regenerating activities claimed for geranium would also make it useful for aged skin. Although the many varieties of geranium—including wild geranium and English geranium—all belong to the same botanical family, their uses may differ. Geranium oil is obtained by steam distillation from the entire plant, and is widely used in perfumery and cosmetics.

Germall II—the trade name for imidazolidinyl urea, a preservative. *See also* imidazolidinyl urea.

germander extract (*Teucrium scorodonia*) (**garlic sage; wood sage**)—credited with astringent and tonic properties. It is useful for skin problems and wounds. The whole herb is used for manufacturing the extract.

GHPT—*see* guar hydroxypropyltrimonium chloride.

ginger root extract (*Zingiber officinale*)—healing, tonic, antiseptic, anti-inflammatory and, potentially anti-oxidant. It is also incorporated into cosmetic formulations for its odor-masking properties. Among ginger's many constituents are aldehydes, gingerol, shogaol, and paradol as well as essential oils, volatile oils, and vitamins A, B_6, and C.

ginkgo biloba extract (**ginkgo extract**)—credited with anti-oxidant properties, it also appears to aid fibroblast cells in the production of collagen and elastin. This ability is attributed to a number of flavonoid fractions, including quercetin, kaempferol, and ginkgetin. Additionally, ginkgo is an anti-inflammatory and may help improve a couperose condition because of a protective effect on vascular walls. Ginkgo was used in folkloric medicine as a blood vessel dilator because of its ability to increase blood flow and stimulate tissue oxygen consumption. It is considered a beneficial anti-aging ingredient. Ginkgo's key constituents include ginkgolide and bilobalide, catechin, tannin, quercetin, and luteolin.

ginkgo extract—*see* ginkgo biloba extract.

ginseng extract (*Panax sp.*)—considered tonic and nourishing because of its vitamin and hormone content. It seems to aid in diminishing wrinkles and helps dry skin. It is also said to promote skin elasticity, perhaps by stimulating sterol and protein production. Other claims include skin rejuvenating, oxygenating, and stimulating properties. Folkloric remedies cite use for boils, bruises, sores, and swellings. This root's active components are called ginsenosides and these are said to be responsible for revitalizing and reactivating epidermal cells. Other important constituents include saponins, mucin, and vitamin B. The extract comes from the root. Ginseng has been associated with many allergic skin reactions.

ginseng root extract—a redundancy because the portion of the plant used therapeutically is the root. *See also* ginseng extract.

ginsenosides Rb$_1$—a manufacturer's composition said to promote elastin synthesis by the dermal fibroblasts. The active components of this mixture are reported as gensenosides from ginseng varieties, including *Panax notoginseng* and *Panax quinquefolium*. This would most likely be used in anti-aging and skin-toning products because of the apparent impact on skin elasticity. *See also* ginseng extract.

glucans—studies indicate an ability to stimulate immune system activity, thereby helping the body fight a variety of infectious diseases caused by bacterial, fungal, viral, and parasitic organisms. Glucans also seem to have anti-tumor properties. *See also* polyglucan.

gluconolactone—used in cosmetics for its anti-acne properties. It can also help improve skin hydration given its water-binding ability. In addition, formulators may select gluconolactone for its action as a product stabilizer (chelating agent). Some studies indicate potential free-radical scavenging capacities as well. These properties would make it particularly relevant for use in making anti-aging, moisturizing, and possibly sun care products.

glucoronic acid—a chelating agent, pH adjuster, and humectant that gives a smooth feel to the skin.

glucosamine hydrochloride (glucosamine HCl)—used to adjust the pH of a formulation. It also has anti-static and hair-conditioning properties.

glucose—has moisture-binding properties and provides the skin with a soothing effect. It is a sugar that is generally obtained by the hydrolysis of starch.

glucose glutamate—a humectant for hand creams and lotions, as well as a skin conditioner and moisturizer that enhances lather in surfactant systems. Glucose glutamate is the ester of glucose and glutamic acid and is considered a non-comedogenic, non-irritating raw material.

glucose oxidase—an enzyme used to help stabilize a formulation. It can also improve skin feel and condition.

Glucoviton—a trade name referring to a mixture of glucoronic acid and Hydroviton.

G

glutamic acid—a moisture binder and an anti-oxidant. Glutamic acid is an amino acid manufactured by means of fermentation, generally from a vegetable protein.

glutamylamidoethyl imidazole—an amino acid with hair- and skin-conditioning properties. Manufacturers cite an ability to optimize skin cell regeneration and cellular defense, as well as an improved vitamin D activity. It would be recommended for use in anti-aging products and those for "tired" or "stressed" skin.

glutaral (glutardialdehyde)—a broad-spectrum preservative that can cause skin irritation. This is an amino acid occurring in green sugar beets.

glutardialdehyde—*see* glutaral.

glutathione—a peptide composed of cysteine, glycine, and glutamate. It is believed to enhance the skin's cellular metabolism and oxygen utilization. It has been found to protect the fibroblast against free radical-induced oxidation and act as a powerful anti-oxidant. Studies indicate that it can inactivate the tyrosinase enzyme and quench free radicals that contribute to tyrosinase and melanin formation, thereby serving as a skin-lightening or de-pigmenting agent. Glutathione is a component of plant and animal tissue, naturally occurring in the body and essential for the proper functioning of the immune system.

glutathione monomethyl ester—an alkyl ester of glutathione. *See also* glutathione.

glutathione peroxidase—helps control inflammation. Its most frequent application is in shaving preparations. Glutatione peroxidase is an enzyme and a natural anti-oxidant.

glycereth-26—*see* glycerin.

glyceridic oil (hydrogenated)—emollient and skin conditioner.

glycerin (glycerol; propanetriol)—a humectant used in moisturizers. It is water-binding and able to draw and absorb water from the air, thus helping the skin retain moisture. Glycerin has been studied extensively for its hydrating abilities. Based on the data available, glycerin has been established as a good skin-moisturizing agent. At least part of its activity is attributed to its facilitating enzymatic reactions in the skin, thereby promoting corneocyte desquamation. Glycerin also improves the spreading qualities of creams and lotions. It is a clear, syrupy liquid made by chemically combining water and fat that is usually derived from vegetable oil. Although glycerin has not been shown to cause allergies, it may be comedogenic and irritating to the mucous membranes when used in concentrated solutions.

G

glycerin monostearate—*see* glyceryl monostearate.

glycerine—*see* glycerin.

glycerol—a glycerin alcohol. *See also* glycerin.

glycerol stearate lipophilic—*see* glycerin.

glyceryl—a glycerin ester. *See also* glycerin.

glyceryl acrylate/acrylic acid copolymer—a synthetic polymer that acts as a humectant and can also control product viscosity.

glyceryl aminobenzoate (glyceryl PABA, glyceryl p-aminobenzoate)— a sunscreen chemical for UVB absorption with an approved usage level of 2 to 3 percent. It is, however, too water soluble to be effectively used in waterproof formulations, and its use raises safety concerns about the presence of benzocane.

glyceryl arachidonate—an emulsifier and emollient with moisturizing properties. It is reportedly used in suntan gels, creams, and lotions.

glyceryl behenate—derived from the glycerides of coconut fatty acids. It acts as an emollient, lubricant, and/or emulsifier in a cosmetic preparation.

glyceryl caprate—an emollient and emulsifier that can be obtained from plants or synthetically manufactured.

glyceryl caprylate—a coemulsifier, solubilizer, and surfactant that promotes absorption and has bacteriostatic action in cosmetic formulations.

glyceryl dibehenate—a glycerin derivative that acts as an emollient and a lubricant.

glyceryl isostearate—*see* glyceryl mono-isostearate.

glyceryl laurate—a coemulsifier for oil-in-water emulsions. It is also a super fattening agent that promotes absorption and has a bacteriostatic effect.

glyceryl linoleate—an emollient with moisturizing capabilities. It is synthetically produced from naturally derived ingredients.

glyceryl mono-isostearate (glyceryl isostearate)—an isostearic acid often incorporated into cosmetic formulations as an emollient.

glyceryl monostearate (glycerin monostearate; glyceryl stearate)—widely used in cosmetics. It is an emulsifying and solubilizing ingredient, dispersing agent, emollient, formula stabilizer, and surface-action agent. Employed in baby creams, face masks, foundation, and hand lotions, it is often derived from hydrogenated soybean oil. Glyceryl monostearate has little or no toxicity. *See also* glyceryl stearate.

G

glyceryl oleate—an emollient and stabilizer derived from olive oil. It is a water-in-oil emulsifier that allows for softer emulsions than glyceryl stearate.

glyceryl PABA—*see* glyceryl aminobenzoate.

glyceryl polymethacrylate—a film former and viscosity-controlling ingredient. Given its film-forming properties it can be used to help retain moisture in the skin.

glyceryl ricinoleate—an emollient and an emulsifier used in the preparation of creams and lotions.

glyceryl stearate—an emulsifier that helps form neutral, stable emulsions. It is also a solvent, humectant, and consistency regulator in water-in-oil and oil-in-water formulations. In addition, it can be used as a skin lubricant and imparts a pleasant skin feel. Glyceryl stearate is a mixture of mono-, di-, and triglycerides of palmitic and stearic acids, and is made from glycerin and stearic fatty acids. Derived for cosmetic use from palm kernel or soy oil, it is also found in the human body. It is very mild with a low skin-irritation profile; however, a slight risk of irritation exists if products contain poor quality glyceryl stearate.

glyceryl stearate citrate—an emulsifier that can also act as an emollient and help improve overall skin condition.

glyceryl stearate lipophilic—*see* glyceryl stearate.

glyceryl stearate SE—self-emulsifying glyceryl stearate. It provides a stable, uniform oil-in-water emulsion. *See also* glyceryl stearate.

glyceryl tribehenate—also known as tribehenin. See also tribehenin.

glyceryl tri-isostearate (triisosteatin)—an emollient and emulsifier.

glyceryl trioctanoate—an emollient with skin-softening abilities.

glycine—an amino acid used as a texturizer in cosmetic formulations. It makes up approximately 30 percent of the collagen molecule.

glycine soya (soja) protein—a multi-functional ingredient that serves as a solvent, emulsifier, surfactant, and skin conditioner. It can also help improve skin moisturization.

glycine soja (soybean) sterols—a phytosterol that acts as an emollient and is used in a wide variety of cosmetic preparations.

glycoceramides—it is suggested that the topical application of glycoceramides helps replenish intercorneal lipids and regulate the skin's ability to bind and retain moisture. In addition, it improves the ability of hydrophilic and hydrophobic materials to traverse the stratum corneum layer (the movement of water into the skin and removal of by-products of cellular metabolism from the skin). This ensures the intercellular regulatory balance and enhances and restores the barrier function. Glycoceramides can be incorporated into emulsions. *See also* ceramides.

glycocitrates—a combination of glycolic and citric acids used instead of AHAs in some preparations. This substitution is based on the premise that glycocitrates are milder than an AHA such as glycolic acid, and that they provide similar results. Their activity does not appear to be scientifically validated in a significant manner.

glycocoll—*see* glycine.

glycogen—a skin-conditioning agent. It is a high molecular-weight polymer distributed through the cell protoplasm.

glycol palmitate—an emulsion stabilizer. It can also make a product more opaque and act as a skin conditioner.

glycol stearate—can be utilized as a detergent, emulsifier, surfactant, thickener, stabilizer, and emollient in cosmetic formulations. It also converts clear cleansers or other preparations to ones that are pearly.

glycolic acid (hydroxyacetic acid)—reduces corenocyte cohesion and corneum layer thickening where an excess buildup of dead skin cells can be associated with many common skin problems, such as acne, dry and severely dry skin, and wrinkles. Glycolic acid acts by dissolving the internal cellular cement responsible for abnormal keratinization, facilitating the sloughing of dead skin cells. It also improves skin hydration by enhancing moisture uptake as well as increasing the skin's ability to bind water. This occurs in the cellular cement through an activation of glycolic acid and the skin's own hyaluronic acid content. Hyaluronic acid is known to retain an impressive amount of moisture and this capacity is enhanced by glycolic acid. As a result, the skin's own ability to raise its moisture content is increased. Glycolic acid is the simplest alpha hydroxyacid (AHA). It is also the AHA that scientists and formulators believe has greater penetration potential largely due to its smaller molecular weight. It is mildly irritating to the skin and mucous membranes if the formulation contains a high glycolic acid concentration and/or a low pH. Glycolic acid proves beneficial for acne-prone skin as it helps keep pores clear of excess keratinocytes. It is also used for diminishing the signs of age spots, as well as actinic keratosis. However, glycolic acid is most popularly employed in anti-aging cosmetics because of its hydrating, moisturizing, and skin-normalizing abilities, leading to a reduction in the appearance of fine lines and wrinkles. Regardless of the skin type, glycolic acid use is associated with softer, smoother,

G

healthier, and younger looking skin. Glycolic acid is naturally found in sugarcane but synthetic versions are most often used in cosmetic formulations. *See also* alpha hydroxyacid.

glycolipids—emollient. They provide a natural layer of protective fats that keep the skin moisturized and in good condition. They are present at much higher concentrations in the skin during infancy and early childhood, but decrease overtime because of oxidative damage.

glycoprotein—a skin-conditioning agent derived from carbohydrates and proteins. In the body, glycoproteins play a significant role in immune response. *See also* glycoproteins (soluble).

glycoproteins (soluble)—a group of proteins found in the intercellular layers, the best known of which is fibronectin. It is found in the cellular matrix of the dermis and plays a role in cell migration during wound healing. The mechanism by which it might provide cosmetic benefits has not yet been clearly established, although it could be related to the role of glycoproteins in immune response. *See also* fibronectin.

glycosaminoglycans—a group of chemically related polysaccharides that are major components of the extra cellular matrix (ECM) and of connective tissues. They are used in cosmetics for their ability to increase hydration and the elasticity and pliability of the skin. Glycosaminoglycans are credited with film-forming, moisturizing, and firming properties. They reportedly leave the skin smooth and with a pleasant, velvety softness and evenness, and minimize wrinkle appearance. They are easily accepted by the skin because of their high charge and affinity. This group of complex materials, formerly identified as mucopolysaccharides, includes such individual components as hyaluronic acid, chondroitin, chondroitin sulfate, chondroitin 6-sulfate, dermatan sulfate, heparin, and heparin sulfate. As proteoglycans, glycosaminoglycans are derived from cartilaginous fish. They can also be derived from various animal proteins as well as synthetically prepared. *See also* mucopolysaccharides.

glycoside/C-$_{12-16}$—a mixture of synthetic fatty alcohols with 12 to 16 carbons in the alkyl chain.

glycosphingolipids—said to replenish the lipids lost from the skin and renew the skin's barrier function and moisture-binding capacity. When incorporated into aftershave preparations, they also seem to help soothe nicks and cuts. Laboratory studies indicate that glycosphingolipids can reduce transepidermal water loss when applied to the skin, even at 5 percent in a typical oil-in-water emulsion. Glycosphingolipids, a compound of lipids and sugars, are a class of molecules embedded in the membranes of cells throughout the body where they act to regulate the interaction of healthy cells with their environment.

glycyrrhetic acid—*see* 18 beta-glycerrhentinic acid.

glycyrrhetinic acid—anti-irritant, anti-allergenic, anti-inflammatory, skin-lightening, and smoothing properties are attributed to this ingredient, which is also a carrier. It is the organic compound derived from glycyrrhizic acid or shredded licorice roots.

glycyrrhizic acid—a hydrolyzed glycyrrhizin. It is credited with anti-inflammatory and anti-allergenic properties. Studies comparing glycyrrhizin with hydrocortisone found glycyrrhizin to be somewhat milder but longer lasting in effectiveness. Once the application of hydrocortisone is suspended, the symptoms return. This does not appear to be the case with glycyrrhizin. It does not have side effects and is chemically stable so it can be safely used on a continuing basis. *See also* licorice extract.

goa powder (*Andira araroba*) (**araroba; bahia powder; brazil powder; goa**)—used in traditional medicine for treating skin diseases, including psoriasis and eczema. It may have applications in cosmetics for dry skin. The powder's primary constituents include alkalis, benzene, chrysarobin (a reduced quinone), and resins. Its activity is attributed to its high chrysarobin content (approximately 80 percent). The *Andira araroba* tree is common to Bahia, Brazil.

goji berry (*Lycium barbarum*)—also known as matrimony vine. It is an anti-oxidant. *See also* matrimony vine.

goldenrod extract (*Solidago sp.*)—considered antiseptic and recommended for use in acne products to discourage the spread of infection through skin pustules. The extract is made from the leaves of various species of *Solidago*.

goldenseal extract (*Hydrastis canadensis*)—reportedly effective in treating eczema, itching, and wounds. Native Americans valued the root for its general ulceration-healing properties. Goldenseal extract's main constituents are the alkaloids berberine, hydrastine, and canadine. The extract is obtained from the plant's rhizomes, which are said to be much more alkaloid-rich than the root.

gotu kola extract (*Centella asiatica*) (**hydrocotyl; Hydrocotylasiatica; Indian pennywort**)—traditionally used for couperose condition. It was also used for soothing and anti-itching treatment in dermatological disorders. Gotu kola is a known inhibitor of keratinocyte proliferation, making it useful in the treatment of

G

severely dry skin such as psoriasis. It may also promote circulation and serve as an anti-cellulite ingredient. In addition, gotu kola is considered healing. It is helpful against sunburns and other superficial, though not extensive, burns. Gotu kola's activity is because of such constituents as phytosterols, glycosides, tannins, and essential oils.

grape—used in extract form, it is described as tonic, with anti-inflammatory, redness-reducing, and decongestant properties. It is also an anti-oxidant. All of these traits make it particularly beneficial in anti-aging, after-sun, and other sun care products. Grape's main constituent is a high proportion of berberin. In addition, grapes contain vitamin C, chlorophyll, and enzymes. The value of these components to the skin is based on the method of extract processing and cosmetic manufacturing.

grapefruit extract (*Citrus paradisi*)—reported as having antiseptic and skin-conditioning properties. It is indicated as beneficial for oily skin. Fresh grapefruit juice contains vitamin C and is very acidic. As such, in high concentrations, it is too caustic to use on the skin and face. There should be no problem, however, at normal use levels. The extract obtained from the juice is preferred over that of the rind, as there is practically no vitamin C available in the rind. Furthermore, unless properly obtained and processed, fertilizers and insecticide residues on the rind may provoke blemishes and allergic reactions in sensitive people. As vitamin C is considered an unstable component, grapefruit extract's value in cosmetics depends on the method of extraction and the product's formulation.

grapefruit oil—used as a fragrance and also as an active component with anti-irritant properties. Grapefruit oil is indicated for work with the lymphatic system.

grapefruit seed extract—said to have anti-bacterial properties. This is the extract from the seeds of the grapefruit. *See also* grapefruit extract.

grapeseed extract—considered a counterirritant with soothing, anti-oxidant, and anti-bacterial properties. Grapeseed extract contains polyphenols and high levels of procyandins. *See also* grape.

grapeseed oil—has moisturizing and nourishing properties because of its high linoleic acid content. Grapeseed oil is the fixed oil obtained by pressing grapeseeds.

G

green apple extract—*see* apple extract.

green clay—*see* clay.

green tea extract (*Camellia sinensis L.*)—a powerful anti-oxidant because of its catechin content, it is also known to be an anti-bacterial, anti-inflammatory, and a stimulant. In clinical studies, green tea demonstrates an ability to prevent or at least postpone the onset of such illnesses as cancer and heart disease. This is attributed to the catechin component's ability to penetrate into a cell, thereby protecting the cell from free radicals and associated damage. Because of its anti-oxidant properties, green tea is usually incorporated into anti-aging formulations. When applied topically, it can also reduce skin swelling. In addition, it can be found in sunscreens, given its ability to extend the product's SPF. The extract and its associated catechins can be obtained from both the plant and its dried leaves. Other constituents of green tea include caffeine and phenolic acids.

guaiac extract (*Guaiacum officinale*)—credited with antiseptic and stimulating properties. The resin, with therapeutic properties, is extracted from the hard wood of the guaiac tree.

guanidine carbonate—used to adjust the pH of a formulation.

guanine—color. It is mixed in water and used primarily in nail polish to achieve a pearlized effect. It has been greatly replaced by either synthetic pearl or aluminum and bronze particles. Guanine is obtained from plant or animal sources.

guar gum—has a coating action on the skin that allows for moisture retention. Often used as a thickener and emulsifier in cosmetic formulations, guar gum is a polysaccharide found in the seeds of the guar plant. It is the nutrient material required by the developing plant embryo during germination. When the endosperm, once separated from the hull and embryo, is ground to a powder form, it is marketed as guar gum.

guar hydroxypropyltrimonium chloride (**GHPT**)—an anti-irritant and anti-inflammatory that is also used as a thickening, conditioning, and anti-static agent. It helps maintain a product's smoothing action. Some manufacturers cite it as also having skin-softening capabilities. It imparts excellent skin conditioning in creams or lotions that otherwise may not be used on the face. It adds lubricity to a product when in contact with the skin. There is some evidence that it can enhance a formulation's viscosity and stability. It is a derivative of guar gum.

guarana seed extract (*Paullinia cupana*)—constituents include theophylline and caffeine, which makes it popular in anti-cellulite products for tonic and draining activity.

gum acacia—*see* acacia.

G

gum Arabic—*see* acacia.

gynostemma pentaphyllum extract—reported as astringent when obtained from the whole plant. An extract from the leaves and stems combined can also have anti-oxidant and emollient properties. It has a high saponin content, which research indicates may be similar to that of ginseng roots. Other constituents include sterols and flavonoids. This is a Chinese herb used in traditional medicine; its common Western name is jiaogulan.

G

H

hamamelis (winterbloom; witch hazel)—*see* witch hazel.

hamamelis (dry) extract—claimed botanical properties include anti-free radical, UVB absorber, healing, soothing, and anti-itching activity. *See also* witch hazel.

hawthorn extract (*Crataegus oxyacantha*)—sources cite it as having active constituents with valuable therapeutic properties such as anti-spasmodic, vasodilator, and sedative. It is obtained from the berries, flowers, and/or leaves of the hawthorn plant.

hayflower extract—reported to activate the circulatory system, have analgesic properties, and provide a tightening effect on the skin. Historically, hayflower extract was used in Europe to stimulate circulation and to treat rheumatic complaints. Its many active constituents include essential oils, vitamin D, amino acids, carotinoids, caffeic acid, 4-methoxycinnnamic acid, and tannin. This extract has a faintly sweet fragrance. Hayflower is not a specific plant but rather a mixture that is formed by the leftover blossoms and leaves in a hayloft.

hazelnut extract—attributed with astringent properties, and to improve the skin's overall look and feel.

hazelnut oil—a carrier oil credited with nourishing properties. As a carrier, it imparts excellent lubricity, pale color, and low odor. This oil is used in products designed for dry skin. It is obtained from the nuts of various species of the hazelnut tree.

HDI/trimethylolhexyllactone crosspolymer—a synthetic polymer that helps prevent a formulation from caking in the case of powder cosmetics.

hectorite—one of the principal constituents of bentonite clay. Used as a thickener and suspending agent in water-based systems in oil-in-water emulsions.

helichrysum oil—*see* everlasting oil.

helichrysumitalicum—*see* everlasting oil.

henna extract (*Lawsonia insermis*)—primarily used as a colorant, it provides a reddish-brown hue to products. It is also a conditioner. Henna's properties are described as antiseptic and astringent. Important constituents include mucins, phytosterols, and naptho-quinones. Generally, the extract is obtained from the leaves.

heptane—a solvent and viscosity-decreasing agent.

hesperidin methyl chalcone—a citrus bioflavonoid. Extracted from the peel of sweet oranges, it has anti-oxidant properties. It is used in eye care preparations for reducing the appearance of dark circles.

hesperitin laurate—anti-oxidant and skin conditioner.

hexadecanol—*see* cetyl alcohol.

hexamidine—generally used as a biocide and preservative. Some initial studies are indicating a potential to increase production of skin lipids, such as cholesterol, sphingolipids, and fatty acids. In turn this would help improve skin moisture content. Further evidence of this may be required.

hexamidine diisethionate—an anti-microbial and preservative targeting fungi and yeast. It may also have some emollient capacities.

1,2-hexanediol—a solvent used to dissolve other compounds in a formulation.

hexanoyl dipeptide-3 norleucine acetate—a peptide that acts as an exfoliant and can help improve the overall condition of the skin.

hexyl cinnamal—also known as hexyl cinnamic aldehyde. It is a fragrance that provides a floral, jasmine-like scent.

hexyl laurate—a mild emollient and a vehicle for lipid-soluble active ingredients. It is non-irritating and practically odorless. It enhances product spreadability and feel on skin. *See also* lauric acid.

hexyl nicotinate—penetrates rapidly and dilates blood vessels, thereby temporarily activating blood circulation. This increased blood flow results in an enhanced supply of oxygen, nutrients, and moisture to the skin cells, along with a faster elimination of wastes by means of the metabolic process.

hexyldecyl stearate—an emollient that has occlusive properties. It could help the skin retain moisture while also promoting greater softness, smoothness, and pliability.

hexylene glycol—could be considered a solubilizer. *See also* polyethylene glycol.

hibiscus extract (*Hibiscus sabdariffa*)—moisturizing and refreshing. It provides a tightening effect without stripping the skin of its natural oils. Hibiscus is a botanical recommended for oily skin because of its high degree of astringency and its toning properties. There are about 200 varieties of this plant, whose extract is obtained from the flowers, which contain a number of vegetable acids and pigments. Use of hibiscus extract is increasing in popularity, although it is more frequently used in hair care preparations. A non-irritating form of pyruvic acid is a key constituent of hibiscus extract.

histidine—a skin-conditioning amino acid. *See also* amino acid.

holy thistle—*see* blessed thistle extract.

homomenthyl salicylate—*see* homosalate.

H

homosalate—a chemical UVB absorber included in the FDA's Category I Sunscreen Chemical list. Its approved usage level is 4 to 15 percent by the FDA and 10 percent by the European Union's Cosmetic Directive.

honey—said to be soothing, softening, and moisturizing. Masks and other cosmetic preparations containing honey create a watertight film on the face and permit the skin to rehydrate itself. Strong anti-bacterial and immunological properties are attributed to honey. Its use in cosmetics can be traced back at least to ancient Egypt and Cleopatra. Honey is composed of a variety of sugars, wax, and other substances, including gluconic, citric, malic, formic, and lactic acids; beta-carotene; enzymes; amino acids; and vitamins. It is a saccharic secretion produced enzymatically from flower nectar that is gathered and stored in honeycombs by honeybees. Honey may cause an allergic reaction in people allergic to pollen.

honey extract—an extract obtained from honey. *See also* honey.

honeydew melon (*Cucumis melo*)—see *Cucumis melo.*

honeysuckle extract (*Lonicera fragrantissima*)—healing, soothing, and anti-inflammatory. Additional uses for external application include cutaneous tonic, protection against sunburn, and overall skin clearing. A dozen or more of the 100 different species of honeysuckle have botanical applications. Apparently, the leaves have more effect than the flowers.

honeysuckle oil—a biological additive with properties similar to those of honeysuckle extract.

hops extract (*Humulus lupulus*)—general effects attributed to hops include sedative, inflammation reducing, and wound healing. Hops are also considered to have preservative value. Their use is claimed effective in acne products. Important constituents include humulone, lupulone, amino acids, chlorogenic acid, rutin, quercetin, flavonoids, and a lupamaric acid. The oil and the bitter principle combine to make hops more useful than chamomile or gentian. Hops extract is made from the cones of the hops vine and can cause allergic reactions.

horse chestnut extract (*Aesculus hippocastanum*)—anti-inflammatory, spasmolytic, and promotes improved circulation. It apparently also has the ability to help reduce the permeability of capillaries. This would make it useful in cases of fragile or broken capillaries. Tannic acid provides horse chestnut extract with toning and astringent properties. Horse chestnut is recommended for use in products designed to stimulate circulation and normalize circulatory disorders, such as creams for improving circulation, and bath salts for the stimulation of the whole organism. Some suppliers cite a recommended dosage of 2 to 5 percent for use in creams and emulsions, and others cite 1 to 10 percent for bath and hair products. Constituents include starch, sugar, protein, tannin, oil, vitamins, phytosterol, and an Aesculus Saponin content. The extract is usually obtained from the seed (fruit).

horseheal—*see* elecampane.

horseradish extract (*Armoracia lapathifolia*)—traditionally used against sunburns and superficial and other non-extensive burns, and to give the skin clarity and freshness. Its antiseptic and skin-clearing properties are linked to its ascorbic acid content. The extract is made primarily from the plant's roots.

horsetail extract (*Equisetum arvense*) (**shave grass**)—stimulating, astringent, soothing, healing, and softening. Horsetail is also described as able to increase the skin's defense mechanism, regulate the skin because of the plant's rich mineral content, and even strengthen connective tissue because of the presence of silicic acid. Some product manufacturers state that when mixed with lady's mantle and eyebright extracts, horsetail extract works to prevent and counteract wrinkles in the eye area. This is an extract of the sterile caules of *Equisetum arvense*, a fern plant whose sprouts have high silicic acid content as well as flavone glycosides and saponin. Amino acids such as citruline, valine, asparaginic acid, lucine, and serine have also been detected as constituents of this extract. The recommended usage level is 1 to 10 percent of a formulation's total composition. It can be beneficial in making both anti-aging and acne products.

hortensis extract—*see* savory.

huang qin extract—a plant extract said to have soothing properties.

hyaluronic acid—a glycosaminoglycan component. Hyaluronic acid occurs naturally in the dermis. It is thought to play a critical role in healthy skin by controlling the physical and biochemical characteristics of epidermal cells. It also regulates general skin activity, such as water content, elasticity, and the distribution of nutrients. Its water-absorption abilities and large molecular structure allow the epidermis to achieve greater suppleness, proper plasticity, and turgor. Hyaluronic acid is a natural moisturizer with excellent water-binding capabilities. In a solution of 2 percent hyaluronic acid and 98 percent water, the hyaluronic acid holds the water so tightly that it appears to create a gel. However, it is a true liquid in that it can be diluted and will exhibit a liquid's normal viscous flow properties. When applied to the skin, hyaluronic acid forms a viscoelastic film in a manner similar to the way it holds water in the intercellular matrix of dermal connective tissues. This performance and behavior suggests that hyaluronic acid makes an ideal moisturizer base, allowing for the delivery of other agents to the skin. Manufacturers claim that the use of hyaluronic acid in cosmetics results in the need for much lower levels of lubricants and emollients in a formulation, thereby providing an essentially greaseless product. Furthermore, its ability to retain water gives immediate smoothness to rough skin surfaces and significantly improves skin appearance. For the benefits of hyaluronic acid to be realized in a cosmetic, the product needs to be applied on a regular basis as it is broken down in skin within 24 to 48 hours of application. Note, this is not the case with hyaluronic acid injections as the technology used is different.

hydrocotyl asiatica—*see* gotu kola extract.

hydrocotyl extract—*see* gotu kola extract.

hydrogen peroxide—a bleaching and oxidizing agent, detergent, and antiseptic. It is generally recognized as a safe preservative, germ killer, and skin bleacher in cosmetics. If used undiluted, it can cause burns of the skin and mucous membranes.

hydrogenated coco glyceride—an emulsifier and emollient, it also has skin-conditioning and water-binding capacities.

hydrogenated polydecene—an emollient that can also serve as a solvent.

hydrogenated polyisobutene—an emollient, which can also control the viscosity of a formulation and improve overall skin feel.

hydrogenated tallow octyldimonium chloride—a conditioner used in clear or emulsion systems. It provides a soft feel and is lubricating in skin care products.

hydrogenated vegetable glyceride—an emollient and emulsifying agent obtained from vegetable oil. It is also used as a stabilizer, a viscosity controller, and to facilitate the spreading of a product. The oil source in this case is not identifiable.

hydrolyzed albumen—*see* hydrolyzed egg.

hydrolyzed algin—a skin conditioner that can help improve skin softness and suppleness.

hydrolyzed animal protein—refers to processed collagen and other animal proteins. The primary function of these proteins is to form a glossy film on the skin. However, depending on the degree of hydrolysis, and thus the size of the final molecule, the action can range from film-forming, in order to reduce moisture loss, to that of individual amino acids, which can penetrate the top layers of the corneum layer. The process of hydrolysis, commonly produced by means of enzyme hydrolysis, breaks the bonds of the larger molecules, making them smaller and smaller until finally one gets the amino acids themselves. Manufacturers hydrolyze the proteins in controlled environments to obtain the desired chain length appropriate for the properties of their formulations. The name listed as such does not indicate any specified level of hydrolysis. *See also* animal protein; collagen; collagen hydrolysates; elastin.

hydrolyzed collagen—*see* collagen hydrolysates.

hydrolyzed corn protein—forms a film on the skin's surface. It is used to reduce loss of the skin's natural moisture. *See also* hydrolyzed vegetable protein.

hydrolyzed egg—a skin-conditioning agent that can aid in skin moisturizing and improve skin texture and feel. It is also used in cosmetics as a natural viscosity controller. *See also* egg protein and egg extract.

hydrolyzed elastin—forms a film on the skin's surface. A processed form of elastin that facilitates its use in skin care formulations. *See also* elastin (hydrolyzed).

hydrolyzed extensin—a skin conditioner used to improve skin softness and suppleness. This is a protein derivative of plant origin.

hydrolyzed fibronectin—a humectant and moisturizing agent for skin creams and lotions. It is a processed form of fibronectin that facilitates its use in skin care formulations. *See also* fibronectin.

hydrolyzed glycosaminoglycans—has hygroscopic properties and a small molecular structure that favors penetration into the outer epidermal layers. This ingredient contains low molecular weight oligosaccharides and can be found in hydrating cosmetics. It is recommended for stressed and aging skin. *See also* glycosaminoglycans.

hydrolyzed golden pea protein—forms a film on the skin's surface. This is a water-soluble liquid protein derivative and a vegetable protein of interest because of its high soluble tyrosine content. Tyrosine is considered to play an important role in stimulating cell growth, and is an integral component of tyrosinase, which is responsible for melanin formation. It is considered by some as the best replacement for hydrolyzed animal protein. *See also* hydrolyzed vegetable protein.

hydrolyzed keratin—a processed form of keratin that facilitates its use in skin care formulations. *See also* hydrolyzed animal protein; keratin.

hydrolyzed lupine protein—may help promote the synthesis of epidermal proteins and lipids. It is also said to limit transepidermal water loss and strengthen the barrier function of the skin. Rich in glutamine peptides and oligosaccharides, it is generally incorporated into repairing, regenerating, and hydrating products. *See also* lupine extract.

hydrolyzed manihot esculenta tuber extract—a botanical with film-forming capacities, helping the skin retain moisture, and which are indicated to also provide a lifting and smoothing effect for the skin.

hydrolyzed milk protein—forms a film on the skin's surface that allows the skin to retain moisture. This is a processed form of milk protein that facilitates and improves performance in skin care formulations. *See also* milk protein.

hydrolyzed mucopolysaccharides—a skin hydrator that helps decrease transepidermal water loss because of its strong water-binding properties. This is a mixture of polysaccharides composed primarily of glucosamine and glucuronic acid, and is derived from the hydrolysis of animal connective tissue. *See also* mucopolysaccharides.

hydrolyzed oat protein—an anti-itching skin protectant with a soothing effect on sensitive skin, its lipid content provides improved lubricating and emollient properties. This is a very smooth vegetable protein, derived by acid, enzyme, or other method of hydrolysis. *See also* hydrolyzed vegetable protein; oat; oat protein.

hydrolyzed potato protein—a vegetable protein that serves as a moisturizing agent. It is reported to have a unique amino acid profile, with reasonable levels of the sulfur-containing amino acids cystine and methionine. This is the hydrolysate of potato protein derived by acid, enzyme, or other method of hydrolysis. *See also* hydrolyzed vegetable protein.

H

hydrolyzed rice bran protein—a skin- and hair-conditioning protein derivative, it can help improve skin softness and pliability. It is obtained through the hydrolysis of rice bran. Its primary constituents include amino acids, peptides, and proteins.

hydrolyzed rice bran protein and glycine soja protein and oxido reductases—a mixture of ingredients that is said to reduce puffiness and dark circles around the eyes. This is a manufactured combination of rice bran protein, soybean protein, and a yeast and enzyme mixture (oxido reductases). *See also* rice bran; soybean protein.

hydrolyzed rice protein—a vegetable protein that serves as a good moisturizing agent. This is the hydrolysate of rice protein derived by acid, enzyme, or other methods of hydrolysis. *See also* hydrolyzed vegetable protein.

hydrolyzed serum proteins—a film-former and skin-conditioning substance that reduces transepidermal water loss and has anti-irritant properties. It is also nourishing to the cells. *See also* hydrolyzed animal protein; serum protein.

hydrolyzed vegetable protein—forms a protein-lipid film on the skin, giving products a moisture-retention capacity. These proteins are obtained from wheat, soybean, corn, peas, or other vegetable source. They are made by the hydrolysate of vegetable protein derived by acid, enzyme, or other method of hydrolysis. Some vegetable proteins have, at least theoretically, a composition that can make them appealing as a replacement for animal protein. However, vegetable proteins generally exhibit a different behavior from animal proteins, which affects the chemical reaction, additive, requirements, and cosmetic product stability.

hydrolyzed wheat protein—offers conditioning, moisturizing, and film-forming properties. It is an effective moisturizer in skin care products, where it helps retain moisture in the skin. It is almost always used as a replacement for hydrolyzed animal protein. It is produced by an enzymatic hydrolysis of wheat gluten. *See also* hydrolyzed vegetable protein.

hydrolyzed wheat protein (AMP isostearoyl)—a skin-conditioning ingredient. This is a neutralized alcohol-soluble wheat protein/fatty acid condensate. It can be found in skin tonics. *See also* hydrolyzed vegetable protein; hydrolyzed wheat protein.

hydrolyzed wheat protein polysiloxane copolymer—upon drying, it forms a protective conditioning film on the skin that reduces water loss. This is a wheat protein attached to silicone, which enhances the effects of protein and silicone on the skin. *See also* hydrolyzed wheat protein.

hydrolyzed wheat protein/PVP crosspolymer—a film former, which can help retain moisture in the skin. It also has hair-conditioning and hair-fixing properties.

hydrolyzed whole wheat protein—a modified form of wheat protein to facilitate its performance and incorporation in skin care formulations. *See also* hydrolyzed wheat protein.

hydrolyzed yeast—the hydrolysate of yeast derived by acid, enzyme, or other method of hydrolysis. *See also* protein; yeast.

hydrotriticum wheat amino acids—an ingredient with good moisture-retention properties. It is reportedly able to penetrate the corneum layers and moisturize from within.

H

hydroquinone—a pigment-lightening agent used in bleaching creams. Hydroquinone combines with oxygen very rapidly and becomes brown when exposed to air. Although it occurs naturally, the synthetic version is the one commonly used in cosmetics. Application to the skin may cause allergic reaction and increase skin sun sensitivity. Hydroquinone is potentially carcinogenic and is associated with causing ochronosis, a discoloration of the skin. The U.S. FDA has banned hydroquinone from OTC cosmetic formulations, but allows 4 percent in prescription products. Its use in cosmetics is prohibited in some European countries and in Australia.

Hydroviton—a trade name for a natural moisturizer derived from rose water, plant sugars, and plant-sourced amino acids. It contains glycerin, sodium lactate, TEA-lactate, serine, lactic acid, urea, sorbitol, lauryl diethylenediaminoglycine, lauryl aminopropylglycinel, and allantoin.

2-hydroxy-ρ-methoxycinnamate—*see* cinoxate.

5-hydroxy-2-hydroxymethyl-gamma-pyridone—a skin-lightening agent apparently 32 times more effective than kojic acid. Indications are that it acts as a tyrosinase inhibitor, with anti-oxidant properties and a capacity to protect against UV radiation.

hydroxyacetic acid—*see* glycolic acid.

hydroxyacetone—*see* dihydroxyacetone.

hydroxycitronellal—used to mask odor.

hydroxydecyl ubiquinone—a potent anti-oxidant. *See* idebenone.

hydroxyethyl acrylate/sodium acryloyldimethyltaurate copolymer—an emulsion stabilizer that can also help increase a formulation's viscosity. In addition, formulators may use it as a dispersing agent and to reduce product transparency.

hydroxyethyl cellulose—a thickener, protective colloid, binder, stabilizer, and suspending agent. It is obtained from wood pulp or chemical cotton by treatment with an alkali. *See also* ethyl cellulose.

hydroxyisohexyl 3-cyclohexene carboxaldehyde—fragrance with a light floral scent. It may cause skin irritation.

hydroxylated lanolin—a modified form of lanolin. It increases the tackiness, stickiness, and emulsifying capacity of lanolin. It is a good suspending agent. It is obtained by the controlled hydroxylation of lanolin. *See also* lanolin.

H

6-hydroxy-5-methoxyindole—said to promote melanin synthesis. Thus it is incorporated into cosmetics to create a tanned look, as with dihydroxyacetone. It is claimed to yield a pigmentation quality equivalent to that obtained from natural tanning.

hydroxy octacosanyl hydroxystearate—a consistency regulating agent for water-in-oil emulsions used to improve the body of an emulsion. It is used in creams, liquid makeup, and lipsticks. This is a synthetic beeswax substitute.

hydroxyphenylpropamidobenzoic acid—a conditioning agent that can help enhance skin softness and smoothness.

hydroxyproline—a skin-conditioning amino acid. It is a component of collagen.

hydroxypropyl methylcellulose—improves foaming properties, lubricity, and formula stabilization. It can help formulators reduce active surfactant concentrations in a product without the loss of the desirable lathering properties, thereby resulting in a milder product. It is mild to the skin and eyes. *See also* cellulose gum.

hydroxypropyltrimonium hydrolyzed wheat protein—enhances skin moisture. This is considered an upgraded version of hydrolyzed wheat protein, particularly with respect to moisturizing properties. It is also a mildness agent for surfactants.

hydroxyproylated y-cyclodextrin—helps prevent skin roughness.

8-hydroxy stilbenes—a skin-lightening compound. It inhibits melanin formation by inhibiting tyrosinase activity. It is not known to cause skin irritation.

6-hydroxy-2,5,7,8-tetramethylchroman-2-carboxylic acid—a free-radical inhibitor, this is a water soluble derivative of vitamin E. Studies indicate it penetrates the skin more effectively than vitamin E, and that as an anti-oxidant it is more effective than BHT. It can be used in moisturizing lotions.

hypericum extract (*Hypericum perforatum*)—*see* St. John's wort extract.

hyssop oil (*Hyssopus officinalis*)—attributed properties include healing, tonic, and stimulating. It can also be used as a fragrance.
Hyssop oil is indicated for dermatitis, eczema, and wounds because of its cicatrizant properties. An infusion of the leaves is reportedly used externally for the relief of muscular rheumatism,
bruises, and discolored contusions. The oil is obtained from the
distillation of the whole plant in flower.

H

Iceland moss extract (*Cetraria islandica*)—used in cosmetics for its tonic properties, it can also be incorporated for its cleansing, emollient, skin-smoothing, and skin-soothing capacities. Despite its name, this plant is not a moss but rather a lichen containing about 70 percent lichen starch, plus fumaric acid, oxalic acid, cetrarin, and licheno-stearic acid.

ichthammol—an anti-microbial. It is a dark sulfonated shale oil obtained via the sulfation and ammoniation of a mineral deposit distillate (shale oil). Its various constituents include saturated and unsaturated hydrocarbons, nitrogen bases, acids, and thiophene derivatives.

ichthyol—*see* ichthammol.

idebenone—an anti-oxidant capable of protecting the skin from a variety of free-radical attacks, including the formation of secondary chemicals that negatively affect skin physiology. It is said to improve intrinsic as well as extrinsic skin damage caused by free-radical formation. Idebenone is a synthetically manufactured form of coenzyme Q10 and has a smaller molecular structure. This allows it to penetrate the skin and apparently the cellular membrane. Clinical studies demonstrate a visible improvement in photodamaged skin, reduced skin roughness and dryness, decreased fine lines and wrinkles, and increased skin hydration. In addition, idebenone helps improve hyperpigmentation because its molecular structure is similar to that of hydroquinone. Although most of the associated benefits are seen primarily in the epidermis, some increase in dermal collagen has also been confirmed. Idebenone has been used for such health-related problems as Alzheimer's and heart disease.

illipe butter—also known as *Shorea stenoptera* seed butter. Emollient and moisturizing, it can promote skin suppleness. Given its high melting point, illipe butter can be used to make a cosmetic preparation, such as lipstick or bar soap, more solid or rigid. Its chemical composition and cosmetic activity are similar to that of cocoa butter. It is found in skin and sun care preparations, massage creams, makeup foundations, lipsticks, and hair conditioners. It is obtained from the nuts of the *Shorea stenoptera* tree, native to Borneo.

illite—a clay similar in structure to montmorillonite. It can be used as an exfoliator and skin softener, and to draw impurities and oil to the skin's surface. It can also serve as an abrasive, an absorbent, to prevent caking and to give a formulation greater bulk. Red and yellow illite clay may also be used as a color additive. Green illite is particularly appropriate in oily skin products. Illite is generally found in masks, body wraps, exfoliators, and cleansers. *See also* montmorillonite.

ilomastat—helps prevent the formation of matrix metalloproteinases. Matrix metalloproteinases are a category of enzymes that contribute to the degradation of the extracellular matrix and its proteins, including collagen. Ilomastat helps prevent the formation of this family of enzymes, which protects the skin's extracellular matrix. It also inhibits certain strains of bacteria and serves as a chelating agent.

imidazolidinyl urea—one of the most commonly used anti-bacterial preservatives given its low sensitizing potential. In 2010, it was the tenth most frequently used preservative in the United States (parabens ranged from first to sixth place). Generally, imidazolidinyl urea is not used alone but as a copreservative with parabens for broad-spectrum activity. Although it may yield low levels of formaldehyde when subjected to destructive methods—such as exposure to high temperatures—under normal use conditions, there is no detection of free formaldehyde release. Of all the formaldehyde-releasing preservatives, imidazolidinyl urea is the one least likely to cause skin sensitization and allergic reactions. *See also* urea.

imidurea—an abbreviated annotation for imidazolidinyl urea. *See* imidazolidinyl urea.

Indian chestnut extract—*see* chestnut extract.

inositol—used in emollients for its ability to hold and retain moisture, it belongs to the vitamin B family. Although found naturally in plant and animal tissue, for commercial use it is isolated from corn.

iodopropynyl butylcarbamate—a preservative with broad fungicidal activity used in skin care products. It is recommended for use in difficult formulation systems.

iris extract (*Iris sp.*)—the juice of fresh iris root employed as a cosmetic and freckle remover. Depending on the part of the plant used—flower, root, or leaf—it can be used for its tonic, perfuming, masking odor, and improving skin condition properties. There are many varieties of iris and most of them have a considerable reputation for their medicinal virtues. The *Iris versicolor* variety, for example, produces an official drug in the *U.S. Pharmacopoeia* and is used in cosmetics for its emollient, masking, and tonic properties.

The extract from the root of the *florentina* variety is used for its tonic and odor-masking properties in bath preparations, moisturizers, night creams, and facial masks.

Irish moss—*see* carrageen extract.

iron oxide (iron oxide black, red, or yellow)—an inorganic compound frequently used to add color to cosmetics. It may have some slight sun screening ability. Iron oxide can vary in color from red to brown, black to orange or yellow, depending on the purity and amount of water added.

isoamyl ρ-methoxycinnamate—also known as isopentyl-4-methoxycinnamate. An organic UV filter and absorber with an approved usage level of up to 10 percent in the European Union.

isoarachidyl neopentanoate—an emollient with SPF-enhancing ability. It is generally used in sunscreen preparations. It is considered to be non-comedogenic.

isobutyl paraben—a preservative.

isocetyl alcohol—a skin conditioner with emollient properties, it may also be used as a viscosity builder within a formulation.

isocetyl stearate—an emollient.

isocream—an emollient. This is a mixture of mineral oil, lanolin, petrolatum, and lanolin alcohol.

isocreme—*see* isocream.

isodecyl citrate—a chemical compound used to inhibit the peroxidation of skin lipids. It is also used in cosmetics as an emollient and to facilitate the incorporation of other, hard to work with, ingredients. Often used in such items as anti-aging creams and lotions, sunscreen preparations, and other skin care cosmetics.

isodecyl isononanoate—an emollient with a very low irritancy level that gives the skin a light, dry feel. It is considered non-comedogenic.

isodecyl neopentanoate—emollient and skin conditioning, it is said to improve skin softness. Some formulators may select it as an alternative to cyclomethicone.

isodecyl oleate—an emollient and moisturizer with wetting and pigment-binding properties.

isodecyl paraben—a preservative.

isododecane—a solvent.

isoeugenol—a volatile oil fraction derived from eugenol. It is also found in ylang-ylang and nutmeg oils. It is used in cosmetics as a fragrance or to mask odor.

isoflavones—a family of phytoestrogens related to flavonoids that appear to have an estrogen-like effect. Clinical studies indicate an anti-aging application, given their ability to inhibit the chemical process leading to collagen degradation in the skin. Some sources cite anti-oxidant and anti-inflammatory properties as well. Among commonly used isoflavones are genistein, genistin, glycitein, glycitin, orobol, and prunetin. Soybeans and other soy-derived products are reported as the richest sources of isoflavones, though they are also obtained from red clover.

isoflavonoids—a family of ingredients derived from isoflavones. Isoflavonoids have demonstrated anti-oxidant properties through UV protection and some might also be immunoprotective. *See also* isoflavones.

isohexadecane—an excellent, non-greasy emollient.

isomerized linoleic acid—a film former it can improve the condition of the skin by helping seal in moisture.

isononyl isononanoate—an emollient and skin conditioner, it improves skin smoothness and softness.

isoparaffinC$_{7-70}$—depending on the carbon length, which can range from 7 to 70 carbons long, isoparaffins are commonly used as solvents. However, several also have emollient properties. *See also* paraffin.

isoprene glycol—a possible substitute for propylene glycol. It has good humectant properties, rubs nicely on the skin, and does not leave a greasy feeling. Isoprene glycol is also compatible with a variety of other organic chemicals commonly used by cosmetic formulators. Tests show good tolerance with respect to toxicity and irritation.

isopropanol—*see* isopropyl alcohol.

isopropyl alcohol—a carrier, anti-bacterial, and solvent for skin care lotions. Isopropyl alcohol is made from propylene, a petroleum derivative.

isopropyl hydroxycetyl ether—an emollient and skin-conditioning ingredient.

isopropyl lauroyl sarcosinate—a neutral amino-acid ester that functions as a skin conditioner.

isopropyl isostearate—an emollient that leaves the skin surface with a smooth and supple finish. It also acts as a binder. Isopropyl isostearate is a derivative of isostearic acid. *See also* stearic acid.

isopropyl jojobate—an emollient and skin conditioner it is the ester of isopropyl alcohol and acids derived from jojoba seed oil. It is odorless and has a lower viscosity level than jojoba oil.

isopropyl lanolate—a skin softener and binder, it aids in the proper spreading of a product. It can also assist in extract penetration, and improve skin feel and texture. It is a lanolin derivative. *See also* lanolin.

isopropyl methoxycinnamate—a sunscreen chemical that acts as a UV absorber.

isopropyl myristate—an emollient, moisturizer, binder, and skin softener that also assists in product penetration. An ester of myristic acid, it is naturally occurring in coconut oil and nutmeg. Although isopropyl myristate is generally considered comedogenic, some ingredient manufacturers clearly specify non-comedogenicity on their data sheets.

isopropyl palmitate—an emollient and moisturizer, it also acts as a binder and solvent. Similar to isopropyl myristate, it is produced from the combination of palmitic acid (coconut or palm oil) and isopropyl alcohol. Enzymes are able to metabolize this ingredient and studies do not show allergic reactions or toxicity. Some sources indicate comedogenicity potential.

isopropyl benzyl salicylate—a UV absorber credited with antioxidant properties serving to prevent lipid peroxidation. It is found often in moisturizers and anti-aging products.

isopropyl paraben—a preservative. *See also* propylparaben and parabens.

isopropyl stearate—a binder, emollient, and moisturizer. It leaves the skin with a smooth and supple finish. *See also* stearic acid.

isosorbide monolaurate—imparts greaseless emollience to creams, lotions, and stock preparations.

isostearamidopropyl PG dimonium chloride—an emulsifier that leaves the skin with a soft, smooth feeling. It is not subject to oxidation or rancidity, and has a very mild toxicological profile.

isostearic acid—an emollient that forms a lipid film on the skin permeable to water vapor, oxygen, and carbon dioxide. It can also serve as a binder in pressed powders, or as a cleansing agent, emulsifier and surfactant in other formulations. Isostearic acid is recommended for use in moisturizing cosmetics. This fatty acid is similar to the waxes secreted by birds for feather maintenance.

isostearyl alcohol—an emollient and viscosity builder derived from isostearic acid. It gives the skin a silky feel after product application.

isostearyl isostearate—an emollient resembling jojoba oil. It leaves an almost imperceptible after-feel. Some sources cite it as comedogenic with a slight irritancy potential. This is a derivative of isostearic acid.

isostearyl neopentanoate—an emollient, binder, and skin-conditioning agent with a moisturizing and softening effect. It has minimal allergenicity potential.

isostearyl stearoyl stearate—an occlusive skin-conditioning agent able to increase the viscosity of a formulation.

isotretinoin—a retinoid derivative with improved bioavailability and percutaneous absorption for acne treatment products.

ivy extract (*Hedera helix*)—said to have a slimming and anti-cellulite effect because of its ability to prevent water accumulation in the skin tissue. Ivy extract is considered anti-bacterial, astringent, tonic, and soothing, particularly in burn cases. Apparently, ivy also has detergent, anti-parasitic, decongestant, and analgesic properties. In addition, ivy is indicated as vasoconstrictive and anti-exudative given its vitamin P content and ability to reduce capillary wall permeability. This extract seems to improve massage tolerance of sensitive skin areas as well. It lowers tissue sensitivity, activates circulation, and helps reduce local inflammation. Ivy extract contains saponins, foaming emulsion stabilizers, and surface-active agents that assist in ingredient penetration and the emulsification of fats. Ivy is effective as a circulation stimulant in shower gels and in bath salts for "orange-peel" and bloated skin. In herbal medicine, a decoction of ivy leaves was traditionally used to treat various skin eruptions and skin ulcers. Fresh ivy leaves were used to dress wounds and pus-exuding sores.

jasmine extract (*Jasminum officinale*)—a fragrance. It also has moisturizing, soothing, and skin-conditioning properties. Some ill-defined and unclear medicinal properties have been attributed to the root extract of several varieties of the 150 jasmine species. These properties include the difficult-to-prove benefit of stimulating the fibroblast with an increase in epidermal cell turnover. Jasmine may cause allergic reactions such as swelling. Jasmine extract is derived from the whole plant. *See also* jasmine oil.

jasmine oil—fragrance. It is credited with moisturizing, soothing, skin-conditioning, and healing properties. Given these properties, it is indicated for dry and sensitive skins, and also for skin with dermatitis. There is no essential oil of jasmine; rather jasmine oil is a volatile oil obtained from the plant's flowers through *enfleurage*, a very time-consuming and costly process. The freshly gathered flowers are sprinkled over oiled glass trays and the flowers are renewed every morning while the plant is in bloom. Finally, the pomade is scraped off the glass, melted at as low a temperature as possible, and then strained. When olive oil is used, the flower petals are placed on coarse cotton cloths previously saturated with the olive oil. The cloths are squeezed under a press, yielding what is termed *huile antique au jasmin*. The oil of jasmine is later separated from the olive oil. This makes jasmine oil one of the most expensive oils available, and can lead to the use of adulterated versions. Its sweet odor is so delicate and unique that until recently, artificial or synthetic production was believed impossible. Today, synthetic otto of jasmine exists. However, a portion of the natural oil must be added to the synthetic mixture for a satisfactory product. Jasmine oil may cause allergic reactions such as swelling, which can last several days.

Job's tears extract—emollient, with anti-inflammatory, tonic, cooling, and calming properties. As a traditional botanical remedy, Job's tears were often used in cases of acne. The plant is a broad-leafed grass native to Southeast Asia.

jojoba oil (*Simmondsia chinensis*)—a moisturizer and emollient. Jojoba oil was traditionally held in high regard by Native Americans of the Sonora Desert for its cosmetic properties.

Mystical properties have been attributed to it for its apparent ability to heal the skin. Jojoba oil reduces transepidermal water loss without completely blocking the transportation of water vapor and gases, providing the skin with suppleness and softness. In addition, it gives cosmetic products excellent spreadability and lubricity. Studies indicate that jojoba oil can penetrate rapidly by absorption via the pores and hair follicles. From these areas, it seems to diffuse into the stratum corneum layer and acts with intercellular lipids to further reduce water loss. Ingredient manufacturers claim that the chemical composition, functionality, blending ability, appearance, and feel of synthetically produced jojoba oil are the same as the natural oil. Jojoba oil is not a primary skin irritant and does not promote sensitization. Although it is generally considered non-comedogenic, laboratory studies indicate slight-to-moderate comedogenicity depending on the potency of the oil. Jojoba oil is derived from the plant seeds.

jojoba esters—an emollient and skin-conditioning agent made from jojoba oil and jojoba wax. *See also* jojoba oil.

jojoba powder—a skin conditioner, it is obtained from the dried and ground jojoba seeds.

jojoba wax—employed as a natural scrub bead in scrub gels, scrub soaps, and exfoliating products. It is also emollient, used to control product viscosity, and helps improve the skin's look and feel. Jojoba wax is a waxy substance obtained from the jojoba seed.

jonquil—*see* narcissus flower extract.

juniper extract (*Juniperus communis*)—a fragrance. It is also considered a mild skin stimulant. Juniper extract is believed to help increase epidermal cell turnover. There are some indications that it could also be beneficial for cellulite treatment.

juniper oil—anti-septic, astringent, cleansing, and toning, if used properly. It is also credited with good penetration capabilities. Juniper oil is considered helpful in treating acne and for oily skin. It is also indicated for dermatitis and eczema. Obtained from the distillation of the plant's small branches, juniper oil can be irritating in improper amounts.

juniper berry oil—effective for treating acne. Juniper berry oil has the same properties as those of juniper oil, but it is extracted from the plant's berry rather than its small branches. A distillation of the berries yields the best quality oil.

K

Kalanchoe daigremontiana **leaf extract**—considered a humectant, with astringent and skin-soothing properties. Product manufacturers indicate that it can impart a softer, smoother, more hydrated aspect to the skin. Its constituents include triterpenes, flavonoids, and steroids. This extract is obtained from the leaves of the *Kalanchoe daigremontiana* plant, a succulent found in tropical and subtropical areas.

kaolin (China clay)—a mixture of various aluminum silicates. It is often used in powders and masks given its absorbent, abrasive, bulking, and opacifying properties. This white, soft powder has good coverage and absorption abilities for both water and oil, making it an appropriate absorber of the oil and sweat secreted by the skin. It adheres well to the skin's surface, yet is easily removed with normal cleansing procedures. Kaolin is considered a non-comedogenic raw material.

kaolin China clay—*see* kaolin.

karite (unsaponifiable)—also known as butyrospermum parkii; shea butter. One of a group of vegetable oils with a small molecular structure that is capable of penetrating and possibly becoming involved in the biochemical process of the dermis. It is considered a biological precursor in ceramide synthesis. Karite contains steroidal and triterpenic structures. It is believed that the unsaponifiable fraction of karite can stimulate the dermal fibroblast to synthesize collagen, elastin, proteoglycans, and glycoproteins. *See also* shea butter.

karite butter—*see* shea butter.

kelp—a marine product derived from the giant Pacific kelp. *See* seaweed extract.

keratin—a surface-protective agent with film-forming and moisturizing action. Keratin is often used in cosmetics for its moisture-retention and protective effect. *See also* protein.

keratin amino acids—a mixture of amino acids obtained from the complete hydrolysis of keratin. Like keratin, keratin amino acids have skin-conditioning properties, and they are also anti-static. *See also* amino acids; keratin.

khus-khus—*see* vetiver oil.

kigelia africana fruit extract—a botanical native to Africa with skin-conditioning properties. It has been used in traditional African medicine to treat eczema, and to firm and tone the skin. Ingredient suppliers also attribute it with anti-oxidant, anti-bacterial, anti-fungal, and anti-inflammatory properties, indicating it for use in anti-aging, post-sun, and skin-firming formulations. Among its constituents are fatty acids, coumarins, caffeic acid, and sterols.

kiwi fruit and powder—the fruit of the kiwi contains a variety of polyphenol anti-oxidants and the seeds can be ground into an abrasive powder that is used in scrubs.

kojic acid—a skin-lightening agent that acts through anti-oxidant activity. Kojic acid is a tyrosinase inhibitor, although it is not as effective as licorice extract. When combined with allantoin and other proper ingredients in sunscreen preparations, the mixture can inhibit UV-caused erythema and accelerate wound healing. It is also found to be skin sensitizing and can be irritating.

kojic acid dipalmitate—classified as an emollient, preparations containing kojic acid dipalmitate are said to inhibit UV-induced erythema. *See also* kojic acid.

kojic acid monostearate—a kojic acid derivative said to inhibit tyrosinase, and thus the formation of melanin. Kojic acid monostearate is used in skin-lightening preparations. *See also* kojic acid.

kola extract (*Cola acuminata*)—largely known for its stimulating, astringent, and healing properties, research has also established anti-inflammatory and anti-irritant properties. This extract may be used for dressing wounds. Kola extract is also somewhat effective for preventing the penetration of certain substances into the viable epidermis. It has a high content of caffeine and other stimulants. The extract is obtained from the kola nut.

krameria triandra root extract—manufacturers note an ability to modulate stress-related hormone production in the epidermis. Therapeutic benefits include anti-inflammatory, free-radical scavenging, anti-aging and an ability to protect against lipid peroxidation. Beneficial for red, chapped, and stressed skin. The plant is native to Peru.

kukui nut oil (*Aleurites moluccana*) (**candlenut**)—the kukui nut tree was used by early Hawaiians to soothe cuts and burns and to help protect the skin from damage because of sun and surf. Kukui nut oil is reported to have excellent penetration properties, to aid in soothing and moisturizing the skin, and relieve chapped skin and irritations. This oil does not leave the skin with a greasy after feel. Kukui nut oil is apparently an excellent treatment for psoriasis and eczema, and is also beneficial for acne and other common skin disorders. In addition, it is a sunscreen solubilizer that reduces the greasy feel often associated with sun products. Studies indicate possible sunscreen capabilities of its own, and when used with other sunscreens, it may enhance a formulation's efficacy. Native to Hawaii, the nuts and kernels are roasted and then pressed for their clear oil, which has a high linoleic and linoleic acid content. It is usually supplemented and stabilized with vitamins A, C, and E.

K

lactamide MEA—a surfactant that can also act as a thickener, foam booster, and stabilizer.

lactic acid (sodium lactate)—a multi-purpose ingredient used as a preservative, exfoliant, moisturizer, and to provide acidity to a formulation. In the body, lactic acid is found in the blood and muscle tissue as a product of the metabolism of glucose and glycogen. It is also a component of the skin's natural moisturizing factor. Lactic acid has better water intake than glycerin. Studies indicate an ability to increase the water-retention capacity of the stratum corneum. They also show that the pliability of the stratum corneum layer is closely related to the absorption of lactic acid; that is, the greater the amount of absorbed lactic acid, the more pliable the stratum corneum layer. Researchers report that continuous use of preparations formulated with lactic acid in concentrations ranging between 5 and 12 percent provided a mild to moderate improvement in fine wrinkling and promote softer, smoother skin. Its exfoliating properties can help in the process of removing excess pigment from the surface of the skin, as well as improving skin texture and feel. Lactic acid is an alpha hydroxy acid occurring in sour milk and other lesser-known sources, such as beer, pickles, and foods made through a process of bacterial fermentation. It is caustic when applied to the skin in highly concentrated solutions. *See also* alpha hydroxy acid.

lactobacillus/**papaya fruit ferment extract**—a papaya extract obtained through a fermentation process using *lactobacillus* as the fermenting agent. *Lactobacillus* is a "friendly bacteria" that is naturally occurring in the body and that is used in the fermentation process for certain foods, such as yogurt and sour milk. *See also* papaya enzyme.

lactobacillus/*Solanum lycopersicum* **(tomato) fruit ferment extract**—considered anti-oxidant, anti-aging, and able to provide long-term skin-conditioning activity. This is a filtrate obtained through a fermentation process using lactobacillus as the fermenting agent. *Lactobacillus* is a "friendly bacteria" that is naturally occurring in the body, and used in the fermentation process for certain foods, such as yogurt and sour milk. *See also* tomato.

lactobacillus/Theobroma cacao **fruit ferment filtrate**—helps reduce inflammation.

lactoperoxidase—a glycoprotein with anti-microbial activity, it is used as a stabilizing ingredient to help improve formulation stability and product shelf-life. It is naturally occurring in milk.

lady's mantle extract (*Alchemilla vulgaris*) (**alchemilla**)—said to have UV-absorption ability for both the UVA and UVB spectrums. Other properties include anti-free radical, healing, and anti-inflammatory. Herbalists considered lady's mantle extract to be one of the best wound-healing herbs, and credit it with an ability to dry wounds, reduce inflammation, and promote quicker healing. Thus, it is considered effective in acne products. The active constituents of this perennial plant include tannins, rendering it effective against irritation, itching, and skin burns. Lady's mantle extract contains silicon/silicic acid, and it is reported that when combined with eyebright and horsetail, they all work synergistically to strengthen the connective tissue.

ladybell root extract (*Adenophora stricta*)—a humectant, helping maintain moisture in the skin. It is said to improve dryness and itching due to extreme climates.

lady's thistle extract—*see* milk thistle.

laminaria saccharina extract—a member of the kelp family. *See also* seaweed extract.

laneth-10—an emulsifier that is particularly effective when working with lanolin, it is also used as a surfactant for improving product spreadability and to control product viscosity. This is the polyethylene glycol ether of lanolin alcohol.

laneth-10-acetate—an emulsifier with emollient properties. This is the acetylated ester of an ethoxylated ether of lanolin alcohol.

lanolide—a vegetable-derived substitute for lanolin. It is considered to be a good lanolin replacement due to given an absence of pesticides, anti-parasitic constituents, and heavy metals, which can be present in lanolin.

lanolin—an emollient with moisturizing properties and an emulsifier with high water–absorption capabilities. It forms a network on the skin's surface rather than a film, as is the case with petrolatum (Vaseline®). While long-term studies associate a low incidence of allergic reactions to lanolin, it remains a controversial ingredient based on a potential pesticide content and potential comedogenicity. There is a move among high-quality lanolin manufacturers to produce low-pesticide lanolin and among high-quality cosmetic formulators and manufacturers to use

L

the purist form available. Lanolin's comedogenicity potential is increasingly debated as some researchers believe it to be inaccurate, especially when lanolin is used in an emulsion. Lanolin is a sheep's wool derivative formed by a fat-like viscous secretion of the sheep's sebaceous glands. Some consider it a natural wax.

lanolin (hydrogenated)—a lanolin derivative. *See also* lanolin.

lanolin USP (modified)—an emollient and an emulsifier. This is a highly purified lanolin that meets USP monograph specifications requiring analysis for trace contaminants. *See also* lanolin.

lanolin acetate—a lanolin derivative. *See also* lanolin.

lanolin alcohol—widely used as an emulsifier and emollient in water-in-oil systems. It absorbs a considerable amount of water that is then slowly released for moisturization purposes. Lanolin alcohol is a mixture of organic alcohols obtained from the hydrolysis of lanolin. It may cause skin sensitivity and allergic reactions.

lanolin oil—a lanolin derivative. This is the liquid fraction of lanolin obtained by physical means from whole lanolin. *See also* lanolin.

lanolin wax—a lanolin derivative. This is the semisolid fraction of lanolin obtained by physical means from whole lanolin. *See also* lanolin.

lanolin derivatives—a mixture of unspecified lanolin-derived products. *See also* lanolin.

lappa extract—*see* burdock extract.

Lapsana cummunis **extract (hawk's bread; crepin)**—skin-protective and anti-oxidant properties are attributed to extracts from the *Lapsana* family, and particularly to the *cummunis* species. Formulations with this extract are credited with anti-aging and anti-wrinkle activity. It has also demonstrated an ability to protect the skin against free-radical damage. It is also an anti-septic and a disinfectant.

lasilium—*see* sodium lacate methylsilanol.

lauramide DEA (lauric acid diethanolamide)—a thickener, foam stabilizer, and viscosity builder in cosmetic formulations. It is added to liquid detergents and lauryl sulfate-type cleansers to help stabilize the lather and improve foam formation.

laurel (*Laurus nobilis*) (bay laurel)—when used in oil form, it is said to have anti-septic and astringent properties. This would make it effective for healing and skin problems. The oil is pressed from the berries and leaves.

laureth-2—a surfactant and emulsifying ingredient. It is the polyethylene glycol ether of lauryl alcohol. Increasing the number of moles (laureth-3, laureth-7, and so on) usually makes the product milder. *See also* lauryl alcohol.

laureth-3—a surfactant, detergent, and emulsifier used in cosmetic preparations. *See also* lauryl alcohol.

laureth-7—a wetting agent also used as an emulsifier, surfactant, detergent, and solubilizer for active substances. *See also* lauryl alcohol.

laureth-12—a surfactant, detergent, and emulsifier in cosmetic formulations. *See also* lauryl alcohol.

laureth-23—an emulsifier used with more frequency in oil-in-water than water-in-oil emulsions, though it is effective in both. It is also an emulsion stabilizer and can act as a surfactant. Laureth-23 may cause very minor irritation to skin and eyes. *See also* lauryl alcohol.

lauric acid (η-dodecanoic acid)—given its foaming properties, its derivatives are widely used as a base in the manufacture of soaps, detergents, and lauryl alcohol. Lauric acid is a common constituent of vegetable fats, especially coconut oil and laurel oil. It may have a synergistic effect in a formula to help fight against micro-organisms. It is a mild irritant but not a sensitizer, and some sources cite it as comedogenic.

lauric acid diethanolamide—*see* lauramide DEA.

lauroamphocarboxyglycinate—an organic cleansing agent that removes oil and dirt, and can boost foam, but that can also be slightly irritating to the skin.

lauroamphodiacetate—a mild cleansing agent.

lauroyl methionine lysinate—a free-radical scavenger used in anti-aging skin care cosmetics.

lauroyl lysine—an amino acid that also serves as a skin-conditioning agent and formulation viscosity controller. *See also* lysine.

lauryl alcohol—used in chemical formulations for a variety of purposes, including as an emulsion stabilizer, a skin-conditioning emollient, and a viscosity-increasing agent.

lauryl aminopropyl glycine—a skin-conditioning agent.

lauryl betaine—a skin-conditioning agent. In hair care, it is used as an anti-static conditioning agent and a foam booster.

lauryl diethylenediamino glycine—a skin-conditioning ingredient that appears to have greater application in hair formulations, where it is reported to work as an anti-static agent.

lauryl glucoside—a mild surfactant.

lauryl lactate—an emollient, detergent/emulsifier, and surfactant used in cosmetic formulations.

lauryl methyl gluceth-10 hydroxypropyl dimonium chloride—has anti-irritant, skin conditioning, humectant, and moisturizing properties.

laurylmethicone copolyol—an emulsifier with excellent waterproof properties when used in the proper concentration and with other emulsifiers.

lauryl PCA—an emulsifier that has good affinity with skin lipids. It can increase a product's moisturizing action by decreasing transepidermal water loss. Lauryl PCA is a lipophilic moisturizer with a delayed and remnant effect. Also used as a thickener or viscosity-control agent, it is derived from natural raw materials. This is the lauric ester of PCA.

lauryl PEG-9 polydimethylsiloxyethyl dimethicone—a skin-conditioning ingredient that is also a surfactant, emulsifier, viscosity controller, and solubilizing agent.

lauryl sarcosine—a surfactant for cosmetic formulations.

lavender flower oil—the principal constituent of lavender is the volatile oil, of which the dried flowers contain 1.5 to 3 percent; fresh flowers yield about 0.5 percent. Lavender flower oil is pale yellow, yellowish-green, or nearly colorless. Oil distilled from the earliest flowers is pale and contains a higher proportion of the more valuable esters. The oil distilled from later flowers has a majority of the less valuable ester and is darker in color. Lavender oil owes its delicate perfume primarily to two of its esters that control the scent. Of these, the principal one is linalyl acetate; the second is linalyl butyrate. Other esters present include geraniol, linalool, and limonene. *See also* lavender oil.

lavender green oil—*see* lavender flower oil; lavender oil.

lavender oil (*Lavandula officinalis*)—a fragrance. Lavender oil is considered an all-purpose oil credited with many therapeutic properties, including anti-allergenic, anti-inflammatory, antiseptic, anti-bacterial, anti-spasmodic, balancing, energizing, soothing, healing, tonic, and stimulating. In addition, it is said to help clean small wounds after washing and regulate skin functions. It may also have insect-repellent properties. Lavender oil works well on all skin types and produces excellent results when used for oily skin as well as in the treatment of acne, burns (sunburns as well as other superficial and non-extensive types), dermatitis, eczema, and psoriasis. Lavender oil is said to normalize any skin type and to stimulate cellular

L

growth and regeneration. When added to other oils, lavender can enhance and balance their effect. Lavender is also claimed to help relieve stress, and as such, is believed to be useful in treating skin problems caused or aggravated by stress. The known use of this oil extends at least to the Roman era, when it was a popular additive to baths. It derived its name from this practice and from the Roman word *lavare*, meaning to wash. The oil's main component is linalool acetate; other actives include geraniol, borneol, ocimene, and pinene. Lavender oil is distilled by using the flower tops and stalks. It is generally considered non-toxic, non-sensitizing, and non-irritating.

lawsone with dihydroxyacetone—one of the 21 FDA-approved sunscreen chemicals and listed as a Category I UVB-absorber. Its approved usage level is 3 percent. Dihydroxyacetone (DHA) alone is used as a self-tanning agent in self-tanning products. DHA and lawsone together act as a sunscreen.

lecithin—a natural emollient, emulsifier, anti-oxidant, and spreading agent, lecithin is a hydrophilic ingredient that attracts water and acts as a moisturizer. Generally obtained for cosmetic products from eggs and soybeans, it is found in all living organisms.

lecithin (hydrogenated)—an emulsifier.

lemon balm—*see* balm mint oil.

lemon bioflavonoids extract—obtained by extraction of oil rind. *See also* bioflavonoids; lemon extract.

lemon extract (*Citrus limonum*)—considered anti-bacterial, antiseptic, astringent, and toning. It is also perfuming. Lemon extract is suggested for treating sunburn, acne problems, and oily skin. This extract contains citric acid and vitamins B and C. It can cause irritation and allergic reactions.

lemon oil—as one of the most versatile essential oils in aromatherapy, it is considered a counterirritant, anti-septic, blood purifier, and lymphatic stimulant. The volatile oil is obtained from the fresh peel of *Citrus limonum* (citrus lemon) that contains an essential oil and a bitter principle. Crystals of the glucoside hesperidin are deposited by the evaporation of the white, pulpy portion when boiled in water. Diluted acids decompose it into hesperidin and glucose. The oil is more fragrant and valuable if obtained by expression rather than distillation. Lemon oil can cause an allergic reaction.

lemon peel—*see* lemon oil.

lemongrass oil (*Cymbopogon citratus*)—considered astringent and tonic, it has also exhibited anti-fungal properties. It is widely used in the perfume and soap industries. Lemongrass oil is the volatile oil distilled from the leaves of the lemon grasses.

lettuce extract (*Lactuca virosa*)—said to have emollient properties in its fresh state, but after processing for use in cosmetics, this property is unlikely to be retained. Herbologists attribute a sedative, narcotic property to lettuce extract. It is obtained from wild lettuce (not the garden and salad variety), a plant growing to a maximum height of 6 feet. The whole plant is rich in milky juice that flows freely from any cut made to it.

leuconostoc/**radish root ferment filtrate**—an anti-fungal and anti-microbial, it can be used when designing preservative systems. It is obtained via the fermentation of radish root by *leuconostoc*, a micro organism.

lichen extract—a preservative that can be used against certain types of bacteria, fungi, and yeast. It also contributes to the activity of other preservatives. Lichen extract is a water-free, natural, active agent extracted from alpine lichen. It is non-toxic and non-irritating to the skin.

licorice extract (*Glycyrrhiza glabra*)—considered an anti-irritant, studies indicate an ability to absorb UVA and UVB rays. Studies also conclude that licorice extract has a depigmenting effect as well as an inhibitory effect on melanin synthesis given its ability to act as a tyrosinase inhibitor. As a depigmenting agent, licorice extract is described as more effective than kojic acid and 75 times more effective than ascorbic acid. The chief constituent of licorice root is glycyrrhizin, present in concentrations that range from 5 to 24 percent depending on the variety of licorice used. A member of the bean family, licorice's pharmacological properties are found in the plant's roots and stem.

licorice root extract—*see* licorice extract.

lily extract—there are almost 100 different known varieties of lilies to which antiseptic and skin-clearing properties are generally ascribed. Herbalists have also credited the Madonna lily variety with soothing and astringent properties. The extract, obtained from the bulbs of this variety, is used primarily for its emollient, healing, soothing, and anti-inflammatory action. The extract from leaves and roots of the white pond lily variety has been described as astringent, healing, and anti-inflammatory.

lime blossom extract—perfuming. It is also an emollient with soothing and anti-septic properties. Lime blossom extract is a source of vitamin C. It can cause adverse reactions when the skin is exposed to sunlight.

lime oil (*Citrus acida, Citrus aurantifolia*)—has similar properties and uses as lemon oil. Lime oil is extracted from lime skin by cold pressure or distillation. *See also* lemon oil.

lime tree extract—the main extract from the lime tree is the one obtained from the blossoms. Some extract may also be obtained from leaves and sap. Lime tree extract is sometimes referred to as linden. *See also* linden extract.

limonene—used as a perfuming ingredient and deodorant, it can also act as a solvent. It is naturally occurring citrus rind and in a variety of essential oils including, grapefruit, lime, peppermint, and sage.

d-limonene—used for perfuming and to mask odor. It is a chemical constituent of citrus oil. *See also* lemon oil; limonene.

linalool—a fragrant component of both lavender and coriander. It can be incorporated into cosmetics for perfuming, deodorant, or odor-masking activity.

linden extract (*Tilia sp.*)—extract from the bark can be used to help problem or blemished skin, and is considered refreshing and soothing. Linden extract can also be obtained from linden blossoms and is credited with anti-septic, skin-clearing, soothing, sedative, circulation-stimulating, hydrating, and astringent properties. Linden extract may be used effectively in creams and emulsions for irritated skin, as well as in bath salts for the relaxation of muscle tension and cold. In oil form, linden may be used to mask odor and as a skin conditioner.

linoleamide DEA—a highly effective thickener. It enhances product slip and feel, and is also a conditioner, stabilizer, and viscosity builder. *See also* linoleic acid.

linoleamidopropyl PG-dimonium chloride phosphate—a vegetable-derived emulsifier. It leaves the skin with a smooth after feel, and is non-irritating.

linoleic acid (**vitamin F**)—also known as omega-6. An emulsifier, it is also cleansing, emollient, and skin conditioning. Some formulations incorporate it as a surfactant. Linoleic acid prevents dryness and roughness. A deficiency of linoleic acid in the skin is associated with symptoms similar to those characterizing eczema, psoriasis, and a generally poor skin condition. In numerous laboratory studies where a linoleic acid deficiency was induced, a topical application of linoleic acid in its free or esterified form quickly reversed this condition. In addition, there is some evidence in laboratory tests that linoleic acid may inhibit melanin production by decreasing tyrosinase activity and suppressing melanin polymer formation within melanosomes. Linoleic acid is an essential fatty acid found in a variety of plant oils, including soybean and sunflower.

linoleic acid ethylester—*see* ethyl linoleate.

linoleic acid triglyceride—an emollient and good penetrating agent, it is not widely used because its unsaturated nature creates rancidity problems.

linolenic acid—also known as alpha-linolenic acid; omega-3. An essential fatty acid found in most drying oils. It is slightly irritating to the mucous membranes. It may be used in a cosmetic preparation for any of the following broad uses: anti-static, cleansing, emollient, skin-conditioning, and surfactant properties.

linolenic acid triglyceride—an emollient of limited use because of potential rancidity problems. It is a good penetrating agent.

linseed oil—its botanical properties are listed as emollient, anti-inflammatory, and healing. Derived from the flax plant seed, the oil is obtained by expression with little or no heat.

lipid concentrate—a vague description, as it does not refer to the lipid's origin or source. Lipids, when added to the skin, are considered moisturizers. They renew the skin's barrier function and reduce moisture loss.

lipo hydroxy acid—also known as LHA. *See also* beta-lipohydroxy acid.

liposomes—extremely small, double layer, hollow, spherical, phospholipid membrane vesicles able to encapsulate water-soluble as well as oil-soluble substances. Their compatibility and affinity with cellular membranes allow them to be easily accepted and metabolized by the skin, and provide the skin with "actives" that would not be so readily accepted otherwise. Liposome effectiveness is measured by their ability to deliver encapsulated actives ingredients to target sites. By varying the type of phospholipids used to make liposomes and/or by attaching certain molecules to the surface of liposomes, they can be engineered to have many useful properties, which include: releasing their active content upon reaching the target site; protecting ingredients from acidic and enzymatic degradation before reaching the target site; protecting compounds from premature oxidation; targeting certain tissues or cell types; acting as time releasers of valuable actives. In addition to their carrier abilities and penetration properties, liposomes provide the upper stratum corneum with a pleasant and smooth feeling. Liposomes are predominantly formed by phospholipids of natural, semisynthetic, and/or synthetic origin. Liposomes have brought to the cosmetic field widespread

L

interest in the concepts of microencapsulation and targeted substance delivery.

liquid paraffin—*see* paraffin.

liquorice extract—*see* licorice extract.

liquorice root extract—*see* licorice extract.

lithium magnesium sodium silicate—used to control a formulation's viscosity and to reduce product density or bulk, for example in depilatory or powder-based products.

live yeast cell derivative—*see* tissue respiratory factor.

lotus leaf extract (*Nelumbo nucifera*)—potentially beneficial in anti-cellulite and slimming products, some studies are also indicating skin-darkening properties, which would make it applicable for self-tanning products. Its constituents include isoflavones.

lovage oil (*Levisticum officinale*)—ascribed properties include cleansing, depurative, and draining. In addition, the roots and fruit have aromatic and stimulant activity. Lovage oil is appropriate for use on oily skin. This oil is produced by distillation of the roots, though the leaves and seeds are also used for therapeutic purposes.

luo han guo extract (*Siraitia grosvenorii*)—also known as monk fruit. Studies indicate anti-oxidant properties, though it is mostly cited as a natural and potent sweetener for foods.

lupine amino acids—reported to have excellent hydrating capabilities, lupine amino acids are often found in moisturizers, cleansers, and washes. They are derived from the seeds of *Lupinus albus*. *See also* lupine extract.

lupine extract (*Lupinus albus*)—research attributes a number of physiological benefits to lupine extract, impacting both the stratum corneum and the epidermis. Generally, lupine extract appears to enhance cellular activity (evidence indicates that it may penetrate down to the basal layer) and thicken the epidermis and stratum corneum. It strengthens the epidermal structure by stimulating the production of epidermal proteins, notably filaggrin (which promotes keratin synthesis) and epidermal lipids, including ceramides, cholesterol, and di- and triglycerides. Studies also indicate an improvement and/or restoration of the stratum corneum's barrier function, resulting in reduced transepidermal water loss. This might be attributed to lupine's ability to promote protein and lipid production. Lupine extract is rich in oligosaccharides and low molecular-weight peptides that are high in glutamic acid. It may be particularly beneficial when used in combination with such moisturizing ingredients

L

as lactic acid. Lupine extract is most likely to be found in skin restructuring, repairing, and hydrating preparations. *See also* lupine amino acids.

lysine—a skin-conditioning amino acid. *See also* amino acid.

lysine PCA—increases cellular oxygen intake and improves moisture. Lysine PCA is also used as a neutralizing agent and pH buffer in skin care formulations.

lysine carboxymethyl cysteinate—a water-soluble amino acid complex with the ability to regulate oil secretion.

lysine lauroyl methionate—an amino acid that acts to improve the skin's look, feel, and overall condition.

L

MI/MCI (methylchloroisothiazolinone)—a preservative that works against bacteria and fungi. It is associated with a sensitizing potential, including allergic reactions, in products intended to stay on the skin (e.g., night creams). Its recommended concentration levels range from 7.5 ppm (parts per million) for leave-on products to 15 ppm for rinse-off preparations such as soaps and cleansers. However, MI/MCI in concentrations as low as 7 ppm may induce sensitization.

macadamia nut oil (*Macadamia integrifolia*)—a carrier and an emollient with excellent spreadability, lubrication, and penetration properties. It is moisturizing, leaves a good, smooth, non-greasy afterfeel, and is very gentle to the skin. Its fatty acid composition is similar to the major fatty acid composition of skin sebum, including some of the acids that are crucial to maintaining the skin's water-barrier functions. Macadamia nut oil is beneficial in skin-softening and nourishing preparations. It is also useful in products for mature and/or dry skin given its palmitoleic acid content (up to 20 percent). Palmitoleic acid is a naturally occurring fatty acid produced by the sebaceous glands, the production of which decreases with age. The nut's weight is 70 to 80 percent oil, specifically triglyceride oil and palmitoleic oil. It is very cosmetically stable with low rancidity, and naturally contains tocopherols. The macadamia (nut) tree is grown primarily in Australia and the Hawaiian Islands.

macadamia ternifolia seed oil—*see* macadamia nut oil.

***Macrocystis pyrifera* extract**—also known as bladder kelp. *See also* kelp; seaweed extract.

madonna lily—*see* white lily bulb extract.

magnesium—plays an important role in various processes within the skin, including amino acid synthesis and protein synthesis (e.g., collagen), and in the metabolism of calcium, sodium, and phosphorus.

magnesium aluminum silicate—a thickener with texture-modification and emulsion-stabilizing abilities, as well as astringent properties. This is refined and purified smectite clay. It is non-comedogenic and non-toxic.

magnesium ascorbyl phosphate (**magnesium-1-ascorbyl-2-phosphate**)—a stabilized, synthetically derived version of vitamin C. It is reported to be as effective as vitamin C in regulating collagen biosynthesis, and as an anti-oxidant. *See also* vitamin C.

magnesium aspartate—used in a cosmetic to improve skin condition, look, and feel. Some manufacturers note an ability to promote the adhesion of basal layer cells to the dermal–epidermal junction and in particular to the collagen found there. It would be used in anti-aging and anti-wrinkle cosmetics. This is the magnesium salt of aspartic acid.

magnesium laureth sulfate—a mild surfactant and cleansing agent.

magnesium silicate—*see* talc.

magnesium sulfate—an inorganic salt used as a bulking agent in cosmetic preparations.

maize germ oil—*see* corn oil.

maize gluten amino acids—*see* corn amino acids.

malachite extract—a mineral mostly composed of copper carbonate hydroxide. Some sources cite anti-oxidant and skin protectant activity, associating its therapeutic attributes with its copper content, but clinical evidence is scarce.

maleated soya bean oil—*see* soybean oil.

malic acid—the third smallest alpha hydroxy acid in terms of molecular size. Although it is used in numerous cosmetic products, particularly those indicating a "fruit acid" content and generally designed for anti-aging, unlike glycolic and lactic acids, its skin benefits have not been extensively studied. Some formulators consider it difficult to work with, particularly when compared to other AHAs, and it can be somewhat irritating. It is rarely used as the only AHA in a product. It is found naturally occurring in apples. *See also* alpha hydroxy acid.

mallow extract (*Malva sylvestris*)—attributed with anti-inflammatory, soothing, refreshing, emollient, and wound-healing properties. Mallow extract has high mucilage content. This permits it to swell and form a soft, soothing, protective gel when put in contact with water. It is beneficial in eye treatment preparations, and could also be useful in moisturizers. The extract is often derived from the leaves and flowers of *Malva sylvestris*, generally known as blue, common, or high mallow, although it can be obtained from other types of mallow such as marsh, musk, dwarf, and tree-sea.

M

Malpighia glabra **fruit extract**—*see* acerola.

malt extract—has rubefacient properties in cosmetics due to the presence of yeast. It is tonic, leaving a feeling of overall well-being on the skin, and is a skin protector. Malt extract is used in face masks and toning lotions as a nutrient and texturizer. This dark syrup is obtained by evaporating an aqueous extract of partially germinated and dried barley seeds.

maltodextrin—a polysaccharide obtained most often from corn, potato, or rice starch. It is considered to be absorbent, and skin conditioning. It can also be employed as an emulsion stabilizer and/or a film former. Maltodextrin is incorporated into a variety of cosmetic preparations, including face powders, makeup, creams, lotions, gels, and soaps.

malva—a traditional emollient and moisturizer. Malva is part of the mallow family. *See also* mallow extract.

mandarin extract—has similar properties to those of orange extract. It is obtained from mandarin orange peel. *See also* orange extract.

mandarin oil—its botanical properties are very close to those of orange, with mandarin's sedative and anti-spasmodic properties being more pronounced. It is expressed from the peel of mandarin oranges.

manganese—as an oligoelement, manganese plays a role in collagen synthesis and skin moisturizing. Patents have been assigned on the use of manganese, zinc, and copper in the treatment of acne and sunburns. It can also be used as a colorant, providing a violet color to a product.

manganese aspartate—a skin conditioner, this is the combination of L-aspartic acid and manganese salt.

manganese gluconate—a skin conditioner used to improve or maintain the skin's texture and feel.

mango (*Mangifera indica*)—associated with various benefits, including anti-oxidant skin-softening and smoothing properties, thanks to natural enzymatic activity. When listed simply as mango, it is difficult to identify which part of the plant is used. This limits a full understanding as to why mango was selected for a cosmetic formula. While mango fruit is considered astringent in a cosmetic, the extract of both the fruit and leaf are skin conditioning. Mango seed is abrasive and hence used in scrubs, while the seed oil is emollient. Thus, more specific information as to the form or portion of the plant used is necessary to determine function in the cosmetic formulation.

M

mango butter—emollient, moisturizing, and anti-inflammatory. It could also promote cellular rejuvenation. Mango butter demonstrates some ability to protect against UV rays and appears to release salicylic acid. Constituents include tocopherol, phytosterols, olein, and fatty acids (including stearic and oleic acids). Mango butter is very stable when exposed to oxygen, and can replace paraffin-based emollients. Studies have indicated overall consumer preference for lotions containing mango butter over those using avocado butter or apricot kernel oil. Obtained from the kernel within the mango stone, it is used in skin care cosmetics, sun and post-sun products, hair conditioners, and shampoos.

mannuronate methylsilanol—*see* sodium mannuronate methylsilanol.

margosa oil—commonly known as neem. It is considered to be a healing oil for its anti-septic and sebum-regulating properties. *See also* neem extract.

marigold extract (*Calendula officinalis*)— has anti-septic, healing, and soothing effects. Traditionally, marigold extract was used to heal skin rashes and to clean minor wounds after washing. It may be used against sunburns and other superficial burns due to some emollient capabilities. It is useful in eye treatment cosmetics. Marigold extract's constituents include flavonoids, oleanoic acid glycosides, carotenoids, and phenolic acid. Marigold's carotenoids include lutein and zeaxanthin. The recommended usage level for this extract is 1 to 10 percent. The extract is obtained from the flowers. *See also* xanthophylls.

marine plasma extract—may help in organizing the structure of connective tissue. It is considered healing due to its iodine content, which is present in a natural form complexed with algal peptides and polysaccharides. This makes it a more active and gentler product when applied to the skin. This extract contains plasma (the fluid part of the tissue from which suspended matter such as cells has been removed), vitamins, polysaccharides, essential sea minerals, and some cellular reagents. Trace minerals also include calcium, iron, magnesium, potassium, sodium, and silicon. Vitamin A, water-soluble vitamin B, vitamin C, pantothenic acid, and niacinamide are also present. Marine plasma extract is a trade name for a mixture that combines brown algae and marine animals. It is obtained by extracting the liquid from the cellular mass of marine organisms. It is not known to cause skin irritation.

M

marine seaweed extract—*see* algae extract; seaweed extract.

marine sediments—an all-encompassing name for an unspecified marine-based compound. *See also* algae extract; marine plasma extract; seaweed extract.

marjoram (*Origanum vulgare*)—described as tonic and anti-fungal. Although there are numerous species of marjoram, sweet marjoram and wild marjoram are the most commonly used in cosmetics, and both have similar properties. *See also* marjoram oil.

marjoram oil—its ascribed botanical properties include antispasmodic, calming, and sedative—indicating applications for sensitive or irritated skin. The oil is obtained through distillation. It may cause skin redness and itching.

marshmallow extract (*Althea officinalis*)—emollient and soothing. It can be pain relieving, especially in the case of burns, sunburns, or scrapes. In traditional medicine, marshmallow extract was used as a soothing and anti-itching agent for dermatological treatments. In folklore, it has been used for rough skin, scruff, dry scabs, burns, scalds, and swelling. *See also* althea extract; mallow extract.

marshmallow root extract—*see* althea extract; marshmallow extract.

marula seed oil (*Sclerocarya birrea*)—humectant and emollient. Comprised primarily of oleic acid, it also contains linoleic, alpha-linolenic, plamitic, stearic, and arachidonic acids.

mastic gum (*Pistacia lentiscus*)—film-forming and odor masking. It can also be used as an adhesive. The oil may be anti-bacterial and anti-fungal as well. The gum is a resin derived from a small tree native to the Mediterranean area.

matricaria extract—an extract of the flowerheads of Matricaria chamomilla. *See also* chamomile extract.

matrimony vine (*Lycium barbarum*)—also known as goji berry, wolfberry. It is credited with astringent, skin-conditioning, anti-oxidant, tonic, and anti-bacterial properties. Constituents include vitamins A, C, and E, and essential fatty acids. In cosmetic preparations, it is either the fruit extract or the seed oil that is used.

***Mauritia flexuosa* fruit oil**—*see* buriti pulp oil.

meadowfoam oil (*Lamnanthes alba*)—a rich emollient. When combined with shea butter, the mixture acts as an emollient and emulsifier, and can serve as a lanolin replacement. This mild, stable oil is resistant to oxidation. It is of much interest to cosmetic formulators because of its "dryness" and quick penetration into the skin. The oil is extracted from the meadowfoam seeds that contain 20 to 30 percent oil by weight. It can be found in massage oils and lotions, facial creams, sunblocks, and shaving preparations among others.

meadowsweet extract (*Filipendula ulmaria, Spirea ulmaria*)—appears to have strong anti-free radical properties, as well as

M

aromatic, astringent, analgesic and topical anti-inflammatory activity. The anti-free radical activity is attributed to its flavonoid and tannin content; the anti-inflammatory and analgesic properties are due to non-volatile salicylate derivatives, including salicylic acid and methyl salicylate. Gallic acid is another constituent. Analgesic, anti-inflammatory, and anti-free radical activity make meadowsweet extract particularly useful in sun care preparations. The word *aspirin* is derived from this plant's Latin name: *a* from acetyl and *spirin* from *Spireae*. Meadowsweet is a perennial plant that grows abundantly at the edges of rivers and ditches in meadows and damp woods.

medlar (*Mespilus sp.*)—a fruit-bearing tree that is related to pear and hawthorn. Constituents are said to include carotenes and vitamins A, B, and C. It is used in anti-aging cosmetics.

melanin—a water-soluble form of melanin is available that can be formulated into a product as a free-radical scavenger. Melanin can be naturally extracted from cuttlefish ink or synthetically produced. Research indicates that when employed as a sunscreen, melanin provides better UVA protection and requires lower usage concentrations than other available sunscreens. Its safety is supported through studies conducted with radioactive melanin, which showed no penetration through human skin.

melhydran—increases the skin's moisture-binding capacities. This is the trade name for a concentrated and purified extract of Provence honey from thyme, lavender, and rosemary. Suppliers recommend it for use in moisturizing, bath, aftershave, sun care, and post-sun products. It can also be synthetically produced.

melaleuca—*See* cajeput oil.

melilot (*Melilotus officinalis*) (**sweet clover; white clover**)—credited with emollient, bactericidal, sedative, and virustatic properties. Traditionally, it was used on a couperose condition. Coumarin is melilot's only important constituent. Its related compounds are hydrocoumaric (melilotic) acid, orthocoumaric acid, and melilotic anhydride (lactone), which is a fragrant oil. There are several species of this perennial herb. The whole herb is used for botanical purposes.

melissa (*Melissa officinalis*)—*see* balm mint extract.

melissa oil—*see* balm mint oil.

melon extract—*see Cucumis melo.*

melon juice—*see Cucumis melo.*

menhaden oil—contains essential fatty acids vital to the metabolism of healthy skin. The oil is obtained from the small North Atlantic menhaden fish, which is a little larger than a herring.

M

menthol—a fragrance. It is also said to be anti-septic, cooling, refreshing, and a blood-circulation stimulant. Menthol gives the skin a "cool" feeling after use. It constitutes almost 50 percent of peppermint oil but can also be synthetically produced through the hydrogenation of thymol. It is non-toxic in low doses, but in high concentrations it can be irritating to the skin, especially the mucous membranes. *See also* mint.

menthol extract—*see* menthol.

menthol methyl lactate—cooling and used also as a fragrance.

menthone glycerin acetal—used for adding fragrance, and to leave the skin feeling refreshed and cool. It is a menthol derivative that can be naturally obtained or synthetically manufactured.

menthoxypropanediol—used to mask odor and leave the skin feeling refreshed, it is a synthetic menthol derivative.

menthyl anthranilate—the only FDA-approved liquid sunscreen chemical with UVA-absorption capabilities. It has an approved usage level of 3.5 to 5 percent. This is a stable ingredient and can be combined with other sunscreen chemicals to increase SPF while providing UVA protection.

menthyl lactate—a fragrance component. This is the ester of menthol and lactic acid.

mercaptopyridine—also known as sodium pyrithione. It is a preservative that is not commoly used.

***Mercurialis perennis* extract (dog's mercury)**—used for its tonic properties. Some manufacturers cite wound-healing capacities as well, which could make it effective in products for problem prone skin. Among its constituents are methylamine, saponins and a volatile oil.

mercurials—a category of preservative with a high sensitizing potential, particularly in products intended to be left on the skin. They are used in minute amounts as a preservative in some eye makeup preparations to inhibit bacterial proliferation.

methanione—can be used as a preservative in emollients. This is a synthetic ingredient with the properties of vitamin K. It is used medically to prevent blood clotting, generally sold as a supplement, and not used in skin care.

methicone—a type of silicone used primarily in the formulation of free-flowing cosmetic powders. Methicone can also be found in cosmetic preparations as a skin surface sealant to reduce transepidermal water loss.

methionin—*see* methionine.

methionine—slows down and normalizes oil gland sebum production. Methionine is also used as a texturizer in cosmetic creams. It is an essential amino acid found in a number of proteins and obtained by means of fermentation.

methoxy PEG-22 dodecyl glycol copolymer—an effective water-in-oil emulsifier with a high water-binding capability. This ingredient has good dermatological and toxicological properties, and is very compatible with other skin care ingredients, facilitating its incorporation into cosmetic preparations.

4-methoxybenzoic acid—*see* anisic acid (ρ-anisic acid).

3,l-methoxypropane-1,2 diol—provides a cool sensation when used in facial masks.

methoxy propyl gluconamide—an alpha hydroxy acid derivative used as a moisturizer and an emollient. Its minimal acidity favors its use on dry and very dry, scaly skin, where other alpha hydroxy acid compounds may not be well tolerated.

methyl dihydroxybenzoate—*see* methyl gentisate.

methyl gentisate—also known as methyl dihydroxybenzoate. It is a skin-lightening ingredient that acts by inhibiting the melanocyte's production of tyrosinase. It can be naturally obtained from gentian root. *See also* gentian.

methyl gluceth-10—a skin humectant and a preservative. This is the polyethylene glycol ether of methyl glucose.

methyl gluceth-20—a humectant skin-conditioning agent.

methyl glucose isostearate—an emulsifier with highly effective moisturizing properties.

methyl glucose sesquistearate—a sucrose-based emulsifier.

methyl hydroxy stearate—an emollient used in moisturizing formulations. This is the ester of methyl alcohol and hydroxystearic acid.

methyl paraben—one of the most frequently used preservatives because of its very low sensitizing potential. It is one of the oldest preservatives in use to combat bacteria and molds. It is non-comedogenic.

methylbenzylidene camphor—also known as 4-methylbenzylidene camphor. A UV filter and absorber not known to cause photo allergies.

methylchloroisothiazolinone—a preservative. *See also* MI/MCI.

methylheptyl isostearate—a skin conditioner with occlusive properties. It can help retain moisture in the skin.

methylisothiazolinone—a preservative. *See also* MI/MCI.

M

methylsilanol elastinate—a protein derivative used as a skin-conditioning agent.

methylsilanol hydroxyproline aspartate—a silicon-based skin-conditioner that also has anti-static properties. Suppliers of this ingredient cite skin regeneration, cell renewal, and healing capacities. As such they indicate it for incorporation into such formulations as those for anti-aging, eye contour, firming, and anti-stretchmark. It is a synthetically manufactured ingredient.

methylsilanol mannuronate—tests indicate that as a result of its cutaneous hydration activity, it increases skin suppleness, moisture, and aids in the reduction of cellulite.

mica—used as a texturizer and coloring agent in cosmetics, it provides a "glimmer" or "shimmering" quality in makeup powders. Mica is the group name for a series of ground silicate minerals with similar physical properties but varied chemical composition. Micas range in color from colorless to pale green, brown, or black.

***Michelia alba* leaf oil**—often used for its fragrance and odor-masking properties. The essential oil derived from the plant's leaves. *Michelia alba* is a member of the magnolia family.

microcrystalline cellulose—provides good slip and softness, and acts as a binder. A cellulose fiber isolated from colloidal crystals. *See also* cellulose.

microcrystalline wax—an emulsifier. This is a beeswax substitute characterized by the fineness of its crystals (in comparison with the larger crystals of paraffin wax). It is derived from petroleum.

micronutrients—*see* trace elements.

milfoil extract (*Achillea millefolium*)—credited with anti-septic and antibiotic properties. *See also* yarrow extract.

milk lipid(s)—emollient and skin conditioning.

milk protein—gives a smooth feel to the skin. Milk protein is composed primarily of casein, which is well absorbed by the skin and gives it a gloss and fine touch by forming a soft film. It has water-retention abilities in the range of 13 percent. Milk protein is obtained from milk. If it is hydrolyzed, it is broken down into smaller pieces and is referred to either as hydrolyzed milk protein, milk amino acids, or casein amino acids. Its constituents include the flavones silybin, silydiamnin, and silychristin.

milk thistle (*Carduus marianus; Silybum marianum*)—credited with wound-healing and free-radial scavenging properties. It is used in toners and aftershave preparations. Among its constituents are essential oils, unsaturated fatty acids, polyacetones, and the silymarin group of flavonoids.

milkweed (*Asclepias syriaca*)—used in traditional medicine for its cicatrizant properties on wounds, and therapeutic value on various skin eruptions, including warts. Constituents include tannins, dextrose (sugar), and such fatty acids as oleic, linoleic, and linolenic acids.

millepertuis oil (*Hypericum perforatum*)—emollient and anti-inflammatory, it is used for sunburns, burns, and bruises. Millepertuis oil is the fixed oil obtained from St. John's wort flowers.

mimosa bark extract—*see* mimosa tenuiflora.

mimosa essence—primarily used as a fragrance, it is also credited with anti-inflammatory and astringent properties. It may produce allergic skin reactions. *See also* mimosa tenuiflora.

mimosa tenuiflora (**mimosa bark extract; tepescohuite**)—attributed with epidermal-tissue regenerating, repairing, antiseptic and protecting properties. It is also credited with helping reduce moisture loss. It can be used effectively in post-sun preparations, baby skin care creams, and protective creams. Mimosa tenuiflora has a high bioflavonoid and tannin content. It also contains zinc, necessary for DNA synthesis and cellular nutrition; iron, vital for oxygen transport and intracellular metabolism; magnesium, for its protective role; copper, for anti-inflammation; and manganese, that is said to stimulate cellular metabolism. The mimosa tenuiflora tree is related to the acacia. The bark is the part that is used. It may produce allergic skin reactions.

mineral oil—an emollient cleanser and demulsifier of dirt trapped in pores. Mineral oil is excellent for use in cleansers. In leave-on cosmetics, its comedogenicity or lack thereof appears related to the level of raw material refinement; therefore, some suppliers state that their product is non-comedogenic. When used in leave-on preparations, mineral oil's occlusive capability is considered to help improve the epidermal barrier function. This is a clear, odorless oil derived from petroleum and is not known to cause allergic reactions.

mineral pigments—provide UV protection. Mineral pigments refer to ingredients such as titanium dioxide or zinc oxide, which are usually incorporated into sunscreens, makeup bases, and daytime moisturizers to enhance the product's sunscreening ability.

M

mineral wax—*see* ozokerite.

mink oil—a gentle and effective emollient with skin-softening abilities. Its occlusive properties give it skin-conditioning qualities as well. It is obtained from the subdermal fatty tissues of the mink.

mint oil (*Mentha sp.*)—cooling, tonic, stimulating, anti-septic, and relaxing properties are attributed to mint. Mint was traditionally used as an adjunct soothing and anti-itching treatment in dermatological disorders, and has been considered to provide relief from scratches and insect bites. In addition, this aromatic herb is widely used as a fragrance. There are about 20 species in the *Mentha* genus growing around the world, including peppermint and spearmint, the two most widely used in skin care preparations. These varieties in particular can also serve as cleansers and decongestants indicated for acne and for dermatitis. Mint oil is produced by distillation of the plant.

mireth-3 myristate—an emollient employed as a skin-conditioning agent.

mistletoe extract (*Phoradendron flavescens; Viscum album*)—anti-spasmodic, healing, and calming properties are attributed to this ingredient. Mistletoe is an evergreen, parasitic plant growing on tree branches where it forms pendent bushes 2 to 5 feet in diameter. The extract is obtained from the plant's berries.

mitracarpus—extracts obtained from plants of the mitracarpus genus (*Rubiaceae* family) are credited with skin-lightening and improving overall complexion. The most common species used include *M. Scaber zucc.*, *M. Villosus*, and *M. verticillatus*. The extract is typically obtained by traditional methods, including maceration. Active components include flavonoid, phenolic, and hydroquinone derivatives.

monoammonium glycyrrhizinate—*see* glycyrrhizinate.

monomethylsilanetril lactate—an alpha hydroxy acid derivative with silicone.

monosodium n-cocoylglutamate—a surfactant.

montmorillonite—used as an abrasive in exfoliants and as a bulking agent in masks. It is also used to increase a formula's viscosity, as an emulsion stabilizer, and as an opacifying agent. Montmorillonite, a complex silicate, is a clay mineral that forms the main ingredient of bentonite and Fuller's earth.

Moringa pterygosperma **extract**—commonly known as the horseradish tree. Extract from the seeds are considered to help improve the skin's overall condition, look, and feel. Oil from this plant is also emollient, helping improve skin pliability.

Morus alba—*see* mulberry extract.

mucopolysaccharides—their strong moisture-binding capacity enhances a formulation's hydrating properties and reduces transepidermal water loss. Studies show that mucopolysaccharides will reduce the amount of moisture lost by the skin and will stimulate its moisture intake. This ingredient exhibits the desirable moisture-binding qualities of healthy skin, giving the skin turgor, increased water content, and elasticity. Mucopolysaccharides are highly effective in skin care products. As a natural skin component, mucopolysaccharides fill the spaces between collagen and elastin protein fibers in the dermis, giving them support and providing lubrication and moisture. *See also* glycosaminoglycans.

mucoprotein (soluble)—*see* protein.

mucus of quince—*see* quince.

mud—a mixture of a powder and a liquid. It is usually applied wet as a facial mask and allowed to dry. If the powder and/or liquid contain therapeutic ingredients, these will interact with the skin. Identifying its therapeutic action requires knowing the nature of the powder and liquid being used. In a mask, it also acts as an occlusive agent for the time the mask remains on the skin. This favors the interaction of ingredients in a cream or other products applied prior to the mud.

mugwort (*Artemisia vulgaris*)—improves skin feel and condition. It is also perfuming. Constituents include volatile oil, cineole, linalool, thujone, glycosides, insulin, and tannin. *See also* wormwood.

mulberry extract (*Morus sp.*)—increasingly used in cosmetics for its skin-lightening properties. Mulberry extract appears to inhibit tyrosinase and oxidation activity. Although there are several mulberry varieties, these properties are attributed to white mulberry (*Morus alba*). Studies have indicated that extract obtained from young twigs (*ramulus mori*) of the white mulberry are particularly potent skin lighteners. White mulberry is the variety originally found in China and used as a food source for silkworms. Mulberry was very highly regarded in ancient times and commonly cultivated throughout Europe for multiple uses, including an expectorant and flavoring agent. It is an official entry in the *British Pharmacopoeia*. Constituents of the berry include glucose, protein, tartaric, and malic acids. *See also* ramulus mori extract.

mulberry glycolic extract—astringent.

mung bean extract (*Phaseolus aureus*)—a botanical used in cosmetic preparations since ancient times. It is credited with anti-inflammatory and some anti-oxidant properties. Its active constituents include vitexin and isovitexin, both flavonoids.

musk rose oil (*Rosa moscata; Rosa moschata*)—*see* rose hip oil.

myristal myristate—an ester of myristyl alcohol and myristic acid. *See also* myristic acid; myristyl alcohol.

M

myristic acid—a surfactant and cleansing agent. When combined with potassium, myristic acid soap provides very good, abundant lather. This is a solid organic acid naturally occurring in butter acids such as nutmeg, oil of lovage, coconut oil, mace oil, and most animal and vegetable fats. Although some sources cite it as having no irritation potential, they do indicate comedogenicity potential.

myristyl ether propionate—an emollient and skin-conditioning agent used in pre-shave lotions and moisturizing preparations.

myristyl alcohol—an emollient often used in hand creams, cold creams, and lotions to give them a smooth, velvety feel. Sources indicate it as being mildly comedogenic and potentially irritating.

myristyl lactate—a light emollient and moisturizer with good spreadability. It leaves a smooth, satiny afterfeel. Sources indicate it as being comedogenic and with a slight irritancy potential. *See also* lactic acid; myristyl alcohol.

myristyl myristate—an occlusive skin-conditioning agent that enhances product spreadability and can reduce a product's transparency. It is particularly useful in emulsions that have to "melt" once they come in contact with the skin. This is an ester formed by the combination of the myristyl alcohol and myristic acid fractions of coconut oil. *See also* myristic acid; myristyl alcohol.

myristyl ocatanoate—a light emollient and moisturizer. It leaves the skin's surface with a smooth and supple finish.

myrrh extract (*Commiphora myrrah*)—attributed with disinfectant, anti-septic, anti-inflammatory, anti-itching, cicatrizant, tonic, stimulant, sedative, and astringent properties. It is also a good fixative. Myrrh extract can be valuable in products designed for acne treatment. Myrrh is a traditional and ancient ingredient for perfumes and incense, and was used by ancient Egyptian women in making facial masks and other cosmetic preparations. Myrrh oil is produced by the distillation of the plant's gum.

myrtle oil—astringent and anti-septic with botanical properties closely resembling those of eucalyptus. It is also used as a fragrance ingredient, and can be a deodorant. Its use is indicated for acne and oily skin. Its constituents include cineol, myrtenol, geraniol, linalool, camphene, and borneol. Myrtle is obtained by distillation of the plant's flowers, leaves, and stems.

M

NaAl silicate—*see* sodium aluminum silicate.

nalidone—a natural moisturizing factor that protects the skin from dehydration and increases its moisture-retention capabilities. This is the trade name for sodium PCA. *See* sodium PCA.

NaPCA—*see* sodium PCA.

narcissus (*Narcissus poeticus*)—a fragrance. It is also used as an antispasmodic and is recommended for use in very low concentrations because its oil has been shown to impair cellular functions when added to *in vitro* cell cultures. In addition, large amounts of the extract may produce headaches. This general name may also include narcissus flower extract and narcissus essential wax. As a wax, it can help thicken an emulsion and is considered tonic.

naseberry (*Manilkara zapotilla*)—also known as sapodilla. It is antioxidant and has anti-aging properties. Its constituents include tannin, fructose, pectin, ascorbic acid, mineral salts, and bioflavonoids, particularly proanthocyanidins, which have emollient, humectant, and anti-oxidant activity. The fruit is the part of the plant that is used.

nasturtium extract (*Tropaeolum majus*)—considered to have disinfectant and rubefactant attributes. It is effective when included in acne treatment products. It may produce allergic reactions.

natrium mud extract—*see* mud.

natural moisturizing factor (**NMF**)—refer to entry in Chapter 4.

neem extract—attributed with anti-bacterial, anti-fungal, and antiseptic properties. It may also act as an insect-repellent and be anti-inflammatory. Neem is an evergreen tree originally found in India.

neopentyl glycol dicaprate—an emollient also used to increase a formulation's viscosity. Primarily used in hand and body preparations.

neopentyl glycol dicaprylate/dicaprate—an emollient and formula viscosity-increasing agent used mostly in the manufacturing of lipsticks.

neopentyl glycol diheptanoate—a skin-conditioning and viscosity increasing agent, it is also emollient.

nerol—a primary alcohol used in perfumes, especially those with rose and orange blossom scents. Nerol is a naturally occurring fraction in oil of lavender, orange leaf, palmarosa, rose, neroli, and petitgrain. It is colorless and has a rose-like scent.

neroli—*see* neroli oil; orange flower oil.

neroli oil—a fragrance. It is used in skin care preparations to stimulate cell regeneration. Given its sedative and soothing properties, it is indicated for sensitive and delicate skin. However, neroli oil appears beneficial for all skin types. True neroli is extracted from bitter orange blossom. This is one of the most expensive oils and, therefore, is widely adulterated with the distillation of other citrus blossoms such as sweet orange, lemon, and mandarin. *See also* orange flower oil.

neroli water—*see* orange flower water.

nettle extract (*Urtica dioica*)—its botanical properties are listed as anti-inflammatory, astringent, bactericidal, healing, mildly deodorant, and stimulating. It is considered effective for treating eczema and sunburn. According to some sources, this is the botanical with the highest vitamin E content, and as such, it would have good anti-oxidant properties. Nettle's important constituents include acetylcholine, amino acids, histamine, carotinoids, and chlorophyll. An analysis of fresh nettle also shows the presence of formic acid, mucilage, mineral salts, ammonia, carbonic acid, and water. The formic acid in nettle, along with the phosphates and a trace of iron, makes it a valuable botanical. There are more than 500 species of nettle growing mainly in tropical countries. The whole herb is employed for therapeutic purposes.

niacin—also known as vitamin B_3. It is a water-soluble conditioning agent that improves rough, dry, or flaky skin, helping smooth the skin and improve its suppleness. Niacin enhances the appearance and feel of hair, by increasing body, suppleness, or sheen, or by improving the texture of hair that has been damaged physically or by chemical treatment. When used in the formulation of skin care products, niacinamide and niacin enhance the appearance of dry or damaged skin by reducing flaking and restoring suppleness.

niacinamide—used as a skin stimulant and skin smoother. It is a derivative of niacin, and part of the vitamin B family. *See also* vitamin B.

niaouli oil—anti-septic, bactericidal, and tonic. Its therapeutic properties indicate possible improvement in circulation, antibody activity, and healing in cases of infected wounds and burns. Some of its medicinal properties and indications are the same as those for eucalyptus. Constituents include alpha pinene, beta pinene, gamma terpineol, limonene, and linalool. Niaouli oil is produced through distillation of the leaves of the *Melaleuca viridifora* plant.

niosomes—non-ionic surfactant vesicles that act as a delivery system and are similar to liposomes. According to manufacturers, niosomes interact well with human skin when topically applied. *See also* liposomes.

nonfat dry milk—soothing and moisturizing. It is often used in facial masks. Non-fat dry milk consists mostly of protein and also contains lactic acid, lactose, vitamins, and minerals. *See also* milk protein.

nonoxynol-1—*see* polyoxyethylene nonylphenyl ether.

nonoxynol-14—a surfactant and emulsifying agent. It is used as a non-ionic surface-active agent and as a dispersing agent in cosmetics.

norvaline—a protein amino acid used as a skin-conditioning and anti-static agent.

nutmeg (*Myristica fragrans*)—studies credit nutmeg extract with a skin-lightening effect based on an ability to inhibit tyrosinase activity. An extract, powder, or oil can be obtained from the nut. However, nutmeg oil, credited with tonic and stimulating properties, is not commonly used in cosmetic preparations as it could cause skin irritation.

Nutrilan—a trade name for hydrolyzed animal protein. Manufacturers claim that this ingredient creates a smooth, velvety feeling on the skin's surface. It contains amino acids present in the skin. Nutrilan is an example of how cosmetic companies can list their ingredients and create ambiguity with respect to identity or source. *See also* hydrolyzed animal protein.

nylon—a commonly known synthetic material used as a fiber in eyelash lengtheners and mascaras, and as a molding compound to shape cosmetics. Nylon gives bulk to a formulation and, when appropriate, provides opacifying properties. It can cause allergic reactions.

nylon 11—a bulking agent used primarily in makeup preparations and in some moisturizers.

nylon 12—a bulking and opacifying agent that provides good feel and good elasticity to moisturizers and makeup preparations, including foundations. Nylon 12 reduces oiliness. It is a polyamide derivative of acid 12-aminododecanioic.

nylon 66—a bulking agent.

oak bark (*Quercus sp.*)—its botanical properties are described as slightly tonic, strongly astringent, and antiseptic. It also reduces inflammation and prevents infection. Oak bark extract appears to have greater therapeutic effects than oak root.

oak bud extract—*see* aleppo gall.

oak root—exhibits soothing and anti-inflammatory properties. Oak root is recommended for sensitive skin, protecting it against unwanted reactions such as swelling or redness. The extract is generally obtained from the younger part of the plant.

oakmoss empuree(*Evernia prunastri*)—a fragrance component derived from any one of several resin-yielding lichens that grow on oak trees.

oat (*Avena sativa*)—contains a colloid that has soothing properties on the skin. Generally speaking, all oat grades enhance emulsion stability, increase viscosity, leave a smooth afterfeel, and provide a source of whole natural vegetable protein. Dermatologists indicate oatmeal-based preparations for irritated skins resulting from sunburn, psoriasis, or allergic dermatitis, as oatmeal seems to reduce irritation and relieve redness and itching. In addition to acting as a soap-free cleanser, oats in the form of bran, flour, or meal provide a gentle base for face masks designed to work with delicate, sensitive skin. Oatmeal masks absorb oil from the skin's surface and reduce the redness of irritated, broken-out skin. Oatmeal soaps are non-irritating and good for people with delicate, sensitive skin.

oat bran—abrasive, absorbent, and can add bulk to a formulation. *See* oat.

oat extract—an extract obtained from the seeds of oats. *See also* oat.

oat flour—an abrasive, absorbent, bulking, and viscosity-increasing substance obtained by finely grinding oat kernels. It is used in a variety of cosmetic preparations including powders, masks, mudpacks, moisturizers, suntan gels, hand and body creams, and soaps. *See also* oat.

oat kernel protein—film-forming and skin conditioning it can help keep moisture in the skin. A protein obtained from the kernels of oats.

oat meal flour—used as an abrasive and bulking agent in paste masks and soaps. It is obtained by grinding oats from which the husks have been removed. *See also* oat.

octadecanol—*see* stearic acid.

octadecene/maleic anhydride copolymer—an emulsion stabilizer, film former, and viscosity-increasing chemical used in cosmetic formulations. It is also used in sunscreens as a waterproofing agent.

octadodecylstearyl stearate—an emollient.

octinoxate—the drug name for the sunscreen chemical generally known as octyl methoxycinnamate and ethylhexyl methoxycinnamate. *See also* octyl methoxycinnamate.

octisalate—a UVB protector. This is the drug name for ethylhexyl salicylate and octyl salicylate. *See also* ethylhexyl salicylate.

octocrylene—a UVB sunscreen with strong water-resistant properties and a rather broad-band absorption range. It exhibits good photostability, and is being evaluated by many companies as an effective SPF booster and waterproofing enhancer. This is an expensive ingredient with an approved usage level of 7 to 10 percent in both the United States and the European Union. Although gaining in popularity among formulators, its cost and usage level can limit use. In addition, some studies are indicating it may cause allergic reactions in skin with a history of photoallergy.

octyl dimethyl PABA (padimate-O; p-aminobenzoic acid)—an FDA-approved sunscreen chemical whose INCI name is now ethylhexyl dimethyl PABA. *See also* ethylhexyl dimethyl PABA.

octyldodecanol—an emollient alcohol with good spreadability and skin-conditioning properties. This is a good vehicle for oil-soluble ingredients. It is also used for perfuming.

2-octyl-1-dodecanol—the chemical name for octyldodecanol. *See also* octyldodecanol.

octyl methoxycinnamate (ethylhexyl methoxycinnamate; ethylhexyl p-methoxycinnamate; 2-ethylhexyl p-methoxycinnamate)—*see* ethylhexyl methoxycinnamate.

octyl p-methoxycinnamate—*see* octyl methoxycinnamate.

octyl palmitate—a non-greasy, non-oily moisturizing ester with good spreadability and good solvency properties.

octyl pelargonate—a light emollient that does not leave a greasy feel on the skin.

octyl salicylate (2-ethylhexyl 2-hydroxybenzoate; 2-ethylhexyl salicylate; ethylhexyl salicylate)—*see* ethylhexyl salicylate.

octyl stearate—an emollient with similar properties to those of octyl palmitate. *See also* stearic acid.

octyl triazone—*see* ethylhexyltriazone.

2-octyldodecyl alcohol—*see* octyldodecanol.

octyldodecyl benzoate—an emollient and a solvent with high spreadability. It leaves a pleasant feel on the skin.

octyldodecyl myristate—an emollient.

octyldodecyl neopentanoate—an emollient with skin-conditioning properties.

octyldodecyl stearate—a non-comedogenic emollient.

octyldodecylstearoyl stearate—a non-comedogenic skin-conditioning agent that provides occlusive properties. It is also used to increase viscosity in cosmetic formulations.

octyl hydroxystearate—an emollient used as a skin-conditioning agent.

old English walnut—*see* walnut.

oleamine—an anti-static agent that can be synthetically manufactured or naturally derived.

oleate sorbitan—*see* sorbitan oleate.

oleic acid—also known as omega-9. Oleic acid can improve the skin-penetration abilities of a preparation's other components. An essential fatty acid, it is obtained from various animal and vegetable fats and oils, and may be mildly irritating to the skin.

oleostearine—acts as a binder and an emollient in cosmetic preparations. This is a mixture of the fatty acid triglycerides remaining after the physical separation of low titre oils from beef tallow, although it can also be synthetically manufactured.

oleth-2, -5, -10, -20, -30—all are emulsifiers and solubilizers, and all are versions of a polyethylene glycol ether of oleyl alcohol. Cosmetic formulators will often select a specific one depending on the formulation's other requirements. For example, oleth-5 is also a spreading agent; oleth-20 is particularly useful as a fragrance solubilizer and can be successfully employed in some clear gel systems; oleth-30 has additional surfactant and cleansing properties. *See also* oleyl alcohol.

oleyl alcohol—an emollient, solvent, viscosity-increasing agent, and carrier employed in a wide variety of cosmetic formulations including makeup, skin care, and hand and body preparations. Oleyl alcohol is an unsaturated fatty alcohol found in fish oils and can also be produced synthetically. According to some sources, it is comedogenic and has a mild irritancy potential.

oleyl betaine—a mild emollient, conditioning surfactant, and formulation thickener. *See also* betain; oleamine.

oleyl erucate—an all-purpose emollient sometimes used as a jojoba oil substitute.

olibanum—*see* frankincense.

olibanum oil—a fragrance component. It is astringent with slight anti-inflammatory properties. *See also* frankincense.

oligo active liposomes—liposomes encapsulated with oligo elements.

oligoelements—refer to entry in Chapter 4. *See also* trace elements.

oligopeptide-34—a skin-conditioning, synthetically manufactured peptide containing 13 amino acids, including arginine, aspartic acid, glutamine, serine, and trypophan.

olive extract—a vague ingredient listing as olive extract can be derived from the olive fruit, flower, bud, bark, or leaf. For example, extract obtained from the bud is noted as anti-oxidant and emollient, whereas extract from the flower or bark is said to improve the condition of the skin.

olive oil (*Olea europaea*)—a carrier oil with excellent lubricity, pale color, and low odor. Olive oil is considered an especially good carrier for essential oils. It is a good emollient and can also be used for perfuming. Its unsaponifiable fraction is described also as a type of precursor, although not a biological one, with some claims of its targeting epidermal keratinocytes and stimulating the synthesis of such substances as collagen, elastin, proteoglycans, and glycoproteins.

olive leaf extract—astringent and anti-septic. It also has vasodialating capacities, as well as being perfuming and skin-conditioning. Olive leaf extract has demonstrated some anti-oxidant and free-radical scavenger activities. Olive leaves contain both bioflavonoids and polyphenols. The extract generally found in anti-aging products.

omega-3—an essential fatty acid. *See also* alpha linolenic acid.

omega-6—an essential fatty acid. *See also* linoleic acid.

omega-9—an essential fatty acid. *See also* oleic acid.

orange essence—used for fragrance.

orange oil (*Citrus aurantium* **[bitter orange] and** *Citrus sinensis* **[sweet orange]**)—primarily used in perfumery. Orange oil's botanical properties in skin care are considered anti-inflammatory, anti-bacterial, anti-spasmodic, and sedative, making it suitable for sensitive, delicate skin.

O

orange flower extract—used in folk medicine as a mild sedative. It is considered effective for dry skin.

orange flower oil—a fragrance that is credited with soothing and calming properties when used in skin care preparations. Orange flower oil should not be confused with orange flower extract. The flowers from the bitter orange tree yield, by distillation, an essential oil known as neroli, which forms one of the principal elements of eau de cologne. A pomade and an oil are also obtained from orange flowers through maceration. The oil from sweet orange blossoms is far less fragrant than that from bitter orange. The flowers are distilled immediately after being gathered. The essential oil, which rises to the surface of the distillate, is drawn off, whereas the aqueous portion is sold as orange flower water. One hundred kilograms of flowers will yield 600 grams of oil by volatile solvents, 400 grams by the maceration method, and only 100 grams by enfleurage.

orange flower water—has similar activity to that of orange oil, but its soothing properties appear to be more pronounced.

orange roughy oil—a fish oil that in skin care preparations demonstrates superior spreading and skin-softening properties. Studies indicate that it has a similar capacity to moisturize dry skin as petrolatum.

orchid extract (*Orchis sp.*)—noted to be soothing and skin conditioning, some sources cite it as having restorative and rejuvenation capacities as well. It is also credited as beneficial for dry skin. The extract is obtained from the tubers of various orchid species.

orizanol (**orysanol**)—a powder obtained from rice germ oil attributed with an anti-oxidizing effect on fats and oils.

orysanol—*see* orizanol.

oxido reductases—a mixture of naturally occurring yeast and enzymes that acts as an anti-oxidant by reducing or blocking oxygen.

2-oxothiazolidine carboxylic acid—a glutathione precursor, this ingredient is being studied for its anti-aging, anti-wrinkle properties. *See also* glutathione.

oxybenzone (**benzophenone-3**)—the drug name for an FDA-approved UV filter and absorber. *See also* benzophenone-3.

oxyquinoline sulfate—a disinfectant and a preservative against fungus growth. It is made from phenols.

ozokerite (**cresin**)—a naturally occurring microcrystalline wax. It regulates formulation viscosity, has suspension properties, and gives products stability. Ozokerite is a hydrocarbon wax derived from mineral or petroleum sources that, when refined, yields a hard white microcrystalline wax known as cresin.

P

PABA—also known as p-aminobenzoic acid. It is a sunscreen chemical with an approved usage level of 5 to 15 percent. It is found to be irritating to sensitive skin, has the potential to cause sensitization, and is considered too water soluble. Once extremely popular, this ingredient has practically disappeared from sunscreen formulations. PABA is a yellowish or colorless acid found in vitamin B complex.

padimate A—*see* pentyl dimethyl PABA.

padimate O—the drug name for ethylhexyl dimethyl PABA, a sunscreen chemical formerly known as octyl dimethyl PABA. *See also* ethylhexyl dimethyl PABA.

padina pavonica extract—also known as peacock's tail algae. It is used to improve the look and feel of the skin and has demonstrated anti-fungal properties in clinical tests unrelated to skin care. It is commonly found in the waters of warm temperate to tropical climates, primarily the Mediterranean. *See also* algae extract.

palm oil (hydrogenated)—a consistency regulator and a formula stabilizer for creams, lotions, makeup, and decorative cosmetics.

palm oil glycerides (hydrogenated)—a coemulsifier, dispersing agent, and consistency regulator in cosmetic formulations. It imparts a pleasant skin feel.

palm kernel glycerides (hydrogenated)—an emulsifier and consistency regulator. It is a mixture of mono-, di-, and triglycerides derived from palm kernel oil.

palm kernel oil—used primarily for making soaps and ointments. It is natural oil obtained from the kernel of *Elaeis guineensis*.

palm kernelamide DEA—a non-ionic surfactant, thickener, foam booster, and formula stabilizer in cosmetic preparations. It is also able to control a formulation's viscosity.

Palmaria palmata extract—also known as dulse. It is skin protecting and skin conditioning. Studies related to food preservation indicate anti-oxidant properties primarily as a free radical scavenger, and an ability to inhibit lipid peroxidation by reducing free radical activity. Palmaria palmata's polyphenol content may be the reason for its anti-oxidant and anti-lipid peroxidation activities. It is extracted from the palmaria palmata algae. *See also* algae.

palmarosa oil (*Cymbopogon martini*)—attributed with soothing, moisturizing, anti-septic, tonic, and cell-regenerating properties. Palmarosa oil is said to have an immediate calming and refreshing effect on the skin. It is indicated for acne skin and dermatitis as well as for dry skin. This oil is widely used in perfumery and cosmetology because its fresh, rose-like scent makes it useful for the adulteration of rose oil, one of the most expensive essential oils. It can also be used to mask odors. Palmarosa oil is obtained by distillation of this flowering grasslike plant.

palmitic acid—one of the skin's major fatty acids produced by the sebaceous glands. In cosmetic preparations, it is used as a formula texturizer. This acid is naturally occurring in allspice, anise, calamus oil, cascarilla bark, celery seed, coffee, tea, and many animal fats and plant oils. It is obtained from palm oil, Japan wax, or Chinese vegetable tallow.

palmitoyl hydroxypropyltrimonium amylopectin/glycerin crosspolymer—a skin conditioner.

palmitoyl oligopeptide—a synthetic peptide used in anti-aging products. It is intended to enhance the appearance of dry, flaky, or damaged skin, and to restore skin suppleness. It is also said to reduce the appearance of wrinkles as well as repair age-related skin problems by stimulating collagen production. It is obtained through a chemical reaction between palmitic acid and a synthetic peptide that contains two or more of the following amino acids: alanine, arginine, aspartic acid, glycine, histidine, lysine porline, serine, or valine.

palmitoyl oligopeptide-3—*see* palmitoyl oligopeptide.

palmitoyl pentapeptide-4—a skin conditioner. Clinical studies by manufacturers credit it with an ability to promote collagen, elastin, and glycosaminoglycan synthesis. This would result in an ability to restore skin thickness, which diminishes with age, and to reduce the appearance of lines and wrinkles. Palmitoyl pentapeptide-4 is a synthetic peptide with serine, threonine, and hexadecanoyl derivatives.

palmitoyl tetrapeptide-3—*see* palmitoyl tetrapeptide-7.

palmitoyl tetrapeptide-7—formerly known as palmitoyl tetrapeptide-3. This peptide appears to improve skin elasticity and firmness. It also hydrates, smoothes, and protects the skin. It can be both obtained from the plant and synthetically derived and is found in a variety of different skin care preparations including eye lotions, moisturizers, and night creams. Palmitoyl tetrapeptide-3 appears to act as an anti-inflammatory. This is attributed to its ability to control the secretion of specific chemicals responsible for skin aging (i.e., cytokines and interleukin-6), and hence it may function in a manner similar to the anti-aging hormone, DHEA. Some studies indicate that palmitoyl tetrapeptide-7 may also act as a UV filter.

pansy extract (*Viola tricolor*)—its botanical properties include soothing, healing, and cleansing. Among pansy extract's active constituents are saponins, salicylic compounds, tannins, and flavonoids (e.g., rutin, violantin, scoparin, vitexine, saponaretin, orientin), volatile oils, and the glycosides of the methyl ester of salycilic acid. It is recommended for use in dry skin preparations and for skin problems of various types.

pantetheine sulfonate—helps improve the overall condition of the skin.

pantethine—an emollient and conditioner, it is often found in hair care preparations.

panthenol (**pro-vitamin B$_5$**)—acts as a penetrating moisturizer. Panthenol appears to stimulate cellular proliferation and aid in tissue repair. Studies indicate that when topically applied, panthenol penetrates the skin and gets converted into pantothenic acid, a B complex vitamin. Such action could possibly influence the skin's natural resources of pantothenic acid. It imparts a non-irritant, non-sensitizing, moisturizing, and conditioning feel and promotes normal keratinization and wound-healing. Panthenol protects the skin against sunburn, provides relief for existing sunburn, and enhances the natural tanning process. Panthenol's humectant character enables it to hold water in the product or attract water from the environment, resulting in a moisturizing effect. It enhances skin suppleness, and claims are that it also acts as an anti-inflammatory agent. It is considered a non-comedogenic raw material.

panthenyl triacetate—a panthotenic acid derivative with vitamin B activity. *See also* pantothenic acid.

pantothenic acid—part of the vitamin B complex. It is considered a biological precursor capable of acting as a bio activator. Pantothenic acid's relatively small molecule facilitates permeation of the epidermis, allowing it to participate in the metabolic process of the dermis. Some studies indicate a benefit when incorporated into products destined for treating eczema, psoriasis, skin inflammation, and skin allergies. It is naturally occurring in liver, eggs, dried brewer's yeast, and royal jelly.

papain—a papaya enzyme able to dissolve keratin. Papain is used in face masks and peeling lotions as a very gentle exfoliant. It can be irritating to the skin but less so than bromelin, a similar enzyme found in pineapples and also used in cosmetics. It is considered a non-comedogenic raw material.

papaya (*Carica papaya*)—considered a cleanser for acne prone skin. Its value resides in its papain enzyme content. *See also* papain.

papaya enzyme extract—used as a gentle exfoliant, it also softens the skin and can help smooth the appearance of fine line and wrinkles. *See also* papain.

paprika—used to stimulate blood circulation in the skin.

parabens—one of the most commonly used group of preservatives in the cosmetic, pharmaceutical, and food industries. Parabens provide bacteriostatic and fungistatic activity against a diverse number of organisms, and are considered safe for use in cosmetics, particularly in light of their low sensitizing potential. An evaluation of preservatives for use in leave-on cosmetic preparations lists parabens among the least sensitizing. The range of concentrations used in cosmetics varies between 0.03 and 0.30 percent, depending on the conditions for use and the product to which the paraben is added. *See also* parabens entry in Chapter 4.

paraffin—used in cosmetics as a beeswax substitute. Paraffin is a solid mixture of hydrocarbons obtained from petroleum, although it can also be obtained from wood or coal. Pure paraffin is harmless to the skin, but the presence of impurities may result in irritation, eczemas, and other skin problems.

Parinari curatellifolia **seed oil**—said to have regenerative, restructuring, and moisturizing capacities, thanks to its eleostearic acid content.

parsley extract (*Petroselinum sativum*)—serves as a deodorant. It is said to have disinfectant, anti-inflammatory, and skin-conditioning properties.

parsley oil—traditionally used for soothing and anti-itching treatment in dermatological disorders. It may also be used as a preservative. Parsley oil is extracted from the plant's seeds that contain an oil called apiol. It may cause allergic reactions in sensitive skin.

parsley seed—*see* parsley oil.

partially hydrolyzed protein—*see* protein.

passion flower extract (*Passiflora sp.*)—its botanical properties are described as anti-spasmodic and calming. Extract specifically from the *incarnata* variety is credited with an ability to protect the skin against harmful external factors (e.g., climate). Its active principle, passiflorine, appears to be somewhat similar to morphine. There are four primary *Passiflora* varieties used in cosmetics: *edulis, incarnata, laurifolia,* and *quadrangularis.* Depending on the variety and the portion of the plant used (flower, fruit, or seed), therapeutic properties can range from improving skin condition to astringent, soothing, refreshing, and skin-protecting. *See also* passion fruit extract and passion fruit oil.

passion fruit extract—an emollient with moisturizing and refreshing properties. Passion fruit extract can be soothing as well as act as a skin conditioner and protector. Some of passion fruit's most important constituents include vitamins, polysaccharides, minerals, and amino acids. A listing of "passion fruit" alone is insufficient to determine the variety used or the associated activity. The extract has an aromatic, fruity, tropical scent. *See also* passion flower extract.

passion fruit oil—seen most often on sun care product labels, the oil extracted from the plant's seed is considered emollient, and, depending on the plant's varietal, it may also offer some skin-protecting capacity.

patchouli lite oil—*see* patchouli oil.

patchouli oil (*Pogostemon patchouli*) (**patchouly**)—its botanical properties are described as astringent, anti-inflammatory, decongestive, and tonic. It can be stimulant in low doses, and sedative at high doses. Its botanical attributes make it useful for acne, aged and chapped skin, and skin redness. In Asia, it was a renowned antidote against insect and snake bites. Also used as a perfume in soaps and cosmetics to impart a long-lasting aroma. This oil has a strong, sweet, musty, and very persistent fragrance. The patchouli leaves are dried and fermented prior to distillation. It may produce an allergic reaction in sensitive individuals.

patchouly—*see* patchouli oil.

PCA (Ajidew; Ajidew A-100; 1-2-pyrrolidone-5-carboxylic acid)—a hygroscopic moisturizing ingredient, it serves as a fine humectant. It is frequently used in moisturizing products.

pea extract (*Piscum sativum*)—clinical evidence points to pea extract's ability to inhibit the degradation of collagen and elastin by the protease enzyme. Some ingredient manufacturers also report that it helps retain water in the skin. These traits would make pea extract beneficial for maintaining skin firmness and moisture, and useful in anti-aging or other skin-firming products. The extract is produced from the whole plant.

peach extract (*Prunus persica*)—used for a variety of functions, including as an abrasive, to add bulk and for moisturizing activity. There are differences based on the portion of the plant employed. For example, an extract from peach leaves is considered emollient and moisturizing, and is credited by herbalists with an ability to help stop bleeding and heal wounds. Extract of peach bud is used for its humectant properties, and peach flower extract is moisturizing. Peach extract is recommended for use in products for dry skin.

peach kernel oil—a carrier credited with emollient, calming, and soothing properties. This oil is expressed from the peach kernels.

peach stones (ground)—used in scrubs as exfoliants.

peacock's tail algae extract—*see* padina pavonica extract.

peanut fat—used to add consistency to cosmetic products. Peanut fat is hydrogenated peanut oil. *See also* peanut oil.

peanut oil—utilized as a skin softener, emulsifier, and emollient. It can also be used as a substitute for more expensive oils such as almond and olive in cosmetic creams. Peanut oil has a higher vitamin A, vitamin E, and nicotinic acid content than other nut oils. It is obtained by pressing the seed kernels.

pearl powder—therapeutic benefits are unclear, though it could be anti-inflammatory and detoxifying, and can be an abrasive. It is found in a variety of cosmetic preparations including shampoo, cleansers, indoor tanning products, moisturizers. Amino acids are among constituents. Pearl powder is the result of grinding dried salt or freshwater pearls and should not be confused with the "pearl" used in color cosmetics, which is usually obtained by using mica, bismuth oxychloride, or other such ingredients.

pectin—used as a thickening agent in cosmetic preparations given its gelling properties. It is soothing and mildly acidic and extracted from apples or the inner portion of citrus fruit rind.

PEG, PEG-4, -8, -14, -20, -32, -75, -100, -150, -200—the acronym for polyethylene glycol. PEGs are compatible with a wide range of ingredients and are blended into a formulation to obtain the desired humectancy, viscosity, or melting point. PEGs make excellent solvents, binders, vehicles, humectants, lubricants, and bases. When a number is associated with the PEG entry, it indicates the number of moles present (the PEG's weight). Although each fundamentally serves the same purpose, a cosmetic chemist might choose one PEG over the other for formulatory requirements. For example, PEG-4 can improve a product's resistance to moisture and oxidation, and is generally used in hair products. Certain types of PEG-8 can be used as a moisture and consistency regulator in creams, lotions, and shaving preparations, and PEG-32 can improve a product's spreadability and skin feel. When they are listed with another ingredient such as PEG-5 stearate, it means that a polyethylene glycol (PEG) chain has been added to the stearic acid to enhance water solubility. *See also* polyethylene glycol.

PEG-2 ceteareth—an emulsifier.

PEG-2 stearate—an emulsifier for creams and lotions. This tan-colored wax is derived from stearic acid. *See also* PEG stearate.

PEG-3 sorbitan oleate, -6 sorbitan oleate—an emulsifying agent. Commonly used in cosmetic, toiletry, and fragrance preparations and in suntan gels.

PEG-3 sorbitan stearate, -6 sorbitan stearate, -60 sorbitan stearate—an emulsifying agent and a popular PEG among cosmetic formulators for use in all cosmetic, toiletry, and fragrance preparations, including suntan gels.

PEG-4 dilaurate—an emulsifier.

PEG-4 laurate—used in cosmetic preparations as an emulsifier and a surfactant.

PEG-5 glyceryl stearate—a surfactant-emulsifying agent used in moisturizing and cleansing products.

PEG-5 soy stearol, -10 soy stearol—emollients, emulsifiers, and emulsion stabilizers used in a wide variety of skin and hair care products. PEG-10 soy stearol also has viscosity-modifying properties. These are derived from the sterols found in soybean oil, and are considered non-comedogenic raw materials.

PEG-5 stearate—listed as particularly applicable for hand and body lotions and creams. *See also* PEG stearate.

PEG-6 beeswax, -8 beeswax, -12 beeswax, -20 beeswax—surfactant-emulsifying agents that can gelate lipids.

PEG-6 caprylic/capric glycerides—an emollient and emulsifying agent that helps preserve the skin's lipid content and keep the skin soft. Studies indicate it is effective on psoriasis because of its ability to soften the scaling skin and improve the action of the active ingredient being applied. Manufacturer test results indicate no primary toxic or allergic reactions and good skin tolerance.

PEG-6 dioleate—a surfactant-emulsifying agent derived from oleic acid. It is used as a carrier or base in lotions and other cosmetic preparations.

PEG-6 isostearate—an emulsifier.

PEG-6 lauramide—an emulsifier.

PEG-6 stearate—used primarily as an emulsifier in the formulation of cleansing products. *See also* PEG stearate.

PEG-7 glyceryl cocoate—a self-emulsifying emollient especially suitable for aqueous formulations.

PEG-7M—a binder, emulsion stabilizer, and viscosity-increasing agent used primarily in soaps and cleansing products.

PEG-8 stearate—an emulsifier and thickening agent generally incorporated into hair care products, hand and body creams, and moisturizing preparations. It is also a superfattening agent for shaving preparations and foam baths. *See also* PEG stearate.

PEG-10 sorbitan laurate, -40 sorbitan laurate, -44 sorbitan laurate, -75 sorbitan laurate, -80 sorbitan laurate—cleansing and solubilizing agents. These are among the most popularly used PEGs because of their mildness. They are incorporated into a variety of preparations including skin care cosmetics, suntan products, toiletries, and fragrances. As a group, they are considered noncomedogenic raw materials.

PEG-12 glyceryl distearate, -23 glyceryl distearate—emollient.

PEG-16 macadamia glyceride—emollient. It is derived from macadamia nut oil glycerides.

PEG-18 castor oil dioleate—an emulsifier for creams and lotions, and a viscosity-increasing agent. It is particularly suitable when animal and vegetable oils are used.

bis-PEG-18 methyl ether dimethyl silane—a surfactant, it can also boost foam and improve the solubility of other substances in a formulation. In addition it acts as a humectant, helping bind or retain moisture.

PEG-20 oleate—an emulsifier derived from oleic acid.

PEG-25 PABA—an ultraviolet-light absorber and filter derived from PABA. It is approved for use up to 10 percent in the European Union.

PEG-30 castor oil, -30 castor oil (hydrogenated), -40 castor oil, -40 castor oil (hydrogenated)—emollients, detergents, emulsifiers, and oil-in-water solubilizers recommended for fragrance oils, and for other oils that may be difficult to solubilize. The -40 castor oil version is a powerful solubilizer for solubilizing essential oils and perfumes in oil-in-water creams and lotions. It is similar to PEG-30 castor oil but denser, being a soft paste rather than a liquid. The hydrogenated version is particularly used as a nonionic emulsifier for essential oils and perfumes.

PEG-30 dipolyhydroxystearate—an emulsifier for oil-in-water preparation.

PEG-30 stearate, -32 stearate—a cleansing and solubilizing agent often suitable for moisturizing preparations. PEG-32 stearate is often used in face and neck preparations as well as moisturizers. *See also* PEG stearate.

PEG-40 ricinoleyl ether—*see* ricinoleth 40.

PEG-40 stearate—a hydrophilic emulsifier, stabilizer, anti-gellant, and lubricant for a variety of skin care products, some hair care preparations, toiletries, and perfumes. *See also* PEG stearate.

PEG-45 palm kernel glycerides—an emollient and emulsifying agent derived from palm kernel glycerides.

PEG-50 lanolin—a surfactant used as a cleansing and solubilizing agent primarily in hair straighteners. It is a lanolin derivative.

PEG-60 glyceryl isostearate—a surfactant-emulsifying agent.

PEG-75 lanolin—an emollient, emulsifier, dispersant, plasticizer, and foam stabilizer. It is a polyethylene glycol derivative of lanolin.

PEG-85 lanolin—a surfactant.

PEG-100 stearate—a stabilizer and emulsifier for creams and lotions. Technically, it is the polyethylene glycol ester of stearic acid containing 100 moles of PEG. It is also a cleansing agent and surfactant utilized in skin care products, some hair care preparations, toiletries, and some perfumes. *See also* PEG stearate.

PEG-120 methyl glucose dioleate—a cleansing agent used in soaps, cleansers, and shampoos.

PEG-150/decyl alcohol/SMDI copolymer—a film former that can also be used to control a formulation's viscosity.

PEG-150 distearate—a surfactant used as a cleansing and solubilizing agent.

PEG-180/laureth-50/TMMG copolymer—a thickener with emulsifying and film-forming properties. It can also add lubricity and humectancy to a product.

PEG-180/octoxynol-40/TMMG copolymer—used to control (generally to increase) product viscosity.

PEG-200 hydrogenated glyceryl palmate—a polymer with cleansing, emulsifying, and solvent action. It is often found in cleansing products for face, body, and hair.

PEG/PPG-17/4 dimethyl ether—a conditioner used to improve the overall look and feel of the skin.

PEG-octanoate—all PEG octanoates are listed as emulsifying agents regardless of the number of PEGs in the formulation.

PEG stearate—all PEG stearates are emulsifying agents. Some are more frequently used or are more suitable for use in particular types of preparations, such as body creams and lotions versus cleansers.

Pelargonium graveolens—*see* rose geranium.

pentaerythrityl distearate—an emulsifier, it can be used to increase a product's viscosity.

pentaerythrityl stearate/caprate/caprylic adipate—an extremely emollient compound with moisturizing and protective properties. It is also a viscosity-building agent.

pentaerythrityl tetraethylhexanoate—an emollient, it is also used to control product viscosity.

pentaerythrityl tetraisostearate—a binder and emulsifier, it can help increase product viscosity. As a surfactant, it aids in improving product spreadability. In addition, it is an emollient and acts as an occlusive agent helping prevent or retard water loss from the skin.

pentaerythrityl tetraoctanoate—a binder and viscosity-increasing agent that also has occlusive properties, thereby helping retain moisture in the skin.

pentasodium ethylenediamine tetramethylene phosphate—a chelating agent similar to EDTA.

pentasodium pentate—an inorganic salt used as a water softener, emulsifier, and sequestering and dispersing agent in cleansing creams and lotions. Prepared from the dehydration of mono- and disodium phosphates, it is moderately irritating to the skin and mucous membranes.

pentyl dimethyl PABA (amydimethyl PABA)—a chemical UVB absorber infrequently used because of the PABA component.

pentylene glycol—an alcohol with humectant and anti-bacterial properties.

peony extract (*Paeonia sp.*)—credited with immunostimulant, anti-inflammatory, anti-oxidant, anti-spasmodic, and antibiotic properties. It is also said to be a circulation stimulant and have general skin-beautifying properties. Clinical studies show peony extract to help improve the acne condition and some skin diseases. Among peony's constituents are flavonoids, tannings, stilbenoids, steroids, paeonols, and phenols.

pepper (*Capsicum annuum*)—depending on the form in which it is used (i.e., extract of the whole plant versus extract of just the fruit, or as juice, powder or resin) a wide range of therapeutic properties are attributed to pepper. Extract from the whole plant can help mask odor, is tonic, and also serves to improve skin condition. In a skin care formulation, extract from the fruit can be used for anti-microbial, anti-oxidant, astringent, and skin-protecting properties. In hair care products, it could be used as an anti-dandruff and hair-conditioning ingredient. The juice, powder, and resin forms are all considered skin conditioning. Among pepper's constituents are carotenoids, capsaicin, volatile oil, organic acids, vitamin C, flavonoids (e.g., rutin), and mineral salts.

peppermint (*Mentha piperita*)—in extract form, it helps relieve skin irritation and itching. Peppermint reduces skin redness due to inflammation or acne, cools by constricting capillaries, and has refreshing and tonic properties.

peppermint oil—credited with refreshing, cooling, bactericidal, and anti-irritant properties. It is also used as a fragrance. Peppermint oil can produce allergic reactions such as hay fever, skin rashes, and irritation, especially if a dressing is applied over the oil. Extracted from the leaves of the peppermint plant, menthol accounts for more than 50 percent of its content. *See also* mint oil.

peptide—*see* peptides entry in Chapter 4.

peptide CLB-253, -CL-2572, -CLF-5—trade names for a series of different peptides found in the products of a particular cosmetic product manufacturer. *See* peptide.

peptones—water-soluble protein derivatives. *See also* protein.

pequi fruit (*Caryocar brasiliense*)—also known as souari nut. A humectant, there are indications that it may have anti-oxidant properties. The constituents of the fruit's pulp include carotenoids, as well as significant levels of oleic and palmitic fatty acids. It can be used in oil form, or as an extract of the fruit and leaves.

PERA—*see* polyethoxylated retinamide.

perfluoropolyether—a liquid polymer able to form a protective and lubricating film on the skin. It is recommended as a skin protectant against aggressive chemicals such as surfactants, alkalis, and organic solvents because it might also help prevent irritant contact dermatitis. This ingredient also enhances product stability and improves product feel on the skin. It is suitable for dry and oily skins given its lipo and hydrophobic properties.

perfluoropolymethylisopropylether—used to stabilize emulsions, reduce skin moisture loss, and provide a product with a silky texture.

perhydroxysqualene (squalane)—an emollient that can be obtained from a variety of sources, including wheat germ, olive and bran oils, and shark liver oil. When obtained from shark liver oil, it must be converted from squalene through a process of hydrogenization.

petitgrain biguarade—*see* petitgrain oil.

petitgrain extract—credited with tonic and anti-septic properties. *See also* petit grain oil.

petitgrain oil—widely used in pharmacy and perfumery for its therapeutic and tonic effect. Its fragrance is fresh, invigorating, and slightly floral with a bitter note. Like neroli, real petitgrain (or petitgrain biguarade) is obtained by distilling the leaves of the bitter orange tree. Petitgrain bergamot, petitgrain lemon, and petitgrain mandarin are also produced. It may be irritating to the skin.

petrolatum (petroleum jelly; Vaseline)—softens and smoothes the skin. It forms a film on the skin's surface, preventing moisture loss caused by evaporation, and protecting against irritation. Its disadvantage lies in the difficulty of effectively and properly removing it from the skin. Studies indicate that petrolatum accelerates the recovery of skin surface lipids, permeating throughout the stratum corneum layer, and allowing normal barrier recovery despite its occlusive properties. Thus it does not form or act as an impermeable membrane. It is a purified mixture of semisolid hydrocarbons from petroleum. Petrolatum imparts a greasier feeling than other emollients and also has the potential for clogging pores and causing comedogenicity. Although it can cause allergic skin rashes, petrolatum is non-toxic to the skin when properly purified and of high grade.

petroleum jelly—*see* petrolatum.

phenethyl alcohol—used to mask odor and also as a preservative. *See also* phenyl ethyl alcohol.

phenol—frequently used for medical chemical face peels. It may trap free radicals and can act as a preservative. Phenol, however, is an extremely caustic chemical with a toxicity potential. It is considered undesirable for use in cosmetics. Even at low concentrations, it frequently causes skin irritation, swelling, and rashes.

L-phenylalanine—an amino acid used as a skin-conditioning agent. It has greater use in hair care than in skin care products.

phenoxyethanol—a broad-range preservative with fungicidal, bactericidal, insecticidal, and germicidal properties. It has a relatively low sensitizing factor in leave-on cosmetics. Phenoxyethanol can be used in concentrations of 0.5 to 2.0 percent, and in combination with other preservatives such as sorbic acid or parabens. In addition, it is used as a solvent for aftershaves, face and hair lotions, shampoos, and skin creams of all types. It can be obtained from phenol.

phenoxyethylparaben—a preservative considered a non-comedogenic raw material.

2-phenyl-5-benzimidazolesulfonic acid—*see* phenylbenzimidazole sulfonic acid.

phenyl dimethicone—an anti-foaming agent and an occlusive skin-conditioning agent. This mixture of linear siloxane polymers is a silicone-derived material. *See also* dimethicone.

phenyl trimethicone—serves as a barrier protecting the skin from excessive water loss. It leaves the skin feeling soft and smooth, adds emolliency to a formulation, and reduces any feeling of tackiness. It can also be used to control or prevent a cosmetic preparation from foaming. It is a form of silicone, which is similar to dimethicone but is compatible with a broader range with organic oils and waxes.

phenylalanine—a conditioning agent with greater application in hair care than in skin care preparations. It is also used in suntan products.

phenylbenzimidazole sulfonic acid (2-phenyl-5-benzimidazole-sulfonic acid; 2-phenylbenzimidazole-5-sulfonic acid, ensulizole)—one of 21 FDA-approved sunscreen chemicals for UVB absorption. It has an approved usage level of up to 4 percent in the United States and up to 8 percent in the European Union. When combined with a proper base, it becomes a water-soluble sunscreen. It exhibits a very effective use level versus SPF relationship when compared to other sunscreen chemicals. In addition, when combined with other UVB absorbers, it seems to significantly boost SPF. It can also help protect a product from deterioration when exposed to UV light. Also considered excellent for use in clear sunscreen gels.

2-phenylbenzimidazole-5-sulfonic acid (2-penyl-5-benzimidazolesulfonic acid)—*see* phenylbenzimidazole sulfonic acid.

phenylethyl alcohol (phenethyl alcohol)—used as a disinfectant, a preservative, and for its fragrance properties. It is a primary component of rose oil, and is also found in oranges, raspberries, and tea.

phosphatides—a primary component of lecithin, phosphatides are organic substances composed of fatty acids, glycerol, and phosphoric acid. Egg yolk and soybean are particularly phosphatide rich. *See also* phospholipids.

phosphatidic acid—one of several minor components of cosmetic and pharmaceutical liposomal membranes.

phosphatidylcholine—a major component of most cosmetic and pharmaceutical liposome structures, derived from commercially available egg yolk or soybean lecithin.

phosphatidyl ethanolamine—a minor component of cosmetic and pharmaceutical liposomal membranes.

phosphatidylinositol—a minor component of cosmetic and pharmaceutical liposomal membranes.

phosphatidylserine—used in the manufacturing of large quantities of liposomes.

phosphoenolpyruvic acid—skin care preparations containing this ingredient are said to improve dry skin given its moisturizing properties and its ability to accelerate cell turnover.

phospholipids (phosphatides)—used topically as a moisturizer and emollient because of their inherent compatibility with skin lipids. In general, natural phospholipids have a short-lived effect when topically applied, and are a primary material in the manufacture of liposomes. Phospholipids are complex fat substances that, together with protein, form the membrane of all living cells. *See also* liposomes.

phosphoric acid—a preservative and an anti-oxidant. It is irritating to the skin in concentrated solutions.

phytic acid—used to help maintain product stability. Its therapeutic activities are said to include skin-lightening, anti-inflammatory and anti-oxidant properties. It is naturally occurring in grains, seeds, and beans.

phytosphingosine—a sphingolipid that can improve the overall condition of skin and hair. Some sources site anti-microbial and anti-inflammatory properties. Research indicates similar activity to retinoic acid, in which case it may be particularly beneficial for aging and photo-aging skin.

phytosterol oleate—*see* phytosteryl canola glycerides.

phytosterols—*see* plant sterols.

phytosteryl canola glycerides—moisturizing and soothing. Ingredient suppliers indicate possible anti-inflammatory properties, as well as potential to improve skin-barrier properties through cholesterol replacement in lipid membranes. It is noted as particularly appropriate for sensitive and aging skin, particularly those that may have lowered lipid contents. This is a combination of phytosterol oleate and canola oil.

phytosteryl macadamiate—an emollient, it improves the overall skin condition. An ester of phytosterol and fatty acids from the macadamia nut, it can also be synthetically manufactured. *See also* macadamia nut oil.

phytosteryl/octyldodecyl lauroyl glutamate—an emollient and an occlusive agent helping retain moisture in the skin. It is found in a wide range of skin care formulations, but appears to be more widely used in color cosmetic products.

pilewort extract (*Ranunculus ficaria*)—also known as lesser celandine. It is used in cosmetic preparations as a skin conditioner and skin freshener.

pine bark extract—used as a solvent. It is also an anti-septic and stimulant. Pine bark extract can cause skin irritation.

pine cone extract—said to be a skin stimulant. This extract is obtained from pine cones. *See also* pine extract.

pine extract (*Pinus sp.*)—the different varieties of pine yield resin in greater or smaller quantities, of which a very small amount is employed for therapeutic purposes, primarily as ointments. Pine's therapeutic properties are described as bactericidal and stimulating to blood circulation. Manufacturers usually specify if the extract is from the pine's bark, cone, or needle. It can be irritating to the skin and cause red splotches.

pine needle extract—recommended for use as a skin stimulant. It is the extract of the needles of various pine species.

pine oil (*Pinus palustris*)—originally used as a solvent and a disinfectant, it is also deodorizing, anti-bacterial and anti-septic. Studies are now showing that certain fractions of pine oil may stimulate fibroblast growth, which would mean an increase in the turnover of epidermal cells. Pine oil is produced by distillation of small pine branches. It may be irritating to the skin and mucous membranes.

pineapple enzyme—used in folkloric medicine as an antiinflammatory. It is currently used in face masks and peeling lotions to remove the top layers of cells. Pineapple's activity is based on bromelin, an enzyme that dissolves keratin. Its important constituents include mucins, amino acids, polysaccharides, minerals, flavonoids, and enzymes. It can be irritating to the skin.

piscine oil, C_{30}-C_{46}—a fish oil used as an emollient.

plant extracts—an all-encompassing and vague term usually used for marketing effect. Its lack of specificity does not allow for the identification of potential benefits, botanical properties, or irritating effects.

P

plant sterols—active principles that can perform a variety of functions, including moisturizing. Used by cosmetic formulators to add a lipophilic property to a formulation,it is often derived from plants associated with oils such as soy and canola seed.

plantain extract (*Plantago sp.*)—credited with cooling, soothing, anti-septic, astringent, and bacteriostatic botanical properties. Its constituents include allatoin, apigenin, ascorbic acid, caffeic acid, cinnamic acid, coumaric acid, salicylic acid, tannin and vanillic acid. This is not the banana-like fruit but rather a green leafy herbaceous plant.

plantain fruit extract—*see* banana fruit extract.

***Plukenetia volubilis* seed oil**—commonly known as Inca peanut, sacha peanut, or mountain peanut. It has emollient and humectant properties, as well as acting as a skin protectant against external aggression. Among its constituents are tocopherol and unsaturated fatty acids, specifically omega 3 (alpha-linolenic acid), omega 6 (linoleic acid), and omega 9 (oleic acid). The plant is native to the Amazon, and oil is obtained from the seeds of the plant.

plum extract (*Prunus domestica*)—benefits and activity can vary according to the part of the plant from which the extract is obtained: flower, fruit, or seed. If the extract is from the flower, it is emollient, softening, and smoothing the skin, and it also helps protect the skin against external aggression; if the extract is from the fruit, it is moisturizing and can help smooth the skin; if the extract is from the seed, it is emollient.

plum seed oil—helps improve the overall skin condition. Some cosmetic manufacturers cite their use of plum oil for its anti-oxidant properties given its vitamin E content, as well as its unsaturated fatty acids (oleic and linoleic acids). It also contains beta-carotene and vitamin B.

pollen extract—softens and smooths the skin, and can protect it against external aggression, for example from harsh climates. It is also credited with anti-inflammatory properties. This is an extract of flower pollen that is composed of a variety of vitamins, essential amino acids, enzymes, lipids, fatty acids, and anti-oxidants.

poloxamer 188—a liquid surfactant polymer.

poloxamer 788—a surfactant polymer. A change in number (e.g., poloxamer 188 versus poloxamer 788) indicates the consistency of the ingredient, generally from liquid to paste to solid. The higher the number, the more solid the consistency.

polyacrylamide—a binder, film former, and fixative with greater use in hair and nail than in skin care preparations. It is used in some hand and body lotions and cleansing creams.

polyacrylamidomethyl benzylidene camphor—a sunscreen chemical that works as a UV filter and absorber. It has an approved usage level of up to 6 percent in the European Union.

polyacrylic acid salt—a binder, emulsion stabilizer, film former, and viscosity-increasing agent primarily used in shampoos.

polyalkoxy ester—a thickener, auxiliary emulsifier, and body agent in cosmetic formulations.

polybutene—a binder and viscosity-increasing agent used more in makeup than skin care preparations. Polybutene is a polymer of one or more butylenes obtained from petroleum oils.

polybutylene terephthalate—a film former and viscosity-increasing agent.

polycaprolactone—a synthetic polymer that acts as a suspending agent.

polydecene—an emollient and skin conditioner.

polydimethyl cyclosiloxane—*see* cyclomethicone.

polyether-1—a thickener with emulsifying properties. It can also provide humectancy and lubricity.

polyethoxylated retinamide (**PERA**)—has characteristics similar to retinoic acid and retinol, improving collagen synthesis and promoting wrinkle reduction. The penetration potential of PERA is said to be three times greater than that of retinol and six times greater than that of retinyl palmitate. PERA is a combination of retinoic acid with polyethylene glycol, and is designed for enhanced stability and skin permeability. It would be incorporated into anti-aging products. *See also* retinoids entry in Chapter 4.

polyethylene—used to regulate viscosity, suspension properties, and general stability in cosmetic formulations. It is derived from petroleum gas or dehydration of alcohol.

polyethylene beads—used in scrubs as replacement for almond particles. Some companies prefer it as they consider it less abrasive for delicate skins.

polyethylene glycol (**PEG**)—a binder, solvent, plasticizing agent, and softener widely used for cosmetic cream bases and pharmaceutical ointments. PEGs are quite humectant up to a molecular weight of 500. Beyond this weight, their water uptake diminishes.

polyethylene glycol monostearate—an emulsifier. *See also* PEG.

polyethylene particles—*see* polyethylene beads.

polyethylene terephthalate—a film former and viscosity-increasing agent. This is a synthetic polymer.

polyglucan (beta-glucan)—reported to enhance the skin's natural defense mechanism, which becomes less effective with age and exposure to UV light. It is also credited with wound-healing properties and it promotes cellular activity; serves as a topical moisturizer with long-lasting moisturizing effects; reduces wrinkles; helps protect the skin from infection; and protects the skin from invasion by toxic agents caused by pollution and injuries due to abrasions, exposure to UV light, and extremes in climatic conditions. In addition to this impressive list, polyglucans are credited with immunostimulatory properties. A polyglucan is a hydrophilic ingredient, able to absorb more than 10 times its weight in water. It can be absorbed into the outer layers of the epidermis, thereby facilitating penetration into the pores and follicular openings of the skin. Once applied on the skin, it forms a protective, hydrated film with superior adhesive properties that does not appear to interfere with normal skin respiration. These film-forming and protective properties are particularly valuable for aging skin suffering from diminished collagen and elastin, as well as impaired hydration and elasticity. Derived from yeast cell walls, polyglucans are compatible for formulation with all normally used skin care and other cosmetic ingredients. *See also* glucans; beta-glucan.

polyglyceryl-2 diisostearate—an emulsifier, it also contributes emollient properties to a formulations, helping increase skin softness.

polyglyceryl-3-beeswax—an emulsifier, this is a beeswax derivative that suppliers cite for use in emulsions, oil gels and color cosmetics (e.g., lipsticks). It is an ester of beeswax with polyglycerin-3.

polyglyceryl-3-dioleate—an emulsifier for water-in-oil emulsions. It is listed as being very suitable for use in baby care products, water-resistant sun-protection products, skin creams, and dry skin treatment products. It is an ester of oleic acid with polyglycerol.

polyglyceryl-3 distearate—an emulsifier used in oil-in-water emulsions.

polyglyceryl-3 methylglucose distearate—an emulsifier and skin conditioner.

polyglyceryl-4-oleate—used as an emulsifier in cosmetic formulations. It may also be used as a lubricant, plasticizer, gelling agent, and dispersant. It is prepared by adding alcohol to coconut oil or other triglycerides.

polyglyceryl-6 distearate—an emulsifier. It can be found in products for sensitive skin, baby products, and sun care products.

polyglyceryl-10 dipalmitate—also known as decaglyceryl dipalmitate. It is an emollient and emulsifier.

polyglyceryl-10 stearate—an emuslifer, it can also help improve the skin's overall look and feel.

polyglyceryl methacrylate—a film former used in moisturizers, skin care products, and fragrance preparations. It is a synthetic polymer.

polyhydroxystearic acid—an emulsifier, also used as a dispersing agent.

polyisobutene (hydrogenated)—an emollient.

polylactic acid (PLA)— a lactic acid polymer that can be used as a filler.

polymethylacrylate—a film former. It is a synthetic polymer used in suntan gels, creams, and liquids as well as a variety of makeup preparations such as blushes, foundations, and powders.

polymethyl methacrylate—a film former, it can help maintain moisture in the skin.

polymethoxy bicyclic oxazolidine—a preservative that is active against yeast, bacteria, and mold. It can be used alone or with parabens, in which case it contributes to the preservative activity. This ingredient can be used in rinse-off and leave-on cosmetics, with manufacturers reporting a good toxicological profile at recommended use levels.

polyoxyethylene cetyl ether—*see* polyoxyethylene compounds.

polyoxyethylene compounds—emulsifiers used in cosmetic formulations. *See also* PEG.

polyoxyethylene 20 monooleate—an emulsifier. *See also* PEG 20-oleate.

polyoxyethylene nonylphenyl ether (nonoxynol-1)—an emulsifier.

polyoxyethylene-21 steryl ether—an emulsifier. *See also* steareth-21.

polyoxyethylene propylene glycol monostearate—an emulsifier.

polypentaerythritol tetralaurate—an emulsifier. It is considered a non-comedogenic raw material.

polypeptides—*see* hydrolyzed animal protein; protein. *See also* peptides in Chapter 4.

polyphenols—a class of natural anti-oxidants found in such substances as green tea, coffee, and grapes.

polyquaternium-10—a cellulose polymer and conditioning agent used in skin-conditioning formulations.

polyquaternium-24—suggested by some companies for use as an SPF enhancer in sunscreen formulations. This is a film former similar to polyquaternium-10, but it gives better skin feel and has a lipophilic character that enables it to act as a secondary emulsifier and help form a thicker, more uniform sunscreen film.

polyquaternium-51—used as a film former and for skin-conditioning properties, including to improve skin feel.

polysaccharide xanthan—*see* xanthan gum.

polysilicone-11—a film former, it can help reduce water evaporation from the skin, maintaining hydration. It is used in skin care preparations as well as color cosmetics and hair care products.

polysorbate 20—a solubilizer, emulsifier, viscosity modifier, and stabilizer of essential oils in water.

polysorbate 40—an emulsifier and stabilizer of essential oils in water. It is also a detergent and employed in a variety of cleansing and moisturizing preparations.

polysorbate 60, -60NF—an emulsifier, wetting agent, and detergent emulsifier for mineral oil, fats, and waxes. It is also a stabilizer of essential oils in water. It is widely used in cosmetic and toiletry preparations.

polysorbate 80, -80 NF—an oil-in-water emulsifier, pigment dispersant, and solubilizer for oils and fragrances. It is used in creams, lotions, and makeup bases.

polysorbate 120—a fragrance solubilizer and an emulsifier used in sunscreen preparations and moisturizing creams and lotions.

polytetrafluoroethylene—*see* PTFE.

polyvinyl acetate emulsion—a binder, emulsion stabilizer, and film-forming substance. *See also* polyvinylpyrrolidone.

polyvinyl alcohol—a binder, film former, and viscosity-increasing agent used primarily in makeup and nail polish preparations.

polyvinylpyrrolidone (PVP)—*see* PVP.

pomegranate extract (*Punica granatum*)—has cleansing, astringent, tonic, and purifying properties. It also is a strong natural antioxidant with skin-protecting and anti-inflammatory properties. Its constituents include polyphenols and anthocyanidins. In addition to pomegranate extract, and depending on a formula's requirements, cosmetic formulators can use bark extract, the fruit juice, the seed, and the seed oil.

pomegranate seed oil—used for its emollient properties. Suppliers indicate that is moisturizing, nourishing and protective, and has soothing, anti-irritant, and anti-inflammatory properties. They cite it as particularly beneficial for aging skin as well as for post-sun treatment. Pomegranate seed oil is considered relatively stable; it is easily absorbed by the skin and does not leave a greasy afterfeel. Among its constituents are ellagic acid and omega 5 (also known as punicic acid), which are both anti-oxidants. In addition, it contains vitamins B_1, B_2, and C, as well as potassium and magnesium. It is apparently expensive to manufacture (approximately 200 pounds of fresh pomegranate produces one pound of pomegranate seed oil). *See* also pomegranate extract.

poplar bud extract—said to be anti-bacterial and support wound-healing. It may also be used topically for treating superficially broken skin as well as sunburn.

poppy seed oil (*Papaver orientale*)—occlusive and emollient. Among poppy seed oil's constituents are found linoleic acid, oleic acid, palmitic acid, and stearic acid.

Portulaca oleracea—commonly known as purslane. Its therapeutic activities are considered to include anti-microbial, anti-fungal, anti-inflammatory, and analgesic (pain-relieving). Used in extract form, its constituents include alkaloids, coumarins, glycosides, omega-3 fatty acids, proteins, and flavonoids.

potassium PCA—a humectant that improves skin moisturization.

potassium alginate—*see* algin.

potassium alum (**alum**)—a cosmetic astringent.

potassium carbomer 941—*see* carbomer entry in Chapter 4.

potassium cetyl phosphate—a surfactant used in the preparation of emulsions.

potassium chloride—a laboratory reagent used to increase product viscosity in cosmetic and pharmaceutical preparations.

potassium citrate—it acts as a buffer, maintaining product pH constant, a pH adjuster and a product stabilizer. This is a potassium salt.

potassium hydroxide—used as an emulsifier in lotions and as an alkali in liquid soaps, protective creams, and shaving preparations. Depending on the concentration used, it can be highly irritating to the skin and/or cause a burning sensation.

potassium myristate—a cleansing and emulsifying agent.

potassium phosphate—a humectant and pH adjuster used in cosmetic formulations. Potassium phosphate is an inorganic salt.

potassium sorbate—a preservative primarily against mold and yeast, and used in concentrations of 0.025 to 0.2 percent. It is non-toxic but may cause mild skin irritation.

potassium stearate—a cleansing and emulsifying agent.

potassium sulfate—a reagent in cosmetics. Potassium sulfate is an inorganic salt with a primary function as a viscosity-increasing agent.

potato extract (*Solanum tuberosum*)—studies indicate it can help in treating severe dry skin conditions such as psoriasis. Psoralen, the relevant fraction of potato extract, appears to prevent keratinocyte proliferation, and is known to inhibit DNA synthesis. Among potato's constituents are vitamins B and C, as well as potassium, magnesium, and zinc.

potato starch (**modified**)—a polysaccharide used as a thickener, it works well in acidic formulations. It is also used as an absorbent and binder. *See also* potato extract.

PPG-2 isoceteth-20 acetate—an emulsifier.

PPG-2 methyl ether acetate—a solvent, it is also used as a formula stabilizer and to improve skin penetration in topically applied acne preparations containing erythromycin.

PPG-2 ceteareth-9—a surfactant and emulsifying agent.

PPG-2-PEG 20 isocetyl acetate—a fragrance solubilizer and oil-in-water emulsifier.

PPG-3 benzyl ether myristate—an emollient that provides silicone-like characteristics to a formulation. It is used to give shine in hair products and gloss to lip products. It can also be found in sun care preparations to improve SPF values.

PPG-4 myristyl ether propionate—an emollient.

PPG-5-ceteth 20—a surfactant and emulsifying agent.

PPG-15 stearyl ether—an emollient and skin-conditioning agent.

PPG-20 methyl glucose ether—an emollient.

PPG-26-buteth-26—a skin conditioner, emulsifier and fragrancing ingredient. Its function in a product will depend on the formulator's need.

PPG-30 cetyl ester, -50 cetyl ester—both are emollients.

pregnenolone hemisuccinate—used topically as an anti-inflammatory and anti-itch agent. It is a corticosteroid. *See also* primula extract.

primrose—*see* primula extract.

primula extract (*Primula officinalis*; *Primula vulagris*) (**primrose**)—traditionally used as an adjunct soothing and anti-itching treatment. It is useful in dry skin preparations. The leaves of some species are known to cause skin irritation sometimes resulting in a form of eczema.

procollagen—water binding and moisturizing. Procollagen is a triple helical molecule of collagen, and is fully soluble and membrane permeable. It is hygroscopic and, as such, is able to bind many times its weight in water. Procollagen is found naturally in the skin as a first stage in the production of collagen. With age, there is a decrease in the skin's procollagen content that may have some correlation to the increased dryness and reduction in elasticity often associated with mature skin.

proline—a skin-conditioning agent. An amino acid found in the collagen molecule. *See also* amino acid.

propanediol—a solvent and used to reduce a formulation's viscosity. It can be synthetically manufactured or naturally derived from certain plants (e.g., from corn).

propanetriol—*see* glycerin.

propolis—once considered a mystical cure for such problems as infections and troubled skin. Chemists recognize propolis as having a potential sun protective function, and many preparations for acne problems also contain propolis as an active substance for its healing, cleansing, and anti-seborrhoeic properties. It is also moisturizing and can help smooth the skin. Propolis is made up of resins, balsam, various waxes, essential oils, pollen, flavonoids, amino acids, vitamins, and minerals. This is a component of beeswax, often referred to by beekeepers as "bee glue." It is collected from trees, shrubs, flowers, and other types of plants visited by bees.

propolis extract HD 10%—*see* propolis.

propyl gallate—an anti-oxidant with preservative properties.

propylparaben—one of the most frequently used preservatives against bacteria and mold. It has a low sensitizing and low toxicity factor, is reputed to be very safe, and considered to be a non-comedogenic raw material. *See also* parabens entry in Chapter 4.

propylene carbonate—used in chemical reactions as a solvent, plasticizer, solubilizer, or dilutent.

propylene glycol—next to water, this is the most common moisture-carrying vehicle used in cosmetic formulations. It has better skin permeation than glycerin, and it also gives a pleasant feel with less greasiness than glycerin. Propylene glycol is used as a humectant because it absorbs water from the air. It also serves as a solvent for anti-oxidants and preservatives. In addition, it has preservative properties against bacteria and fungi when used in concentrations of 16 percent or higher. There is a concern that propylene glycol is an irritant at high concentrations, though it appears to be quite safe at usage levels under 5 percent. *See also* glycerin.

propylene glycol ceteth-3 acetate—an emollient used in moisturizing preparations.

propylene glycol dicaprylate/dicaprate—has very good emollient properties. It also provides a product with good skin coverage, and spreadability and absorption promotion properties. It does not cause skin irritation.

propylene glycol di-isostearate—considered an excellent emollient, it is is similar to jojoba oil.

propylene glycol di-pelargonate—an emollient ester with good skin-penetrating and spreadability properties. It does not leave a greasy feel.

propylene glycol mono-isostearate (propylene glycol iso stearate)—an emollient.

propylene glycol monomethyl ether—a stabilizer and skin-penetration enhancer often found in topical acne preparations in which erythromycin is the active substance.

propylene glycol myristyl ether acetate—a skin-conditioning agent and emollient; also used in lipstick.

protein (partially hydrolyzed protein; peptide; peptone; polypeptide)—its main function is to produce a good film on the skin, thus helping reduce the loss of natural moisture. The films formed by animal proteins, such as collagen and elastin, are not occlusive as may be the case with mineral oil. Rather, they lie on the skin and have an affinity for it. All proteins, whether animal, vegetable, or silk derived, are built up from amino acids linked together to form a polymer. Depending on its source, the molecular weight of naturally occurring proteins may range from several thousands to millions, and the amino acid composition, which also influences the protein's properties, may vary widely. In the case of collagen-derived proteins, attributes include the ability to form clear solutions, contribute viscosity, stabilize oil-in-water emulsions, bind moisture, and form glossy films. The benefits claimed are soft and silky skin feel, increased moisture retention with a related improvement of elasticity, and a decrease in chapping and irritation conditions. Adding protein to skin-cleansing surfactants reduces skin irritation and dryness. Animal-derived collagen protein has been the preferred protein because of performance, ease of availability, and cost. However, because of consumer preferences to move away from animal products, vegetal proteins have been perfected for use in skin care cosmetics. The most popular appears to be wheat-based hydrolyzed protein. Proteins are usually hydrolyzed to achieve lower molecular values, thereby enhancing their moisture-binding properties.

pseudoalteromonas **ferment extract**—a humectant derived from marine bacteria, it can help reduce skin roughness.

pseudocollagen—acts in much the same way as collagen, leaving the skin feeling soft and supple. Pseudocollagen forms a moisture-retentive film on the skin in a similar way to soluble collagen. It represents the pseudocollagenous extract of yeast cells, and is plant derived.

PTFE (polytetrafluoroethylene)—a bulking agent, it is also used in cosmetic preparations to improve the formulation's feel and spreadability. PTFE may also have some waterproofing potential.

pullulan—used as a binder and film former in a variety of formulation categories (skin, make-up and hair), it is a polysaccharide derived from the *Aureobasidium pullulans* yeast.

pumice powder—usually employed in cosmetics for removing rough skin. It is used in hand-cleansing preparations, skin-cleansing grains, powders, and soaps for acne. Because of its abrasive action, daily use is not recommended. If used continuously on dry, sensitive skin, it will most likely cause irritation. It can also be an irritant when used in soapless detergents. Pumice is of volcanic origin and consists primarily of complex silicates of aluminum and alkali metals.

pumpkin (*Cucurbita pepo*)—credited with purative properties. Cosmetic applications include use in acne products and as an anti-seborrheic. Among its constituents are beta-carotene and linoleic acid.

pumpkin enzyme—exfoliating and softening, it can help smooth the appearance of fine line and wrinkles.

pumpkin seed extract—classified as a skin conditioner, ingredient suppliers indicate an ability to promote collagen synthesis, and thus to help improve the appearance of fine lines and wrinkles, skin tone, smoothness, firmness, and elasticity. Supporting clinical evidence is currently scant.

purcellin oil (nonanimal) (cetearyl octanoate)—used as a fixative in perfumes. This is a synthetic mixture of fatty esters designed to simulate the natural oil obtained from the preen glands of waterfowl.

PVP (polyvinylpyrrolidone)—a chemical ingredient that, depending on the formulatory requirement, can act as a binder, viscosity controller, emulsion stabilizer, or film former. Its benefits include water and wear resistance, pigment dispersion, a non-greasy feel, and improved stick integrity. PVP is commonly found in waterproof sunscreens, mascaras, and lipsticks in order to improve their wear.

PVP/eicosene copolymer—a waterproofing polymer with sunscreen absorption properties. *See also* polyvinylpyrrolidone.

PVP/hexdecene copolymer—designed for use in formulations where unique delivery systems are desired. *See also* polyvinylpyrrolidone.

PVP/triacontene copolymer—a PVP with greater waterproofing abilities and significantly improved retention of UV absorbers in sunscreen products than PVP/eicosene. *See also* polyvinylpyrrolidone.

pyridoxine dipalmitate—a skin-conditioning agent used in moisturizing formulations.

pyridoxine hydrochloride—*see* pyridoxine HCL.

pyridoxine HCL—a skin-conditioning agent that is also widely used in hair products.

pyridoxine tripalmitate—soothing to the skin. This is a stable, oil-soluble form of vitamin B_6. It prevents scaling and skin dryness, and is also used as a product texturizer.

pyrrolidonic carbon acid (nalidone)—a natural moisturizing factor that protects the skin from dehydration and increases its moisture-retention capabilities. *See also* sodium PCA.

pyruvic acid—an alpha hydroxy acid that can be irritating and is considered difficult to work with. It has a larger molecular size than the most commonly used AHAs. Sodium pyruvate is more commonly used, and is an organic salt. *See also* alpha hydroxy acid.

Q

Quassia amara—an anti-bacterial. Quassia yields quassin, a bitter alkaloid obtained from the wood of *Quassiaamara*. It is primarily used as a denaturant for ethyl alcohol.

quaternium-15—an all-purpose preservative, it is active against bacteria, mold, and yeast, and used in concentrations of 0.02 to 0.3 percent. Though not a primary skin irritant, quaternium-15 is considered a highly sensitizing preservative when used in leave-on cosmetic preparations. Dermatologists find it to be the most frequent sensitizer among preservatives in the United States. It is probably the greatest formaldehyde releaser among cosmetic preservatives, causing dermatitis in people who are allergic to formaldehyde and even in those who are not. The technical data of some manufacturers indicates, however, that quaternium-15 does not contain or release free gaseous formaldehyde. These would most likely be versions of quaternium-15 that have been specially formulated and adjusted to avoid formaldehyde release. The Cosmetic Ingredient Review (CIR) Panel has concluded that 0.2% or less is a safe and effective use level in cosmetics that eliminates the sensitization potential of the product.

quaternium-18—a surfactant.

quaternium-18 bentonite—a thickener and conditioning agent. It helps control product viscosity.

quaternium-18 hectorite—used as a thickener and suspending agent. It helps control product viscosity. Produced by a reaction of hectorite and the quaternary salt, it is used in concentrations of 1.5 percent. *See also* hectorite.

quercus **extract (English oak extract)**—*see* oak.

quinquina—*see* cinchona extract.

quince extract (*Pyrus cydonia*)—when obtained from the juice of the fruit, it is astringent and tonic. It is considered appropriate for dry skin and in eye treatment preparations. *See also* quince seed.

quince seed—an emollient, emulsifier, and thickening agent, it can also be used as an abrasive. Quince seed extract can also help mask odor. It may cause allergic reactions.

quinine extract—an alkaloid from the bark of *Cinchona officinalis*. *See also* cinchona extract.

ramulus mori extract—credited with strong skin-lightening abilities because of tyrosinase inhibition activities. Even at low concentrations, ramulus mori has demonstrated more efficacious tyrosinase inhibition capacities than kojic acid and arbutin. Studies indicate little to no irritation caused by this extract. Ramulus mori extract is derived specifically from the young twigs of the white mulberry tree (*Morus alba*). These properties would make ramulus mori beneficial in products designed to even skin tone. *See also* mulberry extract.

rapeseed sterols (*Brassica campestris*)—a mixture of at least two of the following sterols: sitosterol, stigmsterol, campesterol, and cholesterol, the primary sterol components of rapseseed. Credited with emollient properties, it can help maintain the skin feeling soft and smooth. In some forms (e.g., PEG-10 rapeseed sterol), it also has cleansing properties. This botanical is related to the cabbage family.

raspberry concentrate (*Rubus idaeus*)—botanical properties are described as astringent and tonic. Raspberry concentrate is also added to cosmetics for its fragrance-enhancing ability. Some sources claim that there is no evidence of raspberries having any external value for enhancing the skin, and that they may increase allergenicity.

raspberry extract—when the extract is obtained from the whole plant it exhibits properties able to protect the skin against harmful external aggressors. Extract from the fruit is considered astringent, tonic, smoothing, as well as keratolytic, helping exfoliate excess dead cells from the surface of the stratum corneum. Among raspberry's constituents are the flavonoids kaempferol and quercetin, tannins, polypeptides, volatile oil, citric and malic acids, and vitamins A, B, C, and E.

raspberry seed oil—attributed with anti-oxidant, free radical scavenging and anti-inflammatory properties. In addition, it is anti-inflammatory, skin conditioning, and emollient, and ingredient suppliers indicate potential UVA and UVB absorption capacities. It is made up of a very high percentage of essential fatty acids (including omega-3 and omega-6), carotenoides, and vitamin E. This is the fixed oil obtained from raspberry seeds.

red algae extracts—*see* seaweed extract.

red clover (*Trifolium pratense*)—depending on the part of the plant used (flower; stem; leaf; flowers, stems, and leaves combined) and the format of the ingredient (extract, powder, juice) properties can range from exfoliant (red clover flower powder), to anti-oxidant (seed extract), to generally improving overall skin condition (general extract). Thus, it can be used for a variety of purposes in any number of formulations. Red clover has been described as beneficial for acne and eczema. Isoflavones are among its constituents. *See also* isoflavones.

red currant (*Ribes rubrum*)—the fruit has astringent properties, while the fruit extract is considered tonic and refreshing. When used in cosmetic preparations, red currant juice can help improve the skin's general condition. Constituents of red current include vitamin C, fruit acids, pectin, and flavonoids.

red poppy extract (*Papaver rhoeas*)—considered soothing and emollient, this extract is obtained either from the flower's petals or from the full flower. When the extract is derived from poppy seeds it is soothing and skin conditioning. Poppy flower water is known to be astringent and able to mask odor.

red vine extract—anti-inflammatory and anti-itching. Traditionally used for broken or fragile capillaries.

red wine—contains tartaric acid, a member of the alpha hydroxy acid family. Red wine can be used in cosmetics for its anti-inflammatory and polyphenol-based anti-oxidant properties. Red wine's therapeutic benefits are more closely linked to its chemical constituents rather than its topical application on the skin. *See also* alpha hydroxy acid; grape.

resin—used to give gloss, flow, adhesion, and water resistance to cosmetics. This is a brittle substance, usually translucent or transparent, that can be found in nature or synthetically manufactured. Among the natural resins are dammar, elemi, and sandarac, which are formed from the hardened secretions of these plants. Toxicity and allergenicity depend on the source used.

resorcinol—in very mild solutions, it is used as an anti-septic and soothing preparation for itchy skin. In slightly higher concentrations, resorcinol removes the top layer of the stratum corneum and is used particularly in cases of acne. In still higher concentrations, it can act as an aggressive surface skin exfoliant. Resorcinol can also be used as a preservative. While it is a beneficial

R

skin care ingredient when used in low concentrations, it causes irritation in higher concentrations with a strong burning sensation and a reddening of the skin. Used in high concentrations as a peel, resorcinol may cause a variety of problems, including swelling. It is is obtained from various resins.

restharrow extract (*Ononis arvensis*; *Ononis spinosa*)—able to control sebum secretion and is soothing to the skin, it is also an emollient that provides relief for skin itching. Traditionally used for relieving the problems of eczema. The extract is obtained from the plant's roots.

reticulin (soluble)—a protein that acts as a protective agent against water loss. It helps increase the water content of the skin's outer layers, plumping up the epidermis and leaving the skin softer and smoother. Unlike proteins of a similar molecular weight, when reticulin dries, it leaves the skin feeling pleasant and without tackiness.

retinaldehyde—a mild retinoid credited with increasing epidermal thickness without producing erythema.

retinoic acid (tretinoin)—a vitamin A derivative. It has demonstrated an ability to alter collagen synthesis, increase dermal hyaluronic acid levels, and stimulate fibroblast growth and the extracellular matrix. It is used for keratinization disorders and for treating acne. Retinoic acid's anti-aging effect has been convincingly documented and it is often used for treating the visible signs of aging, though these results can take approximately 6 months to be visible. It is associated with a number of adverse effects, including irritation, photosensitivity, skin dryness, redness, and peeling. It should also not be used while pregnant. *See also* retinoids in Chapter 4.

retinol—a retinoid considered to be a skin revitalizer. It is reported to enhance skin radiance and treat conditions associated with chronological aging, such as wrinkles and fine lines, as well as dermatological disorders, including acne, follicular and lesion papules, actinic keratosis, oily skin, and rosacea. According to clinical dermatologists, retinol is one of the few substances with a demonstrated ability to reduce and prevent fine lines and wrinkles. It is able to alter the behavior of aged cells so they act in a more youthful manner. It is considered necessary for normal epidermal cell growth and differentiation and stimulates the production of new blood vessels in the skin, improving skin tone. In addition, retinol has anti-oxidant capacities and protects dermal fibers by counteracting the increased activity of enzymes that degrade collagen and elastin when the skin is exposed to UV rays. Retinol can be drying to the skin when used for a prolonged period of time or in concentrations that are too high. A weaker retinoid than retinoic acid, retinol converts to retinoic acid once on the skin. When compared to retinoic acid, retinol has an increased penetration potential and is less irritating, making it an effective ingredient for anti-aging products. The anti-aging benefits of topically treating skin with retinol are based on its penetration ability, which allows it to reach the sites in the skin requiring treatment. When used on sensitive skin for a prolonged period of time or in concentrations that are too high, retinol can cause dermatitis. *See also* retinoids in Chapter 4.

retinyl esters—precursors of retinoic acid. Common retinyl esters include acetate, propionate, and palmitate. When compared to retinol, they have a more difficult time penetrating the skin and they demonstrate a lower clinical effectiveness. However, they are more stable than retinol and hence considered easier to incorporate into a formulation. With the improvements in delivery technology for retinol, and depending on the formulatory needs, manufacturers are increasingly using retinol rather than the retinyl esters, given retinol's greater activity. *See also* retinoids in Chapter 4.

retinyl linoleate—a conditioning agent, this is an ester of retinol and linoleic acid. *See also* retinol; linoleic acid.

retinyl palmitate—a skin conditioner. This retinoid is considered a milder version of retinoic acid, given its conversion properties. Once on the skin, it converts to retinol, which in turn converts to retinoic acid. Physiologically, it is credited with increasing epidermal thickness, stimulating the production of more epidermal protein, and increasing skin elasticity. Cosmetically, retinyl palmitate is used to reduce the number and depth of fine lines and wrinkles, and prevent skin roughness resulting from UV exposure. Secondary reactions such as erythema, dryness, or irritation are not associated with retinyl palmitate. It is even more effective when used in combination with glycolic acid because it achieves greater penetration. In the United States, its maximum usage level in cosmetic formulations is 2 percent. Retinyl palmitate is the ester of retinol and palmitic acid. *See also* retinoids; retinyl esters; vitamin A palmitate; retinoids in Chapter 4.

retinyl palmitate polypeptide—allows for the delivery of vitamin A as a water-dispersable substance. *See also* retinyl esters.

rhodochrosite extract—attributed with anti-oxidant, skin-conditioning, and skin protecting properties. This extract is obtained from rhodochrosite, a rose-colored mineral composed primarily of manganese carbonate.

rhubarb extract (*Rheum palmatum*)—astringent and tonic, rhubarb is also said to act as a tyrosinase inhibitor and have skin-lightening properties. Constituents include gallic acid, emodin, glucosides, tannoids, and resins. The root is used for obtaining extract, powder, tinctures, syrups, and infusions.

riboflavin (Vitamin B$_2$)—used in skin care preparations as an emollient. It can be found in sun care products as a suntan enhancer. Medicinally, it is used for the treatment of skin lesions.

riboflavin tetraacetate—a skin-conditioning agent, it is a vitamin B$_2$ derivative. *See also* vitamin B.

ribonucleic acid (RNA)—a surface film-forming agent with moisturizing action. This is the polyribonucleotide found in both the nucleus and the cytoplasm of cells.

rice amino acids—humectant and skin-conditioning. This is an amino acid complex. Some chemical manufacturers note that it is all natural and derived from vegetables.

rice bran—soothing. It is credited with promoting collagen formation and inhibiting lipid peroxidation in the skin. It is recommended for dry, mature skin. Rice bran is employed in various forms, including extract, oil, and wax. The oil functions as a carrier and an emollient. The germ and bran of unpolished rice contains linolic acid, oleic acid, palmitic acid, vitamin E, and oryzanol.

rice flour—*see* rice starch.

rice oil (*Oryza sativa*)—emollient, it is recommended for combination skin products where the ingredients must not be too aggressive for the dry skin area, and yet should be helpful for the oily T-zone.

rice germ oil—used in cosmetics for its emollient and occlusive properties.

rice starch—emollient and able to form a soothing, protective film when applied to the skin. In addition, rice starch is employed in cosmetic formulations for its absorbent, bulking, binding and viscosity-controlling action. It is used in baby and face powders. Rice starch is a crystalline polymeric compound obtained from grains of rice.

ricinoleamide DEA—an emulsifier with lubricity, and good wetting and softening properties. It can also serve as a foam booster and formula stabilizer when blended with anionic surfactants such as lauryl sulfates.

ricinoleth—a surfactant used as a cleansing, emulsifying, and solubilizing agent.

RNA—*see* ribonucleic acid.

roe extract (*Acipenser stellatus*) (**caviar**)—used in products for oily and mature dehydrated skins in need of revitalization. It has a high and wide-ranging vitamin content that includes vitamins A, B_1, B_2, and B_6, D, and E. Roe extract contains an array of other constituents including cobalt, copper, fluorine, iodine, iron, magnesium, manganese, phosphorus, silicium, and zinc. The amino acids present are glutamic acid, glycine, methionine, lysine, arginine, histidine, and aspartic acid. In addition, roe has essential and sulfured amino acids and unsaturated fatty acids. Usage levels range from 1 to 5 percent depending on the preparation. It is prepared from sturgeon roe.

roman chamomile oil (*Anthemis nobilis*)—the most popular variety of chamomile, it is different from German chamomile (*matricaria*). It is used in cosmetics for its tonic, healing, and fragrancing properties. *See also* chamomile.

rosa mosqueta oil (*Rosa eglanteria*)—*see* rose hip oil.

rose extract (*Rosa sp.*)—credited with astringent, tonic, and deodorant properties. It is also used as a fragrance.

rose geranium oil (*Pelargonium graveolens*)—a volatile oil used for masking odors and perfuming a product. Among rose geranium's constituents are limonene, menthone, linalool, geranyl acetate, citronellol, and geraniol.

rose hip (Rosa canina)—astringent properties are attributed to the rose hip fruit, and the flower is used to mask odor. Rich in vitamin C, this is the seedpod that remains once the rose petals fall from the flower. *See also* rose hip oil.

R

rose hip oil—emollient. It is also wound-healing and anti-septic. Studies indicate an ability to improve skin hydration, and aid in cases of pruritis and xerosis. It also helps regulate oil gland secretion. Rose hip oil is nourishing and rejuvenating and exhibits strong moisture-retention abilities. Its constituents include very high levels of essential fatty acids, and it is a natural source of retinoic acid. It is beneficial for use in sun care products, given its apparent UV-protection abilities. It is also increasingly incorporated into anti-aging and anti-oxidant products. Rose hip oil can be derived from the rose hips of various different rose varietals, including *Rosa canina*, and *Rosa eglanteria*, which is also known as rosa mosqueta.

rose hip powder—incorporated into formulations as a natural abrasive and for its ability to help remove dead surface cells (keratolytic action). Thus, it helps improve the skin's look, feel, and texture.

rose oil—has been credited with anti-septic, disinfectant, slightly tonic, and soothing properties. Some sources also cite moisturizing and moisture-retention abilities. It is found helpful in cases of skin redness or inflammation, and where moisturization and regeneration is needed. Rose oil may be beneficial to all skin types, particularly mature, dry, or sensitive skins. As one of the most expensive essential oils, true rose oil is only used in very high-grade perfumes. Rose oil is almost always adulterated with substances like geranium, lemongrass, palmarosa, and terpene alcohols. However, the process of adulteration has become so refined that it is almost impossible to discover frauds. To produce rose oil, rose buds are picked for only a few hours in the morning, right after the dew, and are immediately distilled. According to some sources, 30 roses are required to make one drop of oil. It is considered the least toxic of all essences. Given the cost and potential of adulteration, rosewater is widely used as a replacement for rose oil in cosmetics and perfumery. Among its rose oil's many constituents are citronellol, geraniol, nerol, linalool, farnesol, and eugenol.

rose petal extract—has mild astringency and tonic value. *See also* rose extract.

rose wax—floral waxes such as rose and jasmine complement the skin's natural lipids and give a formulation wear- and smudge-resistant properties. It can also form an occlusive barrier on the skin's surface, thereby helping retain skin moisture. Rose wax is an almost odorless residue left after the extraction of the oily fractions.

rosemary extract (*Rosmarinus officinalis*)—considered wound-healing, astringent, toning, tonic, refreshing, stimulating, deodorant, anti-septic, reactivating, anti-bacterial, anti-microbial, softening, and invigorating. Rosemary also helps improve blood circulation, thereby aiding in skin regeneration. An alcohol fraction of rosemary extract had demonstrated strong anti-oxidant activity by hindering free-radical–induced reactions. Rosemary adds fragrance to a formulation. Some constituents of rosemary extract include a variety of amino acids, caffeic acid, rosemary acid, and apigenin. The leaf is the part of the plant that is used.

rosemary leaf oil—can be used to tone, refresh, and mask odor in a formulation. It also helps improve the feel of dry or rough skin. *See also* rosemary extract.

rosemary oil—credited with anti-septic properties, it is also used for masking odor and providing fragrance. Rosemary oil is considered beneficial for acne, dermatitis, and eczema. Some reports indicate that rosemary oil may stimulate fibroblast growth with a possible increase in epidermal cell turnover. This would make it useful in products for aging and mature skin. Rosemary oil, obtained through distillation of the herb's flowering tops, is superior to that obtained through distillation of the stems and leaves. The latter process, however, is more common among the commercial oils.

rosewater—credited with soothing, astringent, and cleansing properties. In addition, it can be used as a vehicle for other ingredients and as an eye lotion. Ointment of rosewater is said to have soothing and cooling properties when applied to abrasions and other superficial skin lesions. Rosewater is often mixed with glycerin, which provides moisturization and lubricity.

rosewood oil (*Aniba rosaeodora*)—one of the major perfumery oils used as a middle note. Until recently, it was little used in aromatherapy. Although it does not have major curative power, it is attributed with astringent and tonic properties. In addition, it can help perfume and mask product odor. Some sources cite it as a useful cellular stimulant and tissue regenerator. As such, it would be applicable to sensitive and aged skin, wrinkles, and general skin care. Clinical evidence to support this however is scarce. Its constituents include camphene, geraniol, neral, gernial, linalool, and linalool oxides. It is very mild, safe to use, and is obtained by means of distillation of the chopped wood.

rough horsetail extract (*Equisetum hyemale*)—many properties are attributed to this botanical extract, including tonic, soothing, emollient, cleansing, healing, and nourishing. It is also said to have anti-bacterial and anti-inflammatory properties. *See also* horsetail extract.

R

rowan (*Sorbus aucuparia*)—also known as mountain ash. The extract, which helps maintain good skin condition, is obtained from the tree's fruit. Constituents include vitamins B and C, sorbite, tannin, carotene, flavonoids, fruit acids (e.g., malic acid), mineral salt, and glucose.

royal jelly—the therapeutic value associated with royal jelly in skin care products includes favoring the regeneration of dermal tissue, stimulating cell metabolism, normalizing sebum secretion, providing photoprotection, moisturizing, improving the skin's look and feel, and acting as an anti-septic and an anti-inflammatory. These characteristics are attributed to royal jelly's complex composition, which includes a mixture of proteins, fats, carbohydrates, water, growth factors, and various trace elements. It has a high amino acid content (including aspartic acid, glutamic acid, glycine, and lysine), a high vitamin content (particularly the B family, but also A, C, and D), and is also made up of such minerals as potassium, calcium, and iron. Manufacturers cite royal jelly as particularly appropriate for use in anti-aging products, as well as those for oily skin.

royal jelly extract HD—an extract of royal jelly. *See also* royal jelly.

Russian white oil—*see* mineral oil.

rutin—described as helping to tighten and strengthen skin capillaries, and as such it could help prevent a couperose condition. It also demonstrates anti-oxidant properties. Rutin is a flavonoid found in rue leaves, buckwheat, and other plants.

R

S

saccharide isomerate—a humectant and skin-conditioning agent.

Saccharomyces cerevisiae **extract** (**living yeast**)—healing and protecting. This extract is also credited with the ability to protect against infection and boost immunodefenses. *Saccharomyces* ferment also acts as a stabilizer for other compounds, particularly enzymes and metals. Constituents include the polysaccharides d-mannan and d-glucan. *Saccharomyces cerevisiae* is a yeast traditionally used to help raise bread. Given its ease of use and stabilizing activity, it is increasingly incorporated in skin care products.

Saccharomyces/**copper, -/manganese, -/selenium, -/zinc ferment(s)**—obtained through the fermentation of *Saccharomyces* in the presence of metal ions (i.e., copper, manganese, selenium, or zinc). The yeast (*Saccharomyces*) provides the base onto which the metal is attached. They are all used to promote and maintain a good skin condition, and are found in a wide range of cosmetic products, including facial moisturizers, anti-aging preparations, acne preparations, sun care products, bronzers, and formulations for reducing skin redness. *See also Saccharomyces cerevisiae* extract.

Saccharomyces **lysate extract**—a yeast extract often found in powder form. Manufacturers note a variety of activity, including an ability to stimulate cellular consumption of oxygen, promote cellular proliferation, and stimulate collagen production. It is also said to be anti-inflammatory and promote healing. It could be incorporated into a number of product types, including anti-aging, sun and post-sun products, makeup, and hair care products.

saccharomyces/**xylinum/black tea ferment**—a skin-conditioning ingredient that is found in a variety of skin care preparations, including eye creams.

saccharum officinarum—moisturizing and helps keep the skin feeling smooth and supple. Manufacturers claim it to be beneficial for acne. This is the latin name for sugar cane.

sacred bark—*see* cascara sagrada extract.

safflower oil (*Carthamus tinctorius*)—a carrier oil also considered hydrating to the skin. It consists primarily of linoleic acid triglycerides. Safflower oil is a non-comedogenic raw material obtained from the plant's seeds.

sage extract (*Salvia officinalis*)—considered to have astringent, antibacterial, anti-septic, anti-inflammatory, stimulating, softening, invigorating, and healing properties. Sage extract was traditionally used as a remedy for every type of inflammation. Among its constituents are an essential oil, which contains borneol, cineole, and thujone, as well as tannic acid, oleic acid, fumaric acid, caffeic acid, niacin, nicotinamide, flavones, and glycosides. The extract is obtained from the herb's leaves.

sage oil—credited with depurative and healing properties, and indicated for acne and oily skin. Sage oil is obtained by distillation of sage leaves and flowers. *See also* sage extract.

St. John's wort extract (*Hypericum perforatum*) (**hypericum extract**)— said to have astringent, anti-inflammatory, and possibly soothing properties. St. John's wort offers general skin protection, especially for sensitive skin and areas with burns. This is an herbaceous perennial plant with hypericine as its important constituent, as well as various flavonoids and phenolic acids.

St. John's wort oil—used as an anti-inflammatory. It is beneficial for sensitive and/or rough, chapped skin as well as acne skin or skin suffering from irritation and inflammation. It is also considered effective for improving capillary circulation. In addition, St. John's wort oil is an antibiotic and can act as a natural preservative. This is a deep red oil. *See also* St. John's wort extract.

salicylamide—an analgesic, fungicide, and anti-inflammatory ingredient used to soothe the skin. Salicylamide is an aromatic amide.

salicylic acid—a beta-hydroxy acid with keratolytic and anti-inflammatory activity. It helps dissolve the top layer of stratum corneum cells, improving the look and feel of the skin. Salicylic acid is an effective ingredient in acne products and as such is widely used in acne soaps and lotions. Because it is lipid soluble, it can more easily reduce sebaceous follicle blockage by penetrating the pores and exfoliating the cellular buildup. It is antimicrobial, anti-septic, enhances the activity of preservatives, and can be used to adjust the pH of products. For the treatment of aging skin, it appears to help improve skin wrinkles, roughness, and tone. In addition, it is a useful ingredient for products formulated to treat psoriasis, callouses, corns, and warts—cases where there is a buildup of dead skin cells. When applied topically, it is reported to penetrate 3 to 4 mm into the epidermis. A small amount

S

of salicylic acid can convert to copper salicylate, a powerful anti-inflammatory. Used at high concentrations, salicylic acid may cause skin redness and rashes. This is a naturally occurring organic acid, related to aspirin. It is found in some plants, particularly the leaves of wintergreen, willow bark, and the bark of sweet birch. Salicylic acid is also synthetically manufactured.

salicyloxy-carboxy acid—a general term for a variety of salicyloxy-based compositions (e.g., salicyloxy-propionic acid) that act as skin-conditioning agents. They may also aid in controlling sebum secretion and improve skin feel. Additional properties are noted as anti-aging (the reduction of wrinkles and benefit to photo aging skin); improved skin tone, radiance, and clarity; and promotion of generally healthier, younger-looking skin. It can also reduce or help prevent stickiness and shine within a formulation.

salt—*see* sodium chloride.

sambucus extract—*see* elder extract.

sandalwood oil (*Santalum album*) (**santal; santalum**)—credited with astringent, anti-inflammatory, anti-bacterial, tonic, stimulant, cooling, and soothing properties. It is also considered a good anti-septic in cases of acne and an astringent for oily skin. There are indications that sandalwood oil may promote epidermal cell turnover as some report it stimulates fibroblast growth. Sandalwood could help prevent the skin dryness associated with seborrheic dermatitis, psoriasis, and eczema. In addition, some manufacturers utilize it as a natural colorant to give products a light red or rose tone. Sandalwood oil might produce a rash in hypersensitive people, especially if it is present in high concentrations. It is produced by distillation of the inner wood.

***Sanguisorba officinalis* root extract**—a botanical extract that has skin cleansing, soothing, refreshing, and tonic properties. It is also reported to promote wound healing. According to clinical researchers, its active constituent is reported to be ziyuglycoside.

santal oil—*see* sandalwood oil.

santalum oil—*see* sandalwood oil.

***Sapindus mukurossi* peel extract** (**soapberry**)—said to be skin conditioning and an effective cleanser, it has a high saponins content. This extract is obtained from the peel (shell) of the soap nut tree.

saponaria extract—*see* soapwort extract.

sarcosine—a naturally occurring amino acid that is used in cosmetic formulations as a skin conditioner. There are some studies indicating that it is effective for oily skin. Its chemical name is n-methyl glycine.

S

sarriette oil—a fragrance with healing, tonic, antiseptic, and anti-inflammatory properties. This oil is derived from an herb native to the Mediterranean basin.

sarsaparilla (*Smilax officinalis*)—said to be healing, anti-septic, and beneficial for chronic skin disease, including psoriasis. Its primary constituents include saponins (sarsaponin and parallin) and sterols (sitosterol and stigmasterol). Regardless of the variety of sarsaparilla, in every case the sarsaparilla's root is the part that is used.

sassafras oil (*Sassafras albidum*)—credited with anti-septic, astringent, and stimulant properties. It is composed of approximately 80 percent saprol. Sassafras oil is obtained from the plant's bark and root through a process of steam distillation. It may produce dermatitis in hypersensitive individuals.

savory extract (*Satureja hortensis*)—also called *hortensis*. It is considered anti-septic, antibiotic, and soothing. It can also be used to perfume a formulation or mask odor. The extract from this hardy herb is indicated for acne skin.

saw palmetto fruit extract (*Serenoa serrulata*)—attributed with anti-inflammatory properties.

scabwort—*see* elecampane.

sclareolide—a fragrancing ingredient, it can help mask formulation odors. It is synthetically manufactured.

sclary sage oil—*see* clary sage oil.

sclerotium gum—can be used as a thickener and stabilizer as well as to improve a formulation's skin feel and spreadability.

scurvy grass extract (*Cochlearia officinalis*)—considered tonic and potentially anti-septic. It is a source of vitamin C.

SD alcohol-40—*see* alcohol SD-40.

SD alcohol-40A—*see* alcohol SDA-40.

SD alcohol-40B—the B denotes a specific denaturing method. *See also* alcohol SD-40.

sea clay—*see* clay.

sea lettuce extract (*Ulva lactuca*)—anti-inflammatory and antioxidant. *See also* seaweed extract.

sea minerals yeast derivative—described as supplying essential minerals for cosmetic applications. Marine elements have been used for centuries for their beneficial effects on all epidermal structures. The mixture of sea elements with low-molecular-weight yeast glycoproteins apparently results in a degree of biocompatibility with the skin and acceptance by the epidermal cells.

sea salt—a mild abrasive used in scrubs. Its water solubility allows it to self-dissolve during product use. It is also employed as a dilutant. Because sea salt does not seem to form secondary reactions, it is considered a stable ingredient in cosmetic formulations. In large grains, it is colored and perfumed, and utilized in bath salts. Sea salt may cause dryness.

sea wave—*see* seaweed extract.

sea wrack—*see* seaweed extract.

seabuckthorn berry oil extract (*Hippophae rhamnoides*)—protects the skin against harmful or irritating external factors. Constituents include vitamin C, vitamin E, carotinoids, amino acids, and flavonols. This plant is a shrub native to Europe and Asia.

seawater—healing powers have long been attributed to the sea. Sea water can have an anti-septic and stimulating effect when used to treat wounds or rashes. Used primarily in oligotherapy and thalassotherapy, its cosmetic benefits have yet to be proven.

seaweed (fresh)—has gelatinous properties. It is the major ingredient in the thin, clear masks that peel off in one piece when applied on the skin. This type of mask allows the skin to build up a supply of water, giving it a moist, supple look. Seaweed is also used in face creams and lotions, providing body and substance to products. It is considered good for oily skin.

seaweed extract (*Fucus vesiculosus*) (**algae extract; black tang; bladderwrack; fucus; kelp; laminaria digitata, sea wave; sea wrack**)— used by the Chinese for curing burns and rashes; by the Polynesians for treating wounds, bruises, and swelling; and by mariners who recognized its healing properties. Seaweed is found to be stimulating, revitalizing, and nourishing to the skin due to its iodine and sulfur amino acid content, which also give it anti-inflammatory and disinfectant abilities. Seaweed's moisturizing properties are attributed to its ability to react with protein and form a protective gel on the skin's surface, reducing moisture loss due to evaporation. It has potential tissue renewal action and positive effects on facial wrinkles, probably because of its silicon content. It protects sensitive skin against irritation, making it particularly effective in shaving creams. It is also beneficial for treating mature and drier skins given its smoothing and softening actions. Seaweed extract seems to be effective in treating acne because of its presumed antibiotic properties, which offer the skin protection against infection. Evidence indicates seaweed may help accelerate wound healing, and improve the healing of burns (including sunburns) and other wounds when in the presence of calcium alginate. It can be utilized as a regenerator in cases of suntanned or "orange peeled" skin. It reportedly

S

improves blood circulation in the skin. Due to its alginates, seaweed is also used by formulators as a thickener for gels and emulsions. In cosmetic products, its total percentage of use varies between 2 and 7 percent. The benefits of seaweed and seaweed extracts can be attributed to the plant's wealth of components that include water, mineral matters, lipids, protids, glucids, and sulfuric esters. It is rich in vitamins including vitamins A, B_1, B_2, B_3, B_5, B_{12}, C, D, E, and K. Among its mineral constituents are iodine, calcium, iron, phosphorus, sodium, potassium, zinc, nitrogen, copper, chlorine, magnesium, and manganese. It has trace amounts of various other minerals such as silver, lithium, silicon, bromine, titanium, cobalt, and arsenic. The amino acid content of seaweed is extremely high compared to other plants, and its polysaccharides include fructose, galactose, glucose, mannose, and xylose. Additional constituents include folic acid, choline, alginic acid, uronic acid, alginates, carrageenan, cellulose, proteins, agar-agar, algin, and iodine-protein complexes. There are more than 17,000 seaweed species that are classified according to color: green, blue, red, and brown. The red and brown varieties, the ones most commonly used in cosmetic preparations and generally referred to as seaweed or algae extract, are green when fresh and olive-brown when dry. The thallus is the part that is used for cosmetic purposes.

selenium—a trace mineral used for years in topical preparations for its anti-fungal properties. Selenium has been shown to have other protective effects such as repairing DNA, reducing the DNA-binding of carcinogens, and suppressing gene mutations. In laboratory studies, skin lotions containing selenium compounds have been shown to decrease UV-induced skin damage such as inflammation, blistering, and pigmentation.

senna (*Cassia angustifolia*) (**Indian senna, meca senna, tinnevelly senna**)—used in traditional medicine as a stimulant. Researchers have isolated a beta-glycan fraction, galactomannan, from the plant's seeds. The cosmetic properties ascribed to this fraction are similar to those of hyaluronic acid. These include skin-softening and smoothing properties; a long-term moisturizing effect with an improvement in the stratum corneum's capacity to hold water; film-forming properties demonstrated by a reduction in transepidermal water loss; and a corrective and repairing ability for dry or rough skin. Senna also acts as an emollient without associated oiliness or leaving an occlusive layer. Its high galactomannan concentration makes senna recommended for skin care preparations designed to relieve or repair dry, rough skin, and for anti-aging cosmetics and moisturizers.

S

sericin—a silk protein that can act as a film former in moisturizers, it also helps maintain skin that is smooth and in good overall condition. *See also* silk protein.

serine—a hydrophilic amino acid. Serine helps retain the skin's moisture balance. *See also* amino acid; protein.

serum protein—contains all essential amino acids. By varying the process, it is possible to concentrate fractions that have high specific essential amino acid contents such as methionine and lysine. It is made by a selected fractionation process to isolate the plasma serum proteins present. *See also* amino acid; protein.

sesame amino acids—provides moisturizing properties and has some natural sugars associated with it. This amino acid complex is produced from sesame seed flour.

sesame oil—a commonly used carrier oil for cosmetic products, it has the same emollient properties as other nut and vegetable oils. Sesame oil is useful in suntan lotions as it blocks 30 percent of the sun's burning UV rays. It is derived from sesame seeds.

shaddock extract—astringent and tonic. This extract is obtained from the fruit of *Citrus grandis,* an unusual pear-shaped citrus fruit similar to a grapefruit.

shave grass—*see* horsetail extract.

shea butter—protects the skin from dehydration and external aggressions due to harsh climate, and is attributed with anti-inflammatory activity. It restores skin suppleness, increases moisturization, and can improve the appearance of irritated dry skin. Shea butter is a natural fat obtained from the fruit of the karate tree. *See also* shea butter (hydrodispersable).

shea butter (hydrodispersible)—an excellent emollient for use in creams, lotions, and makeup preparations. It alleviates skin dryness, and has sun-protection and high skin-penetration properties. It is obtained by the hydroxylation of shea butter.

shepherd's purse (*Capsella bursa pastoris*)—traditionally attributed with wound-healing properties. It is also astringent and anti-inflammatory, making it particularly effective in acne preparations. Its constituents include flavonoids (e.g., diosmin), amines, cholene, acetyl cholene, potassium salt, tannin, resin, and silica.

shinleaf extract (*Pyrola elliptica*)—a botanical reported to be tonic and astringent, it can help maintain the balance of normal skin. Constituents are reported to include tannic, gallic, and malic acids, as well as albumen, arbutin, and some volatile oil. This is a member of the wintergreen family.

S

shiitake mushroom extract (*Lentinus edodes*)—a skin conditioner that may also have anti-microbial and anti-bacterial properties. There is some evidence that it can cause skin irritation.

Shorea stenoptera **seed butter**—*see* illipe butter.

silanetriol—a polymer with hair- and skin-conditioning properties.

silica—also known as silicone dioxide. Silica has a variety of applications: to control a product's viscosity, add bulk, and reduce a formulation's transparency. It can also function as an abrasive. In addition, it can act as a carrier for emollients, and may be used to improve a formulation's skin feel. Spherical silica is porous and highly absorbent, with absorption capabilities roughly 1.5 times its weight. A typical claim associated with silica is oil control. It is found in sunscreens, scrubs, and wide range of other skin care, makeup, and hair care preparations. It has been successfully used in hypoallergenic and allergy-tested formulations.

silica dimethyl silylate—used for its anti-caking, anti-foaming, emollient, emulsion stabilizing, viscosity controlling, dispersing, and slip-modifying properties, making it applicable in a wide variety of products, ranging from make-up to skin care to perfumes.

silicon dioxide (*solum diaomeae*)—formulators may select it as an alternative to diatomaceous earth or clay, particularly when developing mineral make-up, pressed or loose powders. It has abrasive, absorbent, and anti-caking properties, and can also reduce the transparency of a formulation. Silicon dioxide is the U.S. name for what is known as solum diatomeae.

silicon glyconucleopeptides—a conditioning agent. This is protein attached to a silicone.

silicon oil—a generic description usually referring to dimethicone.

silicone (*volatile*)—used in face creams to increase the product's protection capabilities against water evaporation from the skin. Silicone polyethers are mainly used in water-based skin care formulations and give improved softness, gloss, and feel. Silicones have been used in cosmetics for more than 30 years. They are minerals able to repel water. Silicones present formulation problems because of poor compatibility with cosmetic oils and emollients. Silicones are not irritating.

silicone wax—improves a formulation's glide on the skin.

silicum—used in scrubbing preparations for its roughness and texture.

silk amino acids—a silk-derived protein resulting from the complete hydrolysis of silk. *See also* amino acids; silk protein.

silk powder—recommended primarily for use in powder make-ups to improve humectancy, oil absorption, and anti-cracking properties. However, a large amount of silk powder may be needed to obtain the desired results. Silk powder is a micronized powder of natural silk protein and is not compatible with all inorganic pigments used in color cosmetics. It is obtained from the secretion of the silkworm. Silk powder may cause allergic skin reactions.

silk proteins—protect the skin from dehydration and leave it with a smooth feel. They are described as very effective for use in eye wrinkle creams. It is being claimed that their low molecular weight allows for penetration in the top layers of the corneum layer.

siloxanetriol alginate—often used in combination with caffeine for use in anti-cellulite products. The siloxanetriol aginate portion provides skin-conditioning properties.

silver—can provide color to a product or serve as a deodorant. This metal is a good example of when nanotechnology may be used to increase an ingredient's compatibility with a cosmetic formulation, and in this form may be also used as a preservative.

silverweed—*see* cinquefoil extract.

slippery elm extract (*Ulmus fulva*)— soothing and emollient. It is found to be beneficial in aftershave preparations and for treating sunburn. *See also* slippery elm bark extract.

slippery elm bark extract—soothing, anti-septic, anti-inflammatory, healing, and moisturizing. The inner bark is considered to have important medicinal value. Microscopic examination of the bark's tissue shows round starch grains and very characteristic twin crystals of calcium oxalate.

soap bark—a natural surfactant used for its cleansing properties. Some sources indicate a high allergenicity potential.

soapwart extract (*Saponaria officinalis*)—credited with cleansing properties given its saponin content. It is also said to be soothing to the skin and to relieve itching. In traditional medicine, it has been used for acne, psoriasis, and eczema. Its constituents include flavonoids and vitamin C. The extract is made primarily from the roots of this herbaceous perennial, though the leaves and stem may be used as well.

sodium acrylate/sodium acryloyldimethyl taurate copolymer—a thickener, gelling agent, and formulation stabilizer.

sodium alginate—*see* algin.

SOD—*see* superoxide dimutase.

sodium acetylated hyaluronate—a humectant that appears to help retain moisture in the skin while also softening the stratum corneum.

sodium aluminosilicate—*see* sodium aluminum silicate.

sodium aluminum chlorohydroxy lactate—a cosmetic astringent. This is an inorganic salt.

sodium aluminum silicate (sodium aluminosilicate; sodium silicoaluminate)—abrasive, it can also reduce the density of a formulation and be used to increase product viscosity.

sodium benzoate—a non-toxic, organic salt preservative that is particularly effective against yeast, with some activity against molds and bacteria. It is generally used in concentrations of 0.1 to 0.2 percent.

sodium bicarbonate (baking soda)—an inorganic salt used as a buffering agent and a pH adjuster, it also serves as a neutralizer. It is used in skin-smoothing powders.

sodium bisulfate—an inorganic salt used as an anti-septic and a pH adjuster in cosmetic creams. Concentrated solutions can produce strong irritation.

sodium bisulfite—a preservative and anti-oxidant, it is most frequently used as a pH adjuster.

sodium borate—a preservative and emulsifier with astringent and anti-septic properties. It is also used as a pH adjuster. Sodium borate is the sodium salt of boric acid. It may cause skin dryness and irritation.

sodium carbomer—an emulsion stabilizer, it can also act as a film former, helping retain moisture in the skin. In addition, it can give a liquid formulation the consistency of a gel, and control product viscosity.

sodium carboxymethyl betaglucan—used as a binder and to control the viscosity of a cosmetic formulation.

sodium cetearyl sulfate—a surfactant used as a cleansing agent, it is also an oil-in-water emulsifier for creams.

sodium chloride (table salt)—used as a preservative, astringent, and anti-septic to treat inflamed lesions. It can also be used to mask odor, reduce product density, and control viscosity. Diluted solutions are not considered irritating.

sodium chondroitin sulfate—described as a skin-conditioning agent, with possible anti-inflammatory properties. It can be found in such products as moisturizers and night skin care preparations. It is a derivative of natural mucopolysaccharides. *See also* mucopolysaccharides.

S

sodium citrate—may be used in cosmetic formulations as an alkalizer and to bind trace metals in solutions (by means of a chelating action). It is the sodium salt of citric acid.

sodium cocoate—a surfactant used as an emulsifying and cleansing agent primarily in bath soaps and cleansers. This sodium salt of coconut acid may also be listed as coconut oil. *See also* coconut oil.

sodium coco hydrolyzed collagen—a surfactant that is non-irritating to the skin or mucous membranes.

sodium cocoyl glutamate—a very mild cleansing agent that lathers slightly. It is derived from coconut fatty acid and glutamic acid, an amino acid. It can be found in cleansers, acne products, body gels, and shampoos.

sodium cocoyl isethionate—a mild, high-foaming surfactant. It leaves the skin with a soft afterfeel.

sodium cocoylsarcosinate—a surfactant used as a cleansing agent.

sodium dehydroacetate—a preservative against bacteria and fungi that is used at concentration levels of 1.0 percent or less. It is useful in combination with parabens. It may cause skin irritation.

sodium dihydroxycetyl phosphate—a surfactant used as a cleansing agent.

sodium glutamate—an amino acid with skin-conditioning, odor-masking, and hair-conditioning action.

sodium hexametaphosphate—a chelating agent and a corrosion inhibitor. This is an inorganic salt.

sodium hyaluronate—used as a humectant to increase moisture in the skin, it may also serve as an emulsifier. Sodium hyaluronate is capable of binding 1,800 times its own weight in water. It is the sodium salt of hyaluronic acid and is the most commonly used form. *See also* hyaluronic acid.

sodium hydroxide—used to adjust a product pH to make it more acceptable to the skin. It is commonly referred to as caustic soda, and often serves as a chemical reagent when making soap. If too concentrated it may cause severe skin irritation.

sodium hydroxymethyl glycinate—an anti-microbial. It is derived from glycine, a naturally occurring amino acid and is used as a preservative in cosmetics.

sodium isostearoyl lactylate—an ester of lactic acid with moisture-retention properties.

sodium lactate—keeps a product's pH from becoming too acidic. It is moisturizing and moisture binding, as well as being a keratolytic,

S

helping exfoliate excess cells from the surface of the stratum corneum. It is also used as a substitute for glycerin. Sodium lactate is naturally occurring in the skin. *See also* lactic acid.

sodium lactate methylsilanol—an additive used in self-tanning preparations. It helps obtain a more uniform color.

sodium laureth-5 carboxylate—a very mild surfactant with good emulsifying properties, and not affected by water hardness. It substantially improves the skin's tolerance to cleansers.

sodium laureth-11 carboxylate—a surfactant. *See also* sodium laureth-5 carboxylate; sodium laureth-13 carboxylate.

sodium laureth-13 carboxylate—an extremely mild surfactant with good emulsifying properties and insensitive to water hardness, it substantially improves the skin's tolerance of cleansers. It is particularly suitable for high-quality formulations, baby shampoos, and products designed for sensitive skin.

sodium laureth sulfate—an emulsifier and versatile surfactant used in personal care products, especially for its cleansing and foaming properties. It enjoys good skin compatibility and is very often found in shower foams, foam bath products, and liquid soaps. It exhibits a mild to moderate skin irritation index in irritation tests, and has been found to be less irritating than sodium lauryl sulfate.

sodium lauroamphoacetate—a mild surfactant that is especially suitable for use in products where skin tolerance is important (e.g., baby and child care products).

sodium lauroyl glutamate—a surfactant with some moisturizing capacities, it can be derived from vegetal raw materials, and therefore may often be found in "natural" or plant-based cosmetics.

sodium lauroyl lactylate—an emulsifier.

sodium lauroyl oat amino acids—a surfactant with skin-cleansing and conditioning properties. It is derived from oat amino acids.

sodium lauryl sarcosinate—a foaming agent used primarily in hair products.

sodium lauryl sulfate—a base surfactant, foaming agent with good foaming properties, dispersant, and wetting agent. Formulators have found it ideal for designing cleansers and soaps packaged with pump dispensers. However, it is considered among the most irritating surfactants associated with skin dryness and redness. Often, it is either replaced by less irritating but related surfactants such as sodium laureth sulfate, or anti-irritant ingredients are incorporated into the formulation together with the sodium lauryl sulfate in order to reduce sensitivity potential.

sodium magnesium silicate—a binder and bulking agent used primarily in makeup products.

sodium mannuronate methylsilanol—a skin-conditioning agent.

sodium metabisulfite—an anti-oxidant and reducing agent.

sodium metaphosphate—can be used to adjust pH levels, thus acting as a buffer.

sodium methylcocoyl taurate—an emulsifier and mild cleansing agent. It is used in cleansing creams, lotions, shampoos, and bath soaps. It is derived from coconut oil.

sodium methyl oleoyl taurate—an emulsifier and a mild cleansing and foaming agent derived from oleic acid.

sodium oleate—a mild cleansing and foaming agent generally used in soaps. It is derived from natural fats and oils.

sodium C_{12-16} olefin sulfonate—a cleansing agent.

sodium C_{14-16} olefin sulfonate—a cleansing agent. It is also a foaming agent and is most likely to be found in cleansers and shampoos.

sodium PCA (Ajidew NaPCA, Nalidone)—a high-performance humectant given its moisture-binding ability. Sodium PCA is a component of the skin's natural moisturizing factor. For cosmetic use, it is derived from amino acids. It is considered a non-comedogenic, non-allergenic raw material recommended for dry, delicate, and sensitive skins.

sodium PCS (Ajidew N-50)—a humectant. *See also* PCA; sodium PCA.

sodium phosphate—helps maintain product pH.

sodium phytate—a chelating agent, it helps to boost a product's stability.

sodium polyacrylate—a suspending agent, stabilizer, and emulsifier.

sodium polyacrylate starch—a thickener and gellant with good pH stability.

sodium polyphosphate—a preservative against bacteria, molds, and yeasts. When used in high concentrations, it can cause skin irritation.

sodium polystyrene sulfonate—a film former. It holds the actives on site and gives the feeling of skin tightening. It is synthetically manufactured.

sodium pyrithione—a preservative that is not commonly used because of some level of toxicity. It is prohibited in Canada, and it is on the EU Annex II list of substances that must not form part of a cosmetic product composition.

S

sodium ricinolate—an emulsifying agent used in certain soaps and medicines. It is a sodium salt of the fatty acids from castor oil.

sodium shale oil sulfonate—found to be anti-inflammatory, anti-bacterial, fungicidal, anti-septic, and have analgesic properties. It is also a surfactant. A naturally occurring, water- and glycerin-soluble substance that is distilled from oil-shale, it is used in products for acne, eczema, and psoriasis. Among its constituents are sulfur, saturated and unsaturated hydrocarbons, nitrogen bases, and thiophene derivatives.

sodium silicoaluminate—*see* sodium aluminum silicate.

sodium stearate—a fatty acid used as a waterproofing agent. Sodium stearate is one of the least allergy-causing sodium salts of fatty acids. It is non-irritating to the skin. *See also* stearic acid.

sodium stearoyl glutamate—an amino-acid–based cleansing agent and oil-in-water emulsifier. It can be obtained from natural or synthetic sources.

sodium stearoyl lactylate—an emulsifier. It can be obtained from natural or synthetic sources.

sodium sulfate—a filler in the manufacturing of synthetic detergents and soaps and a laboratory reagent. It may enhance the irritant action of certain detergents.

sodium sulfite—has anti-septic, preservative, and anti-oxidant properties. Sodium sulfite is also a topical anti-fungal.

sodium tallowate (tallow)—a defoamer, emollient, and intermediate and surface active agent. *See also* tallow.

sodium/TEA lauryl—a moderately irritating surfactant.

sodium tetraborate—*see* sodium borate.

sodium triceth sulfate—a surfactant.

sodium trideceth sulfate—a surfactant used as a cleansing and emulsifying agent. Its activity and irritation potential depends on the formulation's pH.

soluble elastin—*see* tropoelastin.

solum diatomeae (silicon dioxide)—*see* silicon dioxide.

sorbic acid—a broad-spectrum, non-toxic preservative against molds and yeasts with moderate sensitizing potential in leave-on cosmetics. It is used in concentrations of 0.1 to 0.3 percent, and its activity is dependent on the formulation's pH. Sorbic acid is used as a replacement for glycerin in emulsions, ointments, and various cosmetic creams. It is obtained from the berries of the tree commonly known as mountain ash and rowan, and can also be produced synthetically. Sorbic acid can cause irritation.

sorbitan isostearate—an emulsifier used in the preparation of sunscreens, moisturizing creams, and lotions.

sorbitan laurate—an emulsifier in cosmetic creams and lotions as well as a stabilizer of essential oils in water.

sorbitan monostearate—*see* sorbitan stearate.

sorbitan oleate—a mild emulsifier derived from sugar.

sorbitan olivate—an emulsifier.

sorbitan palmitate—an emulsifier with moisture-binding abilities. It also serves as a solubilizer of essential oils in water. It is derived from sorbitol.

sorbitan sesquioleate—a surfactant used as an emulsifying agent. *See also* sorbitol.

sorbitan stearate—an emulsifier for water-in-oil creams and lotions, and a solubilizer of essential oils in water. It results from the reaction of stearic acid with sorbitol and is, therefore, synthetically produced from naturally derived materials.

sorbitan trioleate—an emulsifier. *See also* sorbitol.

sorbitan tristearate—an emulsifier and alternate for sorbitan stearate.

sorbitate stearate—a secondary emulsifier that helps formulate glossy emulsions.

sorbitol—absorbs moisture from the air to prevent skin dryness, and leaves the skin feeling smooth and velvety. However, if the skin's moisture content is greater than that of the atmosphere, it will draw moisture out of the skin, thereby increasing the feeling of dryness. Sorbitol is used by formulators as a replacement for glycerin in emulsions, ointments, and various cosmetic creams. It is obtained from the leaves and in some cases the berries of mountain ash. Sorbitol also occurs in other berries, cherries, plums, pears, apples, seaweed, and algae.

S

sorrel extract (*Rumex acetosa*)—an astringent. Although there are many varieties of sorrel including wood sorrel, French sorrel, and garden sorrel, similar properties are attributed to all. The extract is obtained from the whole herb or just from the leaves.

sour cherry (*Prunus cerasus*)—helps maintain a healthy skin condition. A variety of other therapeutic values are attributed to sour cherry, some of which depend on the portion of the plant used. For example, extract from the whole plant is anti-oxidant, moisturizing, keratolytic, and skin conditioning. Meanwhile, extract obtained just from the fruit is anti-oxidant and skin conditioning but not necessarily moisturizing or helpful in removing dead surface-skin cells. The fruit itself has astringent properties, and the seed oil is both emollient and can mask odor. Sour cherry's constituents include pectin, fruit acids, sugars, flavonoids, vitamins A, B, and C, polyphenols, mineral salts, and trace elements such as selenium.

southernwood extract (*Artemisia abrotanum*)—botanical sources cite it as having moisturizing, anti-septic, and toning properties. The extract is obtained from the whole plant.

soy amino acids—*see* amino acid.

soy bean oil (soybean oil)—often used as a smoothing ingredient. It has a high content of phosphatides such as lecithin, sterols, and vitamins (A, E, and K). It is used in numerous forms, including hydrogenated, maleated, and unsaponified. Considered by some sources to be somewhat comedogenic, soy bean oil does not cause irritation.

soy bean oil (unsaponified)—said to stimulate the synthesis of collagen, elastin, proteoglycans, and structural glycoproteins. It has a small molecular structure and is thought to act more as a hormone-like cellular messenger once it reaches the epidermal keratinocytes and, particularly, the dermal fibroblast. Its action is likely similar action to that of true biological precursors. *See also* isoflavones.

soy bean glycerides (hydrogenated)—can be used for emollient, emulsifying, and surfactant purposes.

soy bean protein—has good anti-irritant properties.

soy germ oil—*see* soy bean oil.

soy oil—*see* soy bean oil.

soy lecithin—a mild re-fattening agent that can be effectively used in facial cleansers formulated for dry skin.

soy phytosterols—anti-inflammatory and conditioning. These sterols are derived from the soy plant. *See also* plant sterols.

soy sterol—an emulsifier, emollient, and emulsion stabilizer. Soy sterol is considered a non-comedogenic raw material.

spearmint oil (*Mentha viridis*)—a cooling, aromatic stimulant described as having cleansing and decongesting properties. It is also astringent, and can add fragrance while helping mask odor. Its use is indicated for acne and oily skin. Its fragrance and therapeutic activity is similar to that of peppermint but fresher and less harsh. *See also* mint oil.

spermaceti—a waxy substance used in the manufacture of cosmetics to thicken the products and give them shine. Spermaceti is non-toxic and non-irritating. Originally obtained from whales as a source of fish oil, it is now synthetically produced and is a cetyl ester. *See also* cetyl esters.

sphingolipids—ceramide precursors with unique moisturizing properties. They appear to work with the cellular system in providing a restorative effect on a damaged or disturbed stratum corneum layer. Sphingolipids may also exhibit cell-regulating functions. Found naturally occurring in both animals and plants, it is difficult to isolate naturally occurring sphingolipids in an efficient and economical manner given their size and quantities available in an organism. The synthesized version does not exhibit exactly the same properties as the natural one, but is generally considered emollient and useful for protecting the skin against external harm (such as environmental pollutants), while also maintaining skin condition. The use of sphingolipids in cosmetics is limited by availability and price. Sphingolipid liposomes are called sphingosomes.

sphingomyelin—can be used as an amphiphilic liposome component in the manufacture of the liposome capsule.

sphingomyelinase—a fluid that can enhance the skin's moisture-retention properties.

spinach (*Spinacia oleracea*)—generally considered beneficial for promoting and maintaining the skin in good condition, it can also be used as a natural colorant. Spinach contains anti-oxidant flavonoids (spinacetin and patuletin), carotenoids, peptides, histamines, oxalic acid, lutein, omega-3 fatty acids, vitamins A, B_2, B_6, C, E, and H, thiamine, niacin, folic acid, and a variety of minerals including copper and zinc.

***Spiraea* extract**—*see* meadowsweet.

spirulina amino acids—an amino acid complex with high moisturizing capabilities derived from *Spirulina platensis*.

spirulina extract—said to have a hydrating effect on the skin's surface layers. Botanical claims also maintain that certain spirulina proteins contribute to the stimulation of the fibroblast and to tissue regeneration. It is also attributed with anti-oxidant ability. Spirulina is a blue-green algae, with constituents that include protein, vitamins B and E, carotenoids, iron, zinc, copper, and gamma linolenic acid.

spruce oil (*Picea excelsa*)—like sandalwood, rosemary, and jasmine oils, spruce oil has been observed to stimulate fibroblast growth. Although the relevance of this observation has not been scientifically established, it has been noticed that stimulation of fibroblast

S

activity could result in an increase in epidermal cell turnover. Spruce oil is produced by distillation of spruce branches.

squalane—an excellent moisturizer and lubricant, it softens and smoothes the skin while also replenishing skin lipids. Its compatibility with skin lipids can be attributed to the fact that human sebum is made up of 25 percent squalane. Squalane has traditionally been obtained by hydrogenation of shark liver oil or other natural oils. Components found in fish oils may reduce skin irritation and allergic responses. It can also be derived from plant sources or synthetically manufactured.

squalane and squalene and glycolipids and phytosterols and tocopharol—a light emollient that contains natural lipids also found in the skin. This is a natural plant cell oil extract, not a mixture as the name suggests.

squalene—like squalane, squalene replenishes skin lipids while softening and smoothing. It helps maintain the skin in good condition. When used in hair care products, it serves as a hair-conditioning and anti-static agent.

starch gum—*see* dextrin.

stearalkonium chloride—an anti-static that can also be used as a surfactant and/or a preservative depending on formulatory requirements.

stearalkonium hectorite—can help control product viscosity and create a gel-like consistency for a liquid formulation.

stearamide DEA (stearic acid diethanolamide)—a thickener and a wax emulsifier used in soaps, creams, and lotions.

stearamidopropyl dimethylamine—a surfactant and conditioner for facial cleansers, hand cleansers, and baby products. It is very mild to the skin and eyes.

stearate—*see* sodium stearate.

stearate SE—*see* sodium stearate.

steareth-2, -7, -10, -20, -21—these are emulsifiers for water-in-oil formulations, adding stability, and preventing the separation of the two phases. They are the polyoxyethylene ether of fatty alcohol. Steareth-10 is used particularly in creams and lotions of high stability though some sources indicate it has a comedogenicity and mild irritancy potential. Steareth-21 may also be used as a surfactant with very minor irritation potential to the skin and eyes.

stearic acid—an emulsifier and thickening agent found in many vegetable fats. Stearic acid is the main ingredient used in making bar soaps and lubricants. It occurs naturally in butter acids, tallow, cascarilla bark, and in other animal fats and oils. Stearic acid may cause allergic reactions in people with sensitive skin and is considered somewhat comedogenic. *See also* essential fatty acid entry in Chapter 4.

stearic acid diethanolamide—*see* stearamide DEA.

stearoxy dimethicone—an emollient and skin-conditioning agent. *See also* dimethicone.

stearyl alcohol—used to create cosmetic emulsions, and for its anti-foaming and lubricating action. Stearyl alcohol is also a viscosity agent and builder. It is a saturated alcohol of high purity.

stearyl acrylate—generally found in combination with other chemicals, it acts as a film former to help maintain moisture in the skin.

stearyl glycyrrhetinate—anti-inflammatory and soothing. This is the ester of stearyl alcohol and glycyrrhetinic acid, where stearyl alcohol helps improve the penetration of the functional component, glycyrrhetinic acid. *See also* glycyrrhetinic acid.

stearyl heptanoate—a non-greasy emollient that produces a highly water-repellent film. Stearyl heptanoate is a natural preen gland wax that can also be synthetically manufactured.

sterols—steroid alcohols that can be used as lubricants in a variety of cosmetic preparations. Such alcohols contain the common steroid nucleus. Sterols are widely distributed in plants and animals, both in the free form and esterified to fatty acids. Cholesterol is a most important sterol and is often used in cosmetic creams. Ergosterol is an important plant sterol.

stinging nettle extract—traditionally used for mild acne conditions. *See also* nettle extract.

stonecrop (*Sempervivum tectorum*)—also known as houseleek; hens and chicks. Anti-inflammatory and astringent, studies indicate anti-oxidant properties as well. Its constituents include carbohydrates, isocitric acid, citric acid, malic acid, free amino acids (asparagine), caffeic acid, and flavonoids. *See also* citric acid, malic acid, flavonoids.

strawberry extract (*Fragaria vesca*)—astringent. The fruit contains a variety of constituents including malic and citric acids, sugar, mucilage, pectin, woody fiber, and water. It also contains ascorbic acid, thereby supporting early claims of bleaching properties. Extract from the fruit was recommended for use on sunburned areas to soothe the skin. Both the leaves and the fruit were in early pharmacopoeias; however, there is no scientific evidence of benefit or harm.

S

sucrose (**table sugar**)—an emollient, mild emulsifier, and humectant. It can be used in place of glycerin.

sucrose cocoate—soothing and anti-irritant. It is also an emulsifying agent.

sucrose cocoate sorbitan stearate—a sucrose-based emulsifier.

sucrose polybehenate—an emollient and emulsifier, this is a film-forming agent that forms semi-occlusive films. It can also be used as a surfactant, and as a skin conditioner. It exhibits good wear and wash-off resistance. Considered a natural ingredient, it is used in skin care creams and lotions.

sucrose polycottonseedate—a skin-conditioner, emollient, and emulsifying agent.

sucrose polysoyate—an emollient and emulsifier.

sucrose stearate—an emollient and emulsifying agent used primarily in makeup preparations. Sucrose stearate enables the formulation of clear gel microemulsion systems with a reduced physiological effect on the skin and eyes.

sucrose tristearate—incorporated into a cosmetic for softening and smoothing, it is also an emulsifier and helps maintain the skin in good condition.

sulfated castor oil—a surfactant used as a cleansing agent.

sulfur—a mild anti-septic used in acne creams and lotions. It stimulates healing when used on skin rashes. Sulfur may cause skin irritation. *See also* sulfur (colloidal).

sulfur (**colloidal**)—reduces oil-gland activity and dissolves the skin's surface layer of dry, dead cells. This ingredient is commonly used in acne soaps and lotions, and is a major component in many acne preparations. It can cause allergic skin reactions.

sulisobenzone—the drug name for benzophenone-4, a sunscreen chemical. *See also* benzophenone-4.

sumac extract (*Rhus glabra*) (**sumach**)—astringent, anti-septic, and tonic properties are attributed to this botanical. It also helps control oil gland secretion. Depending on the variety of sumac employed, extracts for skin problems are either made from the bark or the leaves. They may also be used for eczema and skin diseases. There are several varieties of sumac, some of which are poisonous. Those that are poisonous cause swelling, inflammation, and pain, ending in ulceration at the touch.

sumach—*see* sumac extract.

sunflower oil (*Helianthus annuus*)—commonly used as a carrier oil, it softens and smooths the skin. Sunflower oil has a high linoleic acid and other essential fatty acid content. In addition, it contains lecithin, carotenoids, and waxes. This oil is considered a non-comedogenic raw material.

sunflower seed oil—expressed from sunflower seeds. *See also* sunflower oil.

superoxide dismutase (SOD)—an enzyme that can serve as an inhibitor of free-radical production and as a free-radical scavenger. In cells, it constitutes a natural defense system against activated oxygen species. SOD converts superoxide radicals into hydrogen peroxide, which are then changed into molecular oxygen and water.

superoxide dismutase (polyoxyalkylene-modified)—used in cosmetic preparations to prevent drying and aging of the skin without causing irritation. *See also* superoxide dismutase.

sweet almond oil—an emollient with soothing properties. *See also* almond oil.

sweet clover extract—*see* clover extract.

sweet lime oil—*see* lime oil.

sweet marjoram oil (*Origanum majorana*)—used by formulators for its refreshing action, as well as for its perfuming and odor-masking activity. This is a volatile oil distilled from the plant's leaves. *See also* marjoram.

sweet orange extract—*see* orange extract.

sweet potato extract (*Ipomoea batatas*)—studies are indicating potential wound-healing properties, which could make this extract beneficial for acne products. Constituents include vitamins A and C, and beta-carotene. The extract is obtained from the whole plant.

synthetic spermaceti—*see* cetyl esters; spermaceti.

S

table salt—*see* sodium chloride.

table sugar—*see* sucrose.

talc—adds softness and sliding ability to a cosmetic formulation. It is also used as a bulking and opacifying agent, and as an absorbent in makeup preparations. Talc is an inert powder, generally made from finely ground magnesium silicate, a mineral.

tallow—considered an occlusive skin-conditioning agent. Tallow is used primarily to manufacture soaps. It is the fat derived from the fatty tissue of sheep or cattle and is considered comedogenic.

tallow glycerides—a surfactant used as an emulsifying agent, it is also emollient. It is incorporated more often into makeup than skin care preparations and is a mixture of triglycerides derived from tallow. *See also* tallow.

tamanu oil (*Calophyllum inophyllum*)—emollient, it is attributed with anti-oxidant, anti-microbial, anti-inflammatory, anti-scarring, healing, and astringent properties. It is also a natural UV absorber. Its composition includes neutral lipids, glycolipids, and phospholipids. Tamanu oil can be found in products used to protect the skin against sun exposure (sun and post-sun creams), anti-aging and regenerating creams, acne preparations, and products for dry and very dry skin. The oil is obtained from the seeds of this evergreen tree.

tamarind (*Tamarindus indica*)—astringent and anti-septic. Researchers have isolated xyloglucan from extracts of the plant's seeds. Xyloglucan has demonstrated strong immuno-stimulating properties. It may have some anti-oxidant capabilities as well. Other constituents of this plant include citric, tartaric, and malic acids; potassium bitartrate; polysaccharides; proteins; and lipids. Scientists recommend tamarind for protecting the skin against environmentally induced damage, stimulating skin repair, and for skin with low immune defenses.

tangerine oil (*Citrus reticulata*)—has botanical properties similar to those of orange, though with greater anti-spasmodic and sedative properties. Its fragrance, reminiscent of bergamot, is sweeter than that of orange. *See also* orange oil.

tapioca starch (*Manihot utilissima*)—used as a thickener, it is also soothing. It is derived from cassava.

tarragon (*Artemisia dracunculus*)—said to have tonic and stimulating properties. Its primary active is estragol, a phenol also known as methyl chavicol. Other constituents include cymene and phellandrene.

tartaric acid—the second largest AHA in size (glycolic acid being the smallest AHA and citric acid the largest). It is not frequently used in cosmetic or anti-aging preparations as formulators find it difficult to work with and it can cause irritation to the skin. *See also* alpha hydroxy acid.

TEA (triethanolamine)—an emulsifier and pH adjuster.

TEA-carbomer—used to create a gel formulation and to control viscosity.

TEA-dodecyl benzene sulfonate—a surfactant often mixed with other surfactants as a cleansing agent.

TEA-isostearate—a surfactant used as a cleansing and emulsifying agent.

TEA-lactate—a surfactant.

TEA-laureth sulfate—a surfactant, foaming, and cleansing agent that can also serve as an emollient. It is often used in facial cleansers and other skin-cleansing and bath products.

TEA-lauryl sulfate—a surfactant used as a cleansing agent with a moderate level of skin irritancy.

TEA-oleamide PEG-2 sulfosuccinate—a surfactant with a very low level of skin irritancy.

TEA-oleate—a mild emulsifier and surfactant.

TEA-salicylate—a chemical UVB absorber. This is one of the 21 FDA-approved sunscreen chemicals with an approved usage level of 5 to 12 percent. TEA-salicylate is a water-soluble chemical with limited UV absorption capability. Formulators may also use it as a preservative.

TEA-stearate—a surfactant considered to be a powerful oil-in-water (hydrophilic) emulsifying and cleansing agent. TEA-stearate is also a moisture absorber used in formulating emulsions. It may be irritating to the skin.

tea leaf extract (*Camellia sinensis*)—studies indicate anti-oxidant, anti-microbial, bacteriostatic, anti-allergenic and anti-inflammatory action as well as an ability to strengthen capillaries. In addition, this extract is astringent and tonic, leaving the skin with a feeling of overall well-being. As a humectant it helps hold and retain moisture, and is also emollient thus it improves skin softness and smoothness. Finally, it also helps protect the skin against harsh environmental conditions, such as climate extremes (sun, wind, cold) and it protects a product against UV-induced degradation. Tea, and especially green tea, is noted to be rich in potent anti-oxidants called catechins. It also contains polyphenols, caffeine, theophylline, and aminophylline. Used in almost all categories of cosmetic products, tea extract has been effectively used in eye treatment products to reduce puffiness. Tea, or *Camellia sinensis*, refers equally to black, green, and white teas. Their differences arise from the processing method rather than from the plant itself.

tea tree oil (*Melaleuca alternifolia*) (**Australian tea tree oil**)—considered a natural preservative with anti-septic, germicidal, and expectorant properties. Its anti-microbial activity toward a wide array of bacteria allows it to promote healing. It is becoming recognized as a topical remedy for yeast, fungus, and skin disorders and infections. Tea tree oil exhibits positive benefits against seborrhea, psoriasis (reduces scaling and redness), eczema (stops itching and reduces redness), and dermatitis. It has been used by Australian Aborigines to treat cuts, wounds, and skin infections, and by European explorers as an herbal tea. This oil's ability to dissolve pus without causing visible or apparent damage to the skin's surface was noted by doctors when using it to clean the surface of infected wounds. It is also ideal for aromatherapy, given its low toxicity. Although effectively used on almost any skin type, except sensitive or couperose skins, it is particularly beneficial to acne, problem, and/or congested skins. Tea tree oil is obtained from distilling the tree's leaves to produce a pale yellow to colorless oil that has a camphor-like scent similar to eucalyptus. Studies indicate it to be nontoxic with negligible to no irritancy.

tepezcohuite—*see Mimosa tenuiflora*.

terephthalylidene dicamphor sulfonic acid—an FDA-approved sunscreen chemical with UV-filtering and absorbing capacities. It has an approved usage level of up to 10 percent in the European Union.

Terminalia ferdinandiana **fruit extract**—also known as kakadu plum. It is an anti-oxidant, has skin-bleaching properties and can be effectively used in the treatment of acne. Among its constituents are vitamin C (ascorbic acid), phenolic compounds, anthocyanins, and amino acids. This plant is native to Australia.

4-tertbutyl 4'-methoxydibenzoylmethane—*see* butyl methoxydibenzoylmethane.

tetradibutyl pentaerithrityl hydroxyhydrocinnamate—a stabilizer that protects products from discoloration because of exposure to light, particularly UV.

tetrahexyldecyl ascorbate—an anti-oxidant that inhibits lipid peroxidation (thereby protecting skin lipids from free-radical damage), it is also used for improving and maintaining the skin's overall condition. Manufacturers also cite an ability to lessen UV damage and stimulate collagen. Studies indicate that tetrahexyldecyl ascorbate may promote a more even skin tone by inhibiting pigment production and by providing skin-lightening and brightening characteristics to a formulation. This is an oil-soluble, stable ester of vitamin C. It is considered less irritating than ascorbic acid.

tetrahydroxypropyl ethylenediamine—used as a solvent and preservative. A component of the bacteria-killing substance in sugarcane, it is very alkaline and may be irritating to the skin and mucous membranes. It might also cause skin sensitization.

tetrasodium EDTA—used as a preservative and also as a sequestering and chelating agent in cosmetic solutions.

tetterwort extract (*Sanguinaria canadensis*) (**bloodroot**)—herbal lore cites external application as helpful for treating eczema and other skin problems. It is used for its refreshing, tonic, and cleansing action. The rootstock is the part that is used.

***Theobroma grandiflorum* seed butter**—*see* cupuaçu seed butter.

theophylline—tonic and skin conditioning. Its cosmetic activity is not clearly or definitively established. It is most often found in anti-cellulite products. Theophylline is in the same family of biochemicals as caffeine. It is naturally occurring in tea.

thiamine HCL (vitamin B$_1$)—used as an emollient. *See also* vitamin B.

thioctic acid—also known as alpha lipoic acid. It is an anti-oxidant. *See also* alpha lipoic acid.

thuja extract—credited with healing, anti-septic and anti-irritant properties. It is potentially effective against pigmentation. The oil is obtained by the distillation of small branches and twigs of yellow or white cedar. *See also* cedarwood oil.

thyme extract (*Thymus sp.*)—its botanical properties have been listed as anti-septic, tonic, anti-bacterial, deodorizing, fungicidal, and circulation stimulating. Certain fractions may have collagenase inhibitor abilities. Thyme extract might also have insect-repellent properties. Its active principle is thymic acid, which has disinfectant properties similar to those of carbolic acid. Thyme extract may cause skin irritation.

T

thyme oil—widely used in botanical therapy since antiquity for its warming, stimulating, and cleansing properties, it is also considered a powerful anti-septic and tonic. Thyme oil serves as a natural preservative with anti-bacterial activity against a wide spectrum of bacterial classes. The genus *Thymus* produces a variety of species, subspecies, and chemotypes, many with completely different chemical compositions. This includes citriodora thyme, lemon thyme, and red thyme. Lemon thyme is described as healing and soothing for its use in skin care. The oil is obtained from the herb's branches and flowers.

tilia (linden)—botanical properties are described as anti-septic, soothing, and emollient. *See also* linden extract.

TiO$_2$—*see* titanium dioxide.

tissue respiratory factor (TRF) (live yeast cell derivative)—described by manufacturers as a powerful anti-inflammatory and moisturizing agent that can promote wound healing. TRF is found to deliver its moisturizing, skin-soothing benefits more effectively than the traditional cosmetic raw materials. It also works with the skin to help improve the skin's appearance and overall health. It is obtained by stimulating living cells into producing protective substances. TRF can be described as a glyco-nucleopeptide and has been safely used for more than 40 years. TRF is a trade name. *See also Saccharomyces lysate* extract.

titanium dioxide (TiO$_2$)—one of the 21 FDA-approved sunscreen chemicals with an approved usage level of 2 to 25 percent. When applied, titanium dioxide remains on the skin's surface, scattering UV light. It is often used in conjunction with other sunscreen chemicals to boost the product's SPF value, thus reducing the risk of irritation or allergies attributed to excessive usage of chemical sunscreens. Its incorporation into sunscreen formulations, makeup bases, and daytime moisturizers depends on the particular size of titanium dioxide employed. The smaller the particle size, the more unobtrusive TiO$_2$'s application. Large particles, on the other hand, leave a whitish wash or look on the skin. Some companies list "micro" or "ultra" when referring to the size of the titanium dioxide particle. According to some sources, titanium dioxide could be the ideal UVA/UVB protection component given its chemical, cosmetic, and physical characteristics. Titanium dioxide is also used to provide a white color to cosmetic preparations.

titanium dioxide (micro)—*see* titanium dioxide.

titanium dioxide (ultra)—*see* titanium dioxide.

T

tocopherol (vitamin E)—an anti-oxidant obtained by vacuum distillation of edible vegetable oils. *See also* vitamin E.

tocopherol acetate—an anti-oxidant that helps prevent unsaturated oils and sebum from becoming rancid. It is considered a non-comedogenic raw material. *See also* vitamin E.

tocopherol ester—considered an effective free-radical scavenger.

tocopherol linoleate—a moisturizer. *See also* tocopherol.

tocopherol nicotinate—used as an anti-oxidant and a skin-conditioning agent.

tocophersolan—an anti-oxidant, this is a water-soluble form of vitamin E.

tocopheryl linoleate—used as an anti-oxidant and a skin-conditioning agent.

tocopheryl phosphate—added to a cosmetic formulation for cleansing, emulsifying, and surfactant activity.

tocopheryl sorbate—most likely used as an anti-oxidant. This is a modified form of tocopherol. *See also* vitamin E; vitamin E acetate.

tocotrienols—an anti-oxidant with UV absorption and skin-conditioning activity. This is a form of vitamin E, and studies indicate that it might be more potent than tocopherol. It could be incorporated into anti-oxidant and anti-aging products. Naturally occurring in oils derived from rice bran, barley, wheat, oat, and palm; the highest levels are contained in palm oil.

tomato (*Solanum lycopersicum*)—therapeutic skin care properties depend on the part of the plant that is used. For example, the extract made from the whole plant is astringent, whereas the fruit itself is considered a humectant and emollient. Tomato water has an ability to mask odor. Sources also cite anti-oxidant activity. The common property to all tomato derivatives in cosmetics is skin conditioning. Tomato's constituents include beta-carotene, carotenoids (lycopene), histamine, fructose, glucose, vitamins A, C, and E, mineral salts, and trace elements.

tomato oil—oil derived from the fruit can help improve and maintain a good skin condition in terms of texture, tone, and look. Oil from the seed softens and smooths the skin, in addition to being skin conditioning. Some sources cite it as particularly appropriate for combination skin.

tonka bean (*Dipteryx odorata*) (**tonquin bean**)—aromatic and tonic, it was traditionally used as a fixative in perfume manufacturing. Its primary constituent is coumaric acid. The seed is the part that is used.

T

tormentil extract (*Potentilla tormentilla*)—considered one of the safest and most powerful herbal astringents. It also has mildly antiseptic and anti-inflammatory properties. Used in Old England for sores, wounds, bruises, and infections. Important constituents of tormentil extract include tannin, phytosterols, flavonoids, chinovic acid, tormentoside, and pseudosaponine. The extract is obtained from the plant's root.

tourmaline—used to increase product viscosity, this is a semiprecious stone. There is little clinical evidence supporting therapeutic claims associated with tourmaline.

trace elements (**micronutrients; oligoelements**)—different elements, usually inorganic, are considered essential to plant and animal nutrition in trace concentrations. The value of their topical application through cosmetic preparations is not clear, although some sources indicate a potential moisturization value.

trace element complex—*see* trace elements.

tragacanth gum—an effective emulsifying agent, binder, film former, and viscosity controller, it is also used as a stabilizing ingredient in lotions. Tragacanth gum is derived from the resin of the *Astragalus gummifer* shrub.

***Trametes versicolor* extract**—used in traditional Asian medicine for its detoxifying, anti-bacterial, anti-fungal properties, as well as to boost the immune system. It is also cited as potentially able to boost superoxide dismutase and glutathione peroxidase activity. The extract is obtained from the *Trametes veriscolor* mushroom.

transglutaminase—an enzyme said to activate the skin's physiological functions.

treemoss extract (*Evernia furfuracea*)—a botanical ingredient that helps mask odor in a product.

trehalose—a humectant and moisturizer, it helps bind water in the skin and increase the skin's moisture content. It is a naturally occurring plant sugar.

***Tremella fuciformis* polysaccharide**—it can be used as an emulsion stabilizer, film former, or skin conditioner and is apparently able to help the skin retain moisture. It is also credited with skin-protecting, anti-inflammatory, and anti-allergenic properties. There is some clinical evidence that it may help increase superoxide dismutase activity and thus be effective in anti-aging formulations. This is the polysaccharide fraction derived from the *tremellia fuciformis* mushroom. Its primary constituent is glucoronoxylomannan.

tretinoin—*see* retinoic acid.

tribehenin—also known as glyceryl tribehenate. It is an emollient and skin conditioner.

tricaprylin—a skin-conditioning agent. *See also* caprylic/capric triglyceride.

tricaprylyl citrate—an emollient and skin conditioner.

Trichilia emetica **seed butter** (natal mahogany)—it is considered skin nourishing and revitalizing, with moisturizing and anti-aging activity. It is an emollient and keeps the skin soft and supple.

triclosan—a preservative considered to have a low sensitizing potential in leave-on preparations.

tricontanyl PVP—a film-forming, waterproofing, and wear-proofing agent. It is oil soluble and easily formulated into sunscreens, skin care creams, lotions, and general cosmetic products. Tricontanyl PVP is a very versatile ingredient. When used in sunscreens, it facilitates the formulation of high SPFs without the need to significantly increase the use of sunscreen chemicals. The result is products with higher SPF, lower irritancy potential, and greater cost effectiveness. Tricontanyl PVP is also used as a pigment dispersant in color cosmetics, and is particularly useful when titanium dioxide is used to increase SPF values. Studies indicate little to no photoallergy or toxicity.

tridecyl stearate—a skin-conditioning agent and an emollient.

tridecyl trimelliatate—an occlusive skin-conditioning agent.

triethanolamine—*see* TEA.

triethanolamine oleate—*see* TEA oleate.

triethanolamine salicylate—*see* TEA salicylate.

triethanolamine stearate—*see* TEA stearate.

triethylene glycol—a solvent prepared from ethylene oxide and ethylene glycol.

triglycerides—consistency regulators for creams, lotions, and makeup. Facilitates blending and imparts good flow properties to products. These are the chief constituents of fats and oils. These oils, such as those of almond, safflower, and cocoa butter, are utilized in cosmetics for enhanced lubricity and emolliency of a product. Fatty acids such as caprylic, capric, and lauric react with glycerin to produce triglyceride oils. There are a variety of triglycerides, including caprylic/capric, lauric, myristic, palmitic, and stearic.

triheptanoin—a triglyceride that acts as a surfactant and skin-conditioning agent, it also helps increase product viscosity. Often used in cleansers, face and neck products, moisturizers and lipsticks.

T

triisostearin—*see* glyceryl triisostearate.

triisostearyl citrate—an occlusive skin-conditioning agent. This is the triester of isostearyl alcohol and citric acid.

triisostearyl trilinoleate—a skin-conditioning and viscosity-controlling agent with occlusive properties.

trilaureth-4 phosphate—an emulsifier and a surfactant.

trilinolein—an emollient, it replenishes the lipids present in the stratum corneum, thereby improving skin look, feel, and texture. Depending on a formulator's requirements, it can also be used as a solvent and to control a formula's viscosity.

trimethyl siloxysilicate—in combination with dimethicone, it works as a waterproofing material for sunscreen preparations. It also reduces skin whitening and greasiness commonly associated with high SPF sunscreen formulations.

trisodium ascorbyl palmitate phosphate—an anti-oxidant and anti-wrinkle ingredient, this is a vitamin C derivative with good penetration capacities. According to manufacturers, it helps promote collagen synthesis.

trisodium EDTA—a preservative. *See also* tetrasodium EDTA.

trisodium HEDTA (trisodiumhydroxy EDTA)—a preservative. *See also* tetrasodium EDTA.

trisodium hydroxy EDTA—*see* trisodium HEDTA.

tristearin—an emollient.

tris (tetramethylhydroxypiperidinol) citrate—a UV absorber and light stabilizer, it protects a product from UV-induced degradation.

trolamine—*see* triethanolamine.

tromethamine—can help mask odor in a formulation. It is also used as a buffer, keeping product pH stable.

tropocollagen—sometimes known as soluble collagen. It has excellent moisture-binding properties and forms a moisture-retentive film on the skin. Formulations using tropocollagen instead of regular collagen are reported to provide a smoother, silkier afterfeel on the skin. The fibroblast produces tropocollagen, which is polymerized into collagen. Tropocollagen is obtained from animal connective tissues. *See also* collagen.

tropoelastin (soluble elastin)—the soluble precursor to elastin, it plays a role in elastin production. Apparently it can compensate for the loss of the skin's own elastin. It is reported to be more effective when applied on the skin than regular elastin. *See also* elastin.

tryptophan—one of the 21 amino acids comprising a protein. Tryptophan is a component of the skin's natural moisturizing factors. *See also* amino acid.

turmeric (*Curcuma longa*)—healing, tonic, mildly stimulating, anti-inflammatory, and has blood-purifying properties. It is also used to perfume or mask product odor. This common spice (used frequently in curry) and coloring agent is used in traditional medicine for a variety of curative purposes, including the treatment of eczema, skin infections, ulcers, burns, and rashes. It may have skin-softening properties and could be beneficial in products for acne.

tyramine—clinical studies indicate skin-lightening capacities.

tyrosine—an amino acid. Cutaneous applications may produce an extra reserve of tyrosine in the skin, assisting or "activating" melanin synthesis. This in turn should increase and prolong the effect of the tanning process. Tyrosine's effect is improved if the product contains vitamin B (riboflavin) plus an additional compound referred to chemically as ATP (adenosine triphosphate). Experiments conducted with *l*-tyrosine in the form of water-soluble derivatives found that it penetrates the epidermis to the basal layer where the melanocytes are located. It is used in suntan accelerators and in skin-bronzing cosmetics to accelerate the tanning process.

T

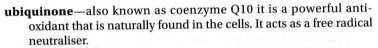

ubiquinone—also known as coenzyme Q10 it is a powerful antioxidant that is naturally found in the cells. It acts as a free radical neutraliser.

ucuuba oil—also known as *Virola sebifera* nut oil. It is attributed with emollient, humectant, skin-conditioning, and anti-septic properties. This nut oil is said to be rich in myristic acid. It is used generally in soaps, cleansers, massage lotions, and hair products. *See also* myristic acid.

***Ulmus davidiana* root extract**—considered anti-inflammatory and moisturizing, with an ability to help improve skin barrier functions. Manufacturers indicate it for use in anti-aging and acne care products. This extract is derived from the root of the Japanese elm.

ultramarine blue—a color additive. It was originally obtained naturally from ground lapis but is now produced synthetically. Ultramarines can also be green, pink, red, or violet, and are synthetic pigments composed of complex sodium aluminum sulfosilicated with the proportions of each element varying in each color. Used primarily in eye shadows, mascaras, and face powders. *See also* color entry in Chapter 4.

ulve extract—*see* seaweed extract.

ulve seaweed—*see* seaweed extract.

***Uncaria gambir* extract**—astringent and potentially anti-oxidant according to some recent studies. The extract might also be used for color. Catechins and caffeic acid are among its constituents.

***Uncaria tomentosa* extract**—also known as cat's claw. It is credited with anti-inflammatory, anti-oxidant, anti-bacterial, and immunostimulant properties. Among its constituents are alkaloids and tannins. The plant is a woody vine, native to the tropical rainforests of Central and South America.

undecylenoyl PEG-5 paraben—a preservative.

urea—incorporated into cosmetics for a variety of purposes, including moisturizing, desquamating, anti-microbial, and buffering. Urea is regarded as a "true" moisturizer rather than a humectant because it attracts and retains moisture in the corneum layer.

It facilitates the natural exfoliation of keratinocytes given its ability to dissolve intercellular cement in the corneum layer. Through its anti-microbial properties that inhibit the growth of micro-organisms in a product, urea can also be part of a larger preservative system. This ingredient's buffering action is attributed to its ability to regulate the hydrolipid mantle. In addition, urea is found to enhance the penetration and absorption of other active ingredients, relieve itchiness, and help leave the skin feeling soft and supple. Anti-inflammatory, anti-septic, and deodorizing actions allow it to protect the skin's surface against negative changes and help maintain healthy skin. Studies show that urea does not induce photoallergy, phototoxicity, or sensitization. The safest concentration of use in skin care preparations is between 2 and 8 percent. High concentrations of urea seem to be unstable when incorporated into skin care preparations and can also cause irritation. Acidic urea solutions can produce burning or stinging sensations.

ursolic acid—helps maintain the look and feel of the skin, acts as a perfume and helps mask odor. Therapeutic benefits in skin care include anti-inflammatory activity. Ursolic acid has demonstrated anti-microbial, anti-bacterial, and anti-fungal action as well.

U

valerian oil (*Valeriana officinalis*)—the therapeutic activities include calming, soothing, and anti-spasmodic. It is also incorporated into cosmetic formulations for perfuming and odor-masking action. Valerian was held in such esteem as a remedy during medieval times that it was called "All Heal." Its composition is complex, with constituents including alkaloids (catinine and valerine), gamma-aminobutyric acid (GABA), volatile oils (particularly valerenic acid to which valerian's sedative properties are attributed), formate, flavones such as hesperidin, and terpenes (e.g., l-camphene, l-limonene, and l-pinene). The oil is present in the dried root in quantities of 0.5 to 2 percent depending on the plant variety and place of growth. It is obtained by steam distillation. Reportedly, it can produce headaches when used frequently and in large quantities.

valeric acid—obtained from valerian extract, which is considered skin conditioning. *See also* valerian oil.

valine—an amino acid used as a skin-conditioning and odor-masking agent. It is more commonly used in hair care preparations than in skin care.

vanilla fruit extract (*Vanilla planifolia*)—vanilla fruit is commonly known as vanilla bean. This extract has skin-soothing, conditioning, protecting, and smoothing properties.

vanilla fruit oil—emollient and skin conditioning, it is obtained from the cured, full-grown, unripe fruit of vanilla. It may cause a skin reaction in overly sensitive skin.

vanilla resinoid—part of a natural preservative mixture that also includes linalool, ex-*bois de rose*, *bois de rose*, lemongrass, cedarwood oil, neroli bigarade petals oil, and other such exotic components.

Vaseline fluid—*see* petrolatum.

veegum—*see* magnesium aluminum silicate.

vegetable oil—a carrier, a skin softener, and an occlusive skin-conditioning agent. Such a listing may refer to a variety of oils alone or in combination, including peanut, corn, sesame, olive, and cottonseed. As the extract type of oil is not specified when listed in this fashion, it is difficult to determine the ingredient's value or any skin reactions that may arise from the ingredient's use. Vegetable oil is an expressed oil of vegetable origin consisting primarily of triglycerides of fatty acids.

vegetable starch—used as a thickening agent.

verbena leaf extract (*Verbena officinalis*)—masking, toning, and refreshing, verbena leaf extract has also exhibited some anti-inflammatory properties. This extract is derived from leaves of verbena plant. Verbena is also called vervain.

verbena oil—also known as vervain oil. It is credited with astringent and anti-spasmodic properties, as well as being a perfuming agent. It is a perennial plant bearing many small, pale lilac flowers.

veronica extract (*Veronica officinalis*)—credited with anti-inflammatory, healing, purifying, tonic, and soothing properties. Some say it promotes healthy tissue growth and a refinement of the pores. There are many species of veronica, with about 20 having been medicinally employed. Regardless of the species, the extract is generally obtained from the plant's flowers, leaves, and stems.

vetiver oil (*Vetiveria zizanioides*) **(khus-khus)**—considered stimulant and tonic, and used in perfumery as well as in cosmetics. The oil, which has an aromatic to harsh woodsy odor, is produced from the roots of a fragrant grass.

violet extract (*Viola sp.*)—traditionally used for soothing and anti-itching skin treatments, and as an anti-septic in skin creams and burn preparations. Violet extract also has cleansing properties. Its important constituents include saponins, anti-septic glycosides (viola quercitin), violine, an alkaloid, salicylic acid, and dye-matter for a blue color. The extract has a slightly sweet, floral scent. Although the violet family encompasses over 200 species, it is the sweet-scented violet that appears to be most appropriate for botanical use. Violet extract may produce a skin rash in those allergic to this particular plant.

vipers bugloss oil (*Echium plantagineum*)—one fraction of this botanical lipid includes stearidonic acid, a fatty acid with known anti-inflammatory properties. Manufacturer studies indicate that it may reduce the skin's inflammatory response to UV rays. It is useful in sunscreens and sun care products, as well as in anti-aging products and anti-inflammatory preparations. Found within the same family as black cohosh and bugbane. *See also* black cohosh extract.

vitamin A—can act as a keratinization regulator, helping to improve the skin's texture, firmness, and smoothness. Vitamin A esters, once in the skin, convert to retinoic acid and provide anti-aging benefits. Vitamin A is believed to be essential for the generation and function of skin cells. Continued vitamin A deficiency shows a degeneration of dermal tissue, and the skin becomes thick and dry. Surface application of vitamin A helps prevent skin dryness and scaliness, keeping the skin healthy, clear, and infection resistant. Its skin regeneration properties appear enhanced when combined with vitamin E. Vitamin A is a major constituent of such oils as cod liver and shark, and many fish and vegetable oils. *See also* retinol; retinoic acid; retinylpalmitate.

vitamin A palmitate—known as a skin "normalizer." It acts as an anti-keratinizing agent, helping the skin stay soft and plump, and improving its water-barrier properties. Because of its impact on the skin's water-barrier properties, it is useful against dryness, heat, and pollution. It is also an anti-oxidant and is suggested for use in sunscreens. Clinical studies with vitamin A palmitate indicate a significant change in skin composition, with increases in collagen, DNA, skin thickness, and elasticity. Vitamin A palmitate's stability is superior to retinol.

vitamin B—literature tends to indicate that B vitamins cannot pass through the layers of the skin and, therefore, are of no value in the skin surface. Current experiments demonstrate, however, that vitamin B_2 acts as a chemical reaction accelerator, enhancing the performance of tyrosine derivatives in suntan-accelerating preparations. *See also* biotin for B_7; panthenol for B_5; pyridoxine tripalmitate for B_6; riboflavin for B_2; thiamine HCL for vitamin B_1.

vitamin C—a well-known anti-oxidant. Its effect on free-radical formation when topically applied to the skin by means of a cream has not been clearly established. The effectiveness of topical applications has been questioned due to vitamin C's instability (it reacts with water and degrades). Some forms are said to have better stability in water systems. Synthetic analogues such as magnesium ascorbyl phosphate are among those considered more effective, as they tend to be more stable. When evaluating its ability to fight free-radical damage in light of its synergistic effect with vitamin E, vitamin C shines. As vitamin E reacts with a free radical, it, in turn, is damaged by the free radical it is fighting. Vitamin C comes in to repair the free-radical damage in vitamin E, allowing E to continue with its free-radical scavenging duties. Past research has indicated that high concentrations of topically applied vitamin C are photoprotective, and apparently the vitamin preparation used in these studies resisted soap and water, washing, or rubbing for three days. More current research has indicated that vitamin C does add protection against UVB damage when combined with UVB sunscreen chemicals. This would lead one to conclude that in combination with conventional sunscreen agents, vitamin C may allow for longer-lasting, broader sun protection. Again, the synergy between vitamins C and E can yield even better results, as apparently a combination of both provides very good protection from UVB damage. However, vitamin C appears to be significantly better than E at protecting against UVA damage. A further conclusion is that the combination of vitamins C, E, and sunscreen offers greater protection than the sum of the protection offered by any of the three ingredients acting alone. Vitamin C also acts as a collagen biosynthesis regulator. It is known to control intercellular colloidal substances such as collagen, and when formulated into the proper vehicles, can have a skin-lightening effect. Vitamin C is said to be able to help the body fortify against infectious conditions by strengthening the immune system. There is some evidence (although debated) that vitamin C can pass through the layers of the skin and promote healing in tissue damaged by burns or injury. It is found, therefore, in burn ointments and creams used for abrasions. Vitamin C is also popular in anti-aging products. Current studies indicate possible anti-inflammatory properties as well. *See also* ascorbic acid.

vitamin C ester—said to promote a visible renewal of the skin's appearance, resulting in skin that looks brighter, firmer, and healthier. This is a general category, however, and the listing does not indicate the form of the ester incorporated into the product. For example, the ester could be either ascorbyl palmitate or magnesium ascorbyl phosphate, where the first has both anti-oxidant and odor-masking properties, while the second is used for anti-oxidant activity but does not provide an odor-masking function.

vitamin D—acts as a keratinization regulator, helping to improve skin feel and firmness with repeated use. This vitamin is absorbed through the skin's outer layers. Studies are indicating that vitamin D is an important factor in epidermal cell turnover. It is generally found in combination with vitamin A, as such a mixture appears to help epithelial growth and promote good skin pigmentation. Like vitamin A, vitamin D is a major constituent of many fish and vegetable oils.

vitamin E (D-alpha-tocopherol; DL-alpha-tocopherol; tocopherol)—considered the most important oil-soluble anti-oxidant and free-radical scavenger. Studies indicate that vitamin E performs these functions when topically applied. It is also a photoprotectant, and it helps protect the cellular membrane from free-radical damage. In addition, vitamin E serves a preservative function given its ability to protect against oxidation. This benefits not only the skin, but also the product in terms of longevity. As a moisturizer, vitamin E is well-absorbed through the skin, demonstrating a strong affinity with small blood vessels and an ability to enhance blood circulation in the skin. It is also thought to improve the skin's water-binding ability. In addition, vitamin E emulsions have been found to reduce transepidermal water loss, thereby improving the appearance of rough, dry, and damaged skin. This vitamin is also believed to help maintain the connective tissue. There is evidence that vitamin E is effective in preventing irritation owing to sun exposure: studies show that vitamin E topically applied prior to UV irradiation is protective against epidermal cell damage caused by inflammation. This indicates possible anti-inflammatory properties. Lipid peroxidation in tissues may be one cause of skin aging. Vitamin E, however, appears to counteract decreased functioning of the sebaceous glands and to reduce excessive skin pigmentation, which is found to increase almost linearly with age. It is available also as a tocopherol-polypeptide complex that delivers the vitamin in a water-dispersable form. In this way, when incorporated into cosmetic formulations, it does not need other compounds to assist in its solubilization. It is useful in anti-aging creams and lotions, and in UV protective products, tocopherol is a naturally occurring vitamin E found in a variety of cereal germ oils including wheat germ oil. It can also be produced synthetically.

vitamin E acetate (tocopherol acetate)—an anti-oxidant with skin-moisturizing activity. Given its free-radical scavenging properties, it is useful in UV protective products. Vitamin E acetate is commonly used to replace vitamin E because it is more stable and is converted to vitamin E by the body. *See also* vitamin E.

vitamin E linoleate—a synthetic version of vitamin E. *See also* tocopheryl linoleate; vitamin E.

vitamin F—used in the treatment and care of dry skin. This is the group name for a family of essential fatty acids comprised of arachidonic, linoleic, and alpha-linoleic acids. *See also* arachidonic acid; linoleic acid.

vitamin H—*see* biotin.

vitamin K—helps promote blood clotting and has been used medically to reduce the possibility of bruising after surgery. It is being incorporated into cosmetic preparations, particularly those used for treating dark circles. It could also be used in acne products, and there are studies underway on its efficacy for the treatment of spider veins.

vitamin P—considered a vascular protector and an anti-inflammatory agent, vitamin P is said to promote capillary health and increase resistance to collagen destruction. Vitamin P is a bioflavonoid that can work in conjunction with vitamin C, helping prevent oxidation of the latter. Vitamin P is found in such food sources as apricots, broccoli, citrus fruit pulp, grapes, prunes, and spinach. *See also* bioflavonoid in Chapter 4.

VP/eicosene copolymer—can be used for a variety of purposes, including binding, film forming, and to control viscosity.

volcanic sand—mildly abrasive it is used in exfoliating products.

V

walnut extract (*Juglans sp.*)—traditionally used for soothing and anti-itching action, as well as against sunburns and other superficial burns. Its fungistatic, anti-septic, and astringent properties can be beneficial in cases of acne and skin diseases. The extract is obtained either from the walnut leaf, which is said to be astringent and cleansing, or from the shell, which is considered astringent and emollient with some odor-masking activity. Tannin is a primary constituent of walnut extract.

walnut leaves (*Juglans regia*)—incorporated into a cosmetic product for astringent, cleansing, scrubbing, skin-conditioning, or soothing purposes. They can also be used as bulking agents and to mask odor. Studies indicate anti-microbial properties as well as a potential ability to impact oxidative stress, thereby functioning as an anti-oxidant. Constituents include tannin, flavonoids, vitamin C, caffeic and ferulic acids, and a volatile oil.

walnut meal—a mild abrasive. *See also* walnut shell powder.

walnut oil—hydrating, toning, anti-inflammatory, nourishing, and emollient. Walnut oil can help maintain skin suppleness. Its constituents include vitamin E, oleic acid, linolenic acid, and a high percentage of linoleic acid (some sources cite up to 60 percent). Its application includes use in moisturizers, eye creams, and body oils.

walnut shell meal—an abrasive. *See also* walnut shell powder.

walnut shell powder—used as an abrasive and bulking agent in cleansers, scrubs, soaps, and masks. It is the powder ground from the shell of English walnuts.

water—listed also as catalyzed, deionized, demineralized, distilled, pure spring, and purified water. Water is an important skin component and is essential for its proper functioning. It is the most common ingredient used in cosmetic formulations and, therefore, is generally listed first on product labels. Water is usually processed to eliminate hardness and minerals, and to avoid product contamination.

water lily extract (*Nymphaea alba*)—soothing. It appears to reduce the temperature and decrease the pain of sun-exposed skin. It is most likely to be incorporated into sensitive skin and post-sun cosmetics. An extract can be obtained from the plant's flower and its root. *See also* lily extract.

watercress extract (*Nasturtium officinale*)—used in folklore for cleansing external ulcers and in night creams for freckles, spots, and acne. An extract derived from both the plant's flower and leaves is credited with helping reduce sebum production. Watercress extract is utilized as a moisture regulator and skin activator for sunburn (and bath) preparations, as well as a perfuming agent. Some clinical studies are indicating anti-oxidant properties through an ability to reduce reactive oxygen species and activity as a free radical scavenger. Important constituents of watercress include minerals, flavonoids, and vitamins. This is a hardy perennial found in abundance near springs and open running watercourses.

W

watermelon (*Citrullus lanatus*)—occasionally referred to as kalahari melon. Its purpose in a cosmetic product will depend on the part and form used. For example, the fruit juice can be used as a humectant, and as a flavoring agent. The seeds and seed powder are abrasive and exfoliant, and the seed oil is emollient. Its constituents include flavonoids, carotenoids, and triterpenoids, which can provide it with anti-inflammatory and anti-oxidant properties. Other constituents include lycopene and vitamin C. Ingredient suppliers and product manufacturers attribute it with skin-regeneration and restructuring properties.

wheat bran extract—considered a moisturizer given its carbohydrate/sugar components. This is the extract from the broken coat material of wheat grains.

wheat germ extract—used in cosmetics because of its high vitamin E content. This extract is obtained from the wheat kernel embryo separated in milling. *See also* vitamin E.

wheat germ glycerides—softens the skin and has good penetration ability. Wheat germ glycerides contain polyunsaturated fats, key for healthy skin. This mixture of mono-, di-, and triglycerides is produced by the transesterification of wheat germ oil, and is commonly used in moisturizers in concentrations of 0.1 to 5 percent. Although some sources indicate it may be irritating, safety tests show it to be non-sensitizing and non-irritating to the skin. It is considered by some to be somewhat comedogenic.

wheat germ oil—an emollient, it helps improve the feel and texture of the skin. The therapeutic benefits associated with wheat germ oil include anti-oxidant and free-radical scavenging properties, given its vitamin E content, as well as regenerating activity.

Additional constituents include vitamins A, B, and D, and lecithin. It is cited as appropriate for use in anti-aging products, as well as for dry skin, sunburned skin, eczema, and on stretch marks. The oil is obtained by the expression or extraction of wheat germ.

wheat germ oil (unsaponifiable)—acts as a hormone-like cellular messenger. Studies indicate that this activity can stimulate the fibroblast to produce collagen, elastin, proteoglycans, and structural glycoproteins.

wheat protein—has elastic and binding properties. It helps to reduce the irritating effect of surfactants and is also known to demonstrate excellent emulsifying action. Given its film-forming abilities on the skin's surface, wheat protein also moisturizes and conditions the skin, increasing skin firmness by helping minimize transepidermal water loss. Some forms of wheat protein are said to be film formers that contract upon drying, causing the flattening out of the skin and a reduction in surface roughness. Wheat protein has an unusually low irritation potential.

wheat protein (soluble)—wheat protein that dissolves in water. It is more commonly used in hair care formulations as a means to introduce protein into the hair shaft and strengthen it. *See also* wheat protein.

wheat starch—used as a demulcent and emollient and in face powders. Wheat starch swells when water is added. It is obtained from wheat.

whey protein—*see* milk protein.

white balsam extract (*Gnaphalium polycephalum*)—a botanical extract with astringent properties.

white clover—*see* melilot.

white dead-nettle—*see* white nettle.

white lily bulb extract (*Lilium candidum*) (**Madonna lily**)—has antiseptic and soothing properties. The roots contain tannin, gallic acid, mucilage, starch, gum, resin, sugar, ammonia, tartaric acid, and fecula. This is a perennial aquatic herb that grows to the surface of the water from a thick horizontal rootstock.

white nettle (*Lamium album*) (**white dead-nettle**)—considered astringent, it is also used to mask odor. It is obtained from the plant's flowers or leaves. *See also* nettle.

white sweet lupine extract—*see* lupine extract.

white tea extract—attributed with a wide variety of properties, it is anti-fungal, anti-microbial, anti-oxidant, and astringent.

Formulators may also use it for fragrancing, as a humectant or as an emollient and to improve overall skin condition. White tea comes from the same plant—*Camellia sinensis*—as green and black tea, and studies are attributing it with a potent anti-oxidant capacity, protecting the skin and the Langerhans cells against oxidative stress. *See also* tea and green tea.

white willow extract (*Salix alba*)—deodorant with tonic and astringent properties. It is used effectively in products for acne and eczema. The extract is obtained from the bark of this large tree. Tannin is a chief constituent, and it contains a small quantity of salicin as well. See also willow extract.

wild alum (*Geranium maculatum*)—astringent and deodorant. It is cited as good for oily skin.

wild basil (*Ocimum gratissimum*)—primarily used as a fragrance component, the essential oil has demonstrated anti-bacterial and anti-fungal properties as well.

wild marjoram—*see* wild Spanish marjoram.

wild pansy extract—*see* pansy extract.

wild Spanish marjoram (**wild marjoram**)—described as having anti-septic and anti-inflammatory properties. *See also* marjoram.

wild thyme extract (*Thymus serpyllum*)—an emollient, tonic, and anti-septic extract traditionally used to clean wounds after washing. It is believed to be less effective than the common variety of thyme. It contains 30 to 70 percent phenols, including thymol and carvacrol. When distilled, some 225 pounds of dried material yield 150 grams of essence. Wild thyme is a perennial herb.

wild yam extract (*Dioscorea villosa*)—helps maintain the skin looking healthy, supple, and in good condition. Given its phtyoestrogen content, sources cited it for use in anti-aging and anti-wrinkle skin care preparations. The root is the part that is used.

willow extract (*Salix sp.*)—described as anti-septic and skin clearing. The roots and leaves have demulcent, tonic, and astringent properties. Apparently, it is very mild, hence its incorporation in lotions and creams for infants.

willow bark extract—a natural source of salicylic acid, beneficial for its exfoliating activity.

winterbloom infusion—*see* witch hazel extract.

witch hazel distillate—an aqueous solution obtained by distillation of *Hamamelis virginiana* twigs. *See also* witch hazel extract.

witch hazel extract (*Hamamelis virginiana*) (**hamamelis; winterbloom**)—traditionally used in the topical treatment of burns, sunburns, skin irritation, insect bites, and bruises. It is credited with anti-inflammatory, astringent, and wound-healing properties. It is often used for its anti-itching, softening, and emollient properties. In addition, anti-free radical activity is now associated with witch hazel, thereby helping counter the damaging effects of UVA, while acting as an absorber of both UVA and UVB. Ideal applications for witch hazel are in sun preparations, after-sun preparations, and creams that strive to regenerate overstrained skin. It can be formulated effectively into gels as an anti-septic preparation for treating impure, greasy skin as well as acne. Some sources cite a recommended dosage of 2 to 5 percent for use in formulations. It is obtained from the leaves and bark of the plant. Its primary constituents are tannins and saponins. Other constituents include volatile oil and gallic acid, with flavonoids also present in the leaves.

W

wood alcohol—*see* alcohol.

wood sage—*see* germander extract.

wool wax alcohols—*see* lanolin alcohol.

wormwood (*Artemisia absinthium*)—attributed actions include perfuming, anti-microbial, and skin conditioning. Given its azulene content, it might also be used for some natural coloring. Among its other constituents are a complex bitter (absinthin), succinic acid, thujyl alcohol, thujyl acetate, thujone, phellandrene, candinene, tannin, and vitamins B and C.

woundwort extract (*Anthyllis vulneraria*)—in herbal medicine, it is considered anti-septic, astringent, and tonic. The extract, obtained from the leaves, has been credited with an ability to stop bleeding and to heal wounds.

xanthan gum (corn starch gum)—serves as a texturizer, carrier agent, and gelling agent in cosmetic preparations. It also stabilizes and thickens formulations. This gum is produced through a fermentation of carbohydrate and *Xanthomonas campestris*.

xanthophylls—a family of biochemicals that are oxygenated derivatives of caratenoids. They can be used as colorants (red to yellow) and for apparent anti-oxidant and anti-free radical properties. Some studies now indicate UV protection capacities as well. Astaxanthin, lutein, and zeaxanthin are examples of xanthophylls. Both lutein and zeaxanthan appear to limit UV-induced skin damage. *See also* astaxanthin.

xylitol—a humectant and skin-conditioning agent. It acts as a humidifier, drawing moisture from the air for skin absorption. Some manufacturers also cite a soothing and anti-microbial action. Xylitol is a naturally occurring sugar in birch bark and a range of fibrous fruits and vegetables, including corn.

xyloglucan—a fraction of tamarind extract. *See also* tamarind.

X

Y

yarrow extract (*Achillea millefolium*) (**Achillea extract; milfoil**)—
attributed with anti-inflammatory and anti-spasmodic effects.
It is famous in traditional medicine for stopping wound bleeding and nosebleeds. Studies indicate an antibiotic activity and an
ability to reduce the blood's clotting time. Yarrow extract is also
described as having astringent, anti-septic, healing, and calming
properties. Considered good in the care of oily and acne skins.
Yarrow's important constituents include flavonoids, amino acids,
sugars, and phytosterols. It grows everywhere: in grass, meadows, pastures, and by the roadside. Since it creeps by its roots and
multiplies by its seeds, yarrow becomes a troublesome weed in
gardens. The whole plant is used in making the extract.

yeast—has a rubefactant effect on the skin, making it good for pale,
yellow skins. It is used in face masks designed to give the skin a
ruddy color. Yeast is a fungus whose usual and dominant growth
form is unicellular. It can cause irritation to dry or sensitive skins.
See also malt.

yeast extract—manufacturers claim it is able to revitalize the skin
with moisture, fight dryness, and give the skin a radiant appearance. In addition, it is claimed that yeast extract has the ability
to minimize the dryness and pain associated with sunburned
and wind-chapped skin; restore the comfort of soft, elastic,
and healthy skin; reduce facial lines; and improve dry skin. Its
constituents include enzymes, vitamins, sugars, and mineral
substances.

yellow toadflax (*Linaria vulgaris*)—also known as wild snapdragon.
It is credited with anti-inflammatory, astringent, cleansing, and
draining properties. Constituents include flavonoids such as
linarin, glycosides, and a variety of organic acids.

yerba mate extract (*Ilex paraguariensis*)—is perfuming and skin-
conditioning. Studies are indicating anti-oxidant, anti-
inflammatory, vasodilating, and lipid-reduction properties.
Among its many constituents are saponins, xanthenes (also
found in coffee and chocolate), polyphenols, minerals, including
aluminum, chromium, copper, iron, nickel, manganese, potas-
sium and zinc, and vitamins A, C, E, B_1, B_2, B_3, B_5, and B complex.

Sometimes it is also called Paraguayan tea. The plant is a member of the holly family and the extract is obtained from its leaves.

ylang-ylang extract—*see* ylang-ylang oil.

ylang-ylang oil (*Cananga odorata; Unona odoratissima*)—mentioned in folklore as a scenting agent and for insect bites. Ylang-ylang is considered relaxing and an excellent anti-stress agent. In addition, it is credited with anti-septic, softening, smoothing, rejuvenating, calming, soothing, and anti-spasmodic properties. It is good for inflamed and/or irritated skin and for controlling acne. Ylang-ylang oil is said to help balance the skin and work to reduce oiliness. Along with its therapeutic effects, ylang-ylang is also believed to be effective for relieving tension. This can be beneficial when working with skin disorders, such as acne and eczema, that can be aggravated by stress. Some sources cite that it takes roughly 100 pounds of blossoms to produce about two pounds of essential oil. This oil is produced by means of steam distillation into a fragrant, yellowish oil of varying grades.

ylang-ylang water—*see* ylang-ylang oil.

yomogi extract—a botanical said to have moisturizing and soothing properties.

yucca—used in cosmetic formulations for masking odor and protecting the skin against aggressive factors (extreme climates, for example). An extract made from the leaves, stems, and roots of the *schidigera* variety is also attributed with cleaning and surfactant action. Some studies indicate anti-inflammatory and anti-oxidant/free-radical scavenging activity. Yucca's constituents include phytoestrogen and a high level of saponins. Generally, the root or the stalk is the part that is used. However, the flower can also be used and is said to have anti-fungal properties.

Z

zinc—described as an oligo element, trace element, or micro nutrient. Zinc is believed to accelerate wound healing. It is also considered an anti-oxidant, offering protection against UV radiation. It appears to favor the sulfur uptake in sulfurated amino acids and facilitates the incorporation of cysteine, an amino acid, into the skin. It also has a synergistic effect with vitamins A and E. Zinc is a component of more than 70 metal enzymes. It promotes collagen synthesis in the dermis and keratinization of the corneum layer. Zinc is useful for acne treatments because it lowers sebaceous secretion, and is also used in the treatment of psoriasis.

zinc aspartate—a skin-conditioning agent. Zinc aspartate is the zinc salt of aspartic acid.

zinc gluconate—helps maintain the skin in good condition and acts as a deodorant by preventing the growth of micro-organisms, such as bacteria, fungi or yeast, in a formulation. Zinc gluconate could also be effectively used in anti-acne products. *See also* zinc.

zinc glycinate—used to adjust a product's pH, or maintain its pH at a desired level.

zinc oxide—has been used to protect, soothe, and heal the skin. Zinc oxide provides an excellent barrier to the sun and other irritants. It is somewhat astringent, anti-septic, and anti-bacterial. When used in sunscreen preparations, it provides both UVA and UVB protection, and can contribute to and/or increase SPF. At the appropriate particle size, zinc oxide is transparent in the visible light spectrum but opaque in the UVC ranges, thereby avoiding a whitening effect when incorporated into sunscreen preparations. Zinc oxide is included on the FDA's list of approved sunscreen chemicals. It demonstrates an impressive synergistic effect when combined with organic sunscreens. Zinc oxide is also used when a white color is desired for a product. It is obtained from zinc ore, a commonly found mineral, and is relatively non-allergenic.

zinc pyrithione—a preservative against bacteria, fungi, and yeast. It is unstable in light and in the presence of oxidizing agents. Zinc pyrithione is useful in gels, creams, heavy lotions, and talcum powder.

zinc stearate—used in cosmetic formulations to increase adhesive properties. It is also used as a coloring agent. This is a mixture of the zinc salts of stearic and palmitic acids.

zinc sulfate—a cosmetic astringent and biocide produced through the reaction of sulfuric acid with zinc. It can cause irritation to the skin and mucous membranes, and may cause an allergic reaction.

zingiber cassumunar **(bengal ginger, cassumunar ginger)**—also known as plai. The root may be used either in extract, oil, or powder forms to mask odor, maintain skin condition, and serve as a humectant. The extract obtained from the plant's leaves and flowers is said to help improve skin feel. Studies indicate antioxidant and anti-inflammatory properties as well. The essential oil has exhibited anti-fungal and anti-microbial capacities. *See also* ginger root extract.

Z

PART III

Botanical Latin Names

Botanical Latin Names

A

Acacia senegal—acacia
Achillea millefolium—milfoil, yarrow
Adenophora stricta—lady bell
Aesculus hippocastanum—horse chestnut
Agrimonia eupatoria—agrimony
Alchemilla vulgaris—alchemilla, lady's mantle
Aleurites moluccana—kukui nut oil
Allium sativum—garlic
Aloe vera—aloe vera
Alternifolia sp.—see *Melaleuca alternifolia*
Althaea officinalis—marshmallow
Andira araroba—goa; goa powder
Anemone sp.—anemone
Angelica sp.—angelica
Aniba rosaeodora—rosewood
Anthemis nobilis—Roman chamomile
Anthyllis vulneraria—woundwort
Arctium lappa—burdock
Arctostaphylos uva-ursi—bearberry
Areca catechu—areca nut palm, betel nut palm
Armoracia lapathifolia—horseradish
Arnica montana—arnica
Artemisia absinthium—wormwood
Artemisia abrotanum—southernwood
Artemisia dracunculus—tarragon
Avena sativa—oat

B

Bambusa arundinacea—bamboo
Bellis perennis—daisy
Berberis vulgaris—barberry
Bertholletia excelsa—Brazil nut
Beta vulgaris—beet
Betula sp.—birch
Bixa orellana—annatto
Borago officinalis—borage
Boswellia thurifera—frankincense
Brassica campestris—field mustard; rapeseed

C

Calamintha officinalis—calamint
Calendula officinalis—calendula; marigold
Calophyllum inophyllum—tamanu
Camellia sinensis L.—tea
Cananga odorata—ylang-ylang
Capsella bursa pastoris—shepherd's purse
Capsicum sp.—pepper
Carduus marianus—milk thistle
Carica papaya—papaya
Caryocar brasiliense—pequi
Caroba balsam—carob
Carthamus tinctorius—safflower
Carum carvi—caraway
Caryophyllus aromaticus—clove
Cassia angustifolia—senna
Castanea sativa—chestnut
Centaurea cyanus—cornflower
Centella asiatica—gotu kola
Certraria islandica—Iceland moss
Chondrus crispus—carrageen, Irish moss
Chrysanthemum parthenium—feverfew
Cimicifuga racemosa—black cohosh

Cinchona ledgeriana—cinchona
Cinnamomum camphora—camphor
Cinnamomum zeylanicum—cinnamon
Citrullus lanatus—watermelon; kalahari melon
Citrus acida—lime
Citrus aurantifolia—key lime
Citrus aurantium—bitter orange
Citrus bergamia—bergamot
Citrus limonum—lemon
Citrus nobilis—mandarin orange
Citrus paradisi—grapefruit
Citrus reticulata—tangerine
Citrus sinensis—sweet orange
Cochlearia officinalis—scurvy grass
Cola acuminata—kola tree
Coleus barbatus—coleus
Commiphora meccanensis—balm of Gilead
Commiphora myrrha—myrrh
Commiphora opobalsamum—balm of Gilead
Coriandrum sativum—coriander
Corylus avellana—hazel
Crataegus sp.—hawthorn
Cucumis sativus—cucumber
Cupressus sp.—cypress
Cucurbita pepo—pumpkin
Curcuma longa—turmeric
Cymbopogon citratus—lemongrass
Cymbopogon martini—palmarosa
Cymbopogon nardus—citronella
Cynara scolymus—artichoke

D

Daucus carota—carrot
Dioscorea villosa—wild yam
Dipteryx odorata—tonka bean
Dryopteris sp.—fern

E

Echinacea angustifolia—echinacea; coneflower
Echium plantagineum—vipers bugloss oil
Elettaria cardamomum—cardamom
Equisetum arvense—horsetail
Equisetum hyemale—rough horsetail
Eucalyptus globulus—eucalyptus
Eugenia caryophyllus—clove
Euphrasia officinalis—eyebright
Euterpe oleracea—açai
Evernia furfuracea—treemoss
Evernia prunastri—oakmoss

F

Fagus sylvatica—beech
Filipendula ulmaria—meadowsweet
Foeniculum vulgare—fennel
Fragaria vesca—strawberry
Fraxinus excelsior—ash
Fucus vesiculosus—fucus seaweed
Fumaria officinalis—fumitory

G

Galium aparine—cleavers
Gentiana sp.—gentian
Geranium maculatum—cranesbill
Geum urbanum—avens
Ginkgo biloba—ginkgo
Glycyrrhiza glabra—licorice
Gnaphalium polycephalum—white balsam
Guaiacum officinale—guaia

H

Hamamelis virginiana—witch hazel
Harpagophytum procumbens—devil's claw
Hedera helix—ivy
Helianthus annuus—sunflower
Hibiscus sp.—hibiscus
Hippophae rhamnoides—seabuckthorn
Hordeum vulgare—barley
Humulus lupulus—hops
Hydrastis canadensis—goldenseal
Hydrocotyle asiatica—gotu kola
Hypericum perforatum—St. John's wort
Hyssopus officinalis—hyssop

I

Ilex paraguariensis—yerba mate
Inula helenium—elecampane
Ipomoea batatas—sweet potato
Iris sp.—iris

J

Jacaranda procera—carob
Jasminum officinale—jasmine
Juglans sp.—walnut
Juniperus communis—juniper

L

Lactuca virosa—lettuce
Laminaria digitata—seaweed
Lamium album—white nettle, blind nettle

Limnanthes alba—meadowfoam
Laurus nobilis—laurel
Lavandula officinalis—lavender
Lawsonia inermis—henna
Lentinus edodes—shiitake mushroom
Levisticum officinale—lovage
Lilium candidum—white lily
Linaria vulgaris—common toadflax; yellow toadflax
Lonicera fragrantissima—honeysuckle
Lycium barbarum—boxthorn, goji berry, matrimony vine, wolfberry
Lycopodium clavatum—clubmoss

M

Macadamia integrifolia—macadamia nut tree
Malva sylvestris—mallow
Manihot utilissima—tapioca
Matricaria chamomilla—German chamomile
Medicago sativa—alfalfa
Melaleuca alternifolia—tea tree
Melaleuca leucadendron—cajeput
Melilotus officinalis—melilot
Melissa officinalis—balm mint
Mentha sp.—mint
Mentha piperita—peppermint
Mentha viridis—spearmint
Mercurialis perennis—dog's mercury
Monarda didyma—bee balm
Morus sp.—mulberry
Musa sp.—banana
Myrica cerifera—bayberry
Myristica fragrans—nutmeg
Myrospermum toluiferum—balsam of tolu
Myroxylon pereirae—balsam of Peru

N

Narcissus poeticus—narcissus; poet's daffodil
Nasturtium officinale—watercress
Nelumbo nucifera—lotus
Nymphaea alba—water lily

O

Ocimum basilicum—basil
Ocimum gratissimum—wild basil
Oenothera biennis—evening primrose
Olea europaea—olive
Ononis arvensis—field restharrow
Ononis spinosa—spiny restharrow
Onopordum acanthium—cotton thistle
Orchis sp.—orchid
Origanum majorana— marjoram; sweet marjoram
Origanum vulgare—oregano
Oryza sativa—rice

P

Padina pavonica—peacock's tail
Paeonia officinalis—peony
Panax sp.—ginseng
Papaver sp.—poppy
Papaver rhoeas—red poppy
Passiflora sp.—passion flower
Pelargonium sp.—geranium
Petroselinum sativum—parsley
Phaseolus aureus—mung bean
Phaseolus vulgaris—bean
Phoradendron flavescens—American mistletoe
Picea excelsa—spruce

Pimenta acris—bay leaf
Pimpinella anisum—anise
Pinus sp.—pine
Pisum sativum—pea
Pistacia lentiscus—mastic
Plantago sp.—plantain
Pogostemon patchouli—patchouli
Potentilla anserina—cinquefoil
Potentilla tormentilla—tormentil
Primula officinalis—primula; cowslip
Prunus amygdalus amara—bitter almond
Prunus amygdalus dulcis—sweet almond
Prunus cerasus—sour cherry
Prunus domestica—plum
Prunus persica—peach
Pyrola elliptica—shinleaf
Pyrus cydonia—quince
Pyrus malus—apple

Q

Quercus sp.—oak

R

Ranunculus ficaria—pilewort
Rhamnus purshiana—casacara sagrada
Rheum palmatum—rhubarb
Rhus glabra—sumac
Ribes nigrum—black currant
Ribes rubrum—red currant
Ricinus communis—castor oil plant
Rosa sp.—rose
Rosa canina—hip rose, dog rose
Rosa eglanteria—rosamosqueta
Rosa moschata—musk rose

Rosmarinus officinalis—rosemary
Rubus idaeus—raspberry
Rubus villosus—blackberry
Rumex acetosa—sorrel
Ruscus aculeatus—butcher's broom

S

Salix sp.—willow
Salvia officinalis—sage
Salvia sclarea—clary sage
Sambucus sp.—elder
Sanguinaria canadensis—bloodroot, tetterwort
Santalum album—sandalwood
Saponaria officinalis—soapwort
Sassafras albidum—sassafras
Satureja hortensis—savory
Sclerocarya birrea—marula
Scrophularia nodosa—figwort
Sempervivum tectorum—hens and chicks; houseleek; stonecrop
Silybum marianum—lady's thistle
Simmondsia chinensis—jojoba
Siraitia grosvenorii—luo han guo, monk fruit
Smilax officinalis—sarsaparilla
Solanum lycopersicum—tomato
Solanum tuberosum—potato
Solidago sp.—goldenrod
Sorbus aucuparia—mountain ash; rowan
Spinacia oleracea—spinach
Spiraea ulmaria—meadowsweet
Stachys officinalis—betony
Styrax tonkinensis—benzoin
Symphytum officinale—comfrey
Syzygium aromaticum—clove

T

Tamarindus indica—tamarind
Taraxacum officinale—dandelion
Taraktogenos kurzii—chaulmoogra
Terminalia ferdinandiana—kakadu plum
Teucrium scorodonia—germander
Theobroma grandiflorum—cupuaçu
Thuja occidentalis—cedar
Thymus sp.—thyme
Thymus serpyllum—wild thyme
Tilia sp.—linden
Trifolium sp.—clover
Trifolium pratense—red clover
Trigonella foenumgraecum—fenugreek
Tropaeolum majus—nasturtium
Turnera aphrodisiaca—damiana
Tussilago farfara—coltsfoot

U

Ulmus sp.—elm
Ulmus fulva—slippery elm
Unona odoratissima—ylang-ylang
Urtica dioica—nettle

V

Vaccinium sp.—blueberry
Vaccinium myrtillus—bilberry
Valeriana officinalis—valerian
Vanilla planifolia—vanilla
Verbena officinalis—vervain
Veronica officinalis—veronica, gypsyweed
Vetiveria zizanioides—vetiver, khus-khus

Viola sp.—violet
Viola tricolor—pansy
Virola sebifera—ucuuba
Viscum album—European mistletoe

Zingiber officinale—ginger